Pediatric Nutrition Handbook

Second Edition

Author: Committee on Nutrition
American Academy of Pediatrics

Gilbert B. Forbes, M.D. Editor
Calvin W. Woodruff M.D., Associate Editor

American Academy of Pediatrics
P.O. Box 927, 141 Northwest Point Road
Elk Grove Village, Illinois 60007

Library of Congress Catalog Card No. 85-070202

ISBN No. 0-910761-06-X

Quantity prices on request. Address all inquiries to:
American Academy of Pediatrics
P.O. Box 927, 141 Northwest Point Road
Elk Grove Village, Illinois 60007

COMMITTEE ON NUTRITION
1982-1985

PREFACE

This second edition of the *Pediatric Nutrition Handbook* represents the combined efforts of the Committee on Nutrition of the American Academy of Pediatrics, the Technical Advisory Group, liaison representatives from other interested groups and Academy committees, and consultants. The Committee on Nutrition hopes this handbook will provide a source of information on current nutrition science as it pertains to infants and children.

Space considerations have precluded exhaustive reviews of the various topics; and the material contained in the handbook, although as complete as possible, cannot be construed as designed to cover every nuance, every opinion, every possible hazard or benefit of the modern nutrition scene. Other sources should be consulted for detailed information on the treatment of nutritional illnesses and on inborn errors of metabolism.

The Committee on Nutrition presents this volume for what it is—a handbook for physicians and others who deal with the health and welfare of infants and children.

For the Committee on Nutrition
Gilbert B. Forbes, M.D., Editor
Calvin W. Woodruff, M.D.,
Associate Editor

ACKNOWLEDGEMENT

Several chapters are adapted from statements by the Committee on Nutrition, and other chapters are edited versions of material from the first edition of the handbook. Some of the material was developed by individual Committee members; other materials were prepared by expert consultants. Contributions are not individually acknowledged because the Committee reserved the right to modify and edit contributions and accepts responsibility for the final document. The Committee gratefully acknowledges the contributions of the primary authors and the assistance of the referees who reviewed individual chapters and the entire document. The assistance of Jean D. Lockhart, M.D., Director, Department of Maternal, Child, and Adolescent Health, of the Academy also is gratefully recognized and appreciated.

Technical Advisory Group

George A. Purvis, Ph.D., Chairman, Fremont, Michigan
John D. Benson, Ph.D., Columbus, Ohio
David A. Cook, Ph.D., Evansville, Indiana
Richard C. Theuer, Ph.D., Fort Washington, Pennsylvania
Rudolph Tomarelli, Ph.D., Radnor, Pennsylvania

Other Contributors

Steven M. Adair, D.D.S., Rochester, New York
H. Peter Chase, M.D., Denver, Colorado
Peter R. Dallman, M.D., San Francisco, California
Purnima Desai, M.D., Valhalla, New York
Harry L. Greene, M.D., Nashville, Tennessee
J.C. Haworth, M.D., Winnipeg, Manitoba, Canada
William C. Heird, M.D., New York, New York
Walter T. Hughes, M.D., Memphis, Tennessee
William J. Klish, M.D., Houston, Texas
Ruth A. Lawrence, M.D., Rochester, New York
Barbara Lipinski, M.S., R.D., Rochester, New York
Bo Lönnerdal, Ph.D., Davis, California

Charles D. May, M.D., Quechee, Vermont
Buford L. Nichols, M.D., Houston, Texas
Donough O'Brien, M.D., Denver, Colorado
William K. Schubert, M.D., Cincinnati, Ohio
Gary E. Stahl, M.D., Philadelphia, Pennsylvania
Raj N. Varma, Ph.D., Mobile, Alabama
John B. Watkins, M.D., Philadelphia, Pennsylvania
Bernard Weiss, Ph.D., Rochester, New York

Contents

Tables

Feeding Normal Infants and Children

Chapter 1

BREAST FEEDING

The Committees on Nutrition of the American Academy of Pediatrics and the Canadian Paediatric Society have strongly recommended breast feeding for full-term infants. The success of adequate lactation will depend in large part on the attitude of professional personnel, a hospital climate which is conducive to breast feeding, and the realization that, although it is a natural function, many mothers need instruction and support.

Prenatal Considerations

The successful management of lactation begins during pregnancy. The pediatrician should plan to discuss feeding plans along with other issues of infant care during a prenatal office visit. Mothers who wish to breast feed should be encouraged to do so, and they should be taught the details of breast-feeding procedures at prenatal visits or during prenatal classes. Breast care should be discussed, including the avoidance of soaps and ointments (the glands of Montgomery in the areola provide the best lubrication for the areola and nipple throughout pregnancy and lactation); and the breast should be examined to identify any problems of the nipple, areola, or breast itself. For example, if there are inverted or flat nipples, the mother should be instructed how to use a shield inside her brassiere in the last months of pregnancy to facilitate eversion. Elaborate exercises and preparations are not necessary for the average woman.

Initiating Lactation

The physician should ensure that nursing mothers receive appropriate professional counseling during their hospital stay. The early days of lactation, which usually take place in the hospital, frequently are critical to the establishment of a good milk supply and effective let-down reflex. The mother should be offered the opportunity to nurse her infant as soon after delivery as possible. She should be offered as much assistance as necessary in positioning herself comfortably and facilitating the infant's proper grasp of the breast. Enough of the areola should be in the infant's mouth to permit the tongue to stroke the areola over the collecting ductals against the hard palate in the act of sucking. This will provide a good seal and proper emptying or milking of these ampullae (see Figures 1 and 2). After a brief (3 to 4 minute) suckling period, the suction should be broken by the mother slipping her clean finger into the corner of the infant's mouth. The infant is then repositioned on the second breast. The mother probably will need assistance in turning over and in moving the infant. A brief suckling period is initiated on the second side. An infant with good Apgar scores will be alert and attentive and should root, grasp, and suckle well.

After the mother and infant are in the postpartum unit, they should not be separated during the first 24 hours, if possible. Breast feedings should continue when the infant is wakeful and at least every 4 to 5 hours to stimulate milk production. This may require feedings as frequently as every 2 hours. Although the length of a feeding should be modified at first to avoid excessive suckling, which may precipitate sore or cracked nipples, more liberal feeding times are associated with greater milk production and an increased likelihood for long-range, successful breast feeding. Sore nipples also may be caused by poor positioning of the infant, this can be prevented by holding the infant in different positions at different feedings. Each feeding should include nursing on both sides to en-

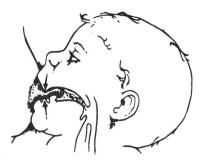

Figure 1. Position of the nipple in the infant's mouth during feeding.

hance the stimulation of milk production. If the mother is unable to move and turn easily, she will require assistance from the staff. Whether the mother lies down or sits up to nurse depends on which position is more comfortable for her. Rocking chairs should be provided for all postpartum rooms to enhance comfort and relaxation during feedings. Usually alternating the side which is used to initiate the feeding and equalizing the time spent at each breast over a day's feedings is wise. By the third postpartum day, a feeding may take 10 minutes or more on each side. Recommendations should be based on individual need and not dictated by protocol or nursery policy.

Breast and Nipple Care

The mother should buy a sturdy, well fitting nursing brassiere and wear it in the hospital to support the breasts, which may engorge shortly after delivery. Because the vascular supply increases and the blood flow is increased 10-fold, there may be some discomfort unless adequate breast support is provided. Frequent, short feedings facilitate establishment of lactation through the early postpartum period. Warm or cold compresses may be used between feedings if the breasts are uncomfortable. Mothers usually prefer to wear a nursing brassiere 24 hours a day in the early months of lactation.

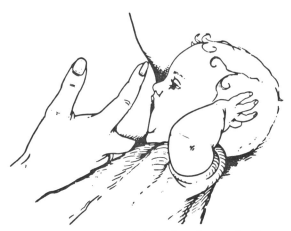

Figure 2. Position of the infant during feeding.

Nipples should be kept dry. No ointments or lotions are needed unless an infection has been diagnosed, then specific medication should be prescribed. Plastic brassiere liners hold moisture and may cause tissue irritation in the first week. If irritation develops, dry heat is effective and can be provided with a lamp (such as that used for the perineum on postpartum hospital wards; 60 watt bulb in shielding frame) placed 1½ to 2 ft away for 20 minutes after each feeding. At home, the mother may wish to use a hair dryer set on low heat and held 6 in. or more from the breast for 10 to 15 minutes after each feeding. The warm air currents are especially soothing. The milk which may dry on the breast also may assist healing. In some countries mother's nipples and areola are deliberately coated with a little milk and allowed to dry as a treatment for soreness.

Care of the Mother and Infant at Home

Support of the lactating woman, especially after discharge home, is critical. She should be encouraged to keep in touch with her physician if questions arise. Having a support person at home to "mother" the mother and support her psychologically is important and frequently means the difference between success and failure.

It may be necessary to prescribe rest for the mother, including a daily nap. Fatigue is a common contributor to problems in breast feeding.

The mother should be cautioned to avoid excessive caffeine from hot and cold beverages and herb teas, which are apt to include theobromine, caffeine, belladonna, or other less well-known stimulants. She also should be encouraged to discuss drug intake with her physician.

A number of drugs are excreted in human milk, but only a few are thought to be contraindications to breast feeding. These include drugs which suppress immune function, radioactive isotopes, some antithyroid drugs and sulfonamides, and, of course, those which act to suppress lactation such as bromocriptine and chlorothiazide. The Committee on Drugs of the Academy has compiled a list of drugs which have not been reported to cause problems in the infant when administered to the lactating mother.[1] Each situation has to be judged on its own merits, based on dose schedule for the mother, feeding pattern of the infant, and the infant's total diet and age. The levels of benzene hexachloride and polychlorobiphenyls are higher in the milk of women who consume contaminated fresh water fish regularly.

Bottle Feedings and Supplements

Under normal conditions, bottle feeding should not be offered to an infant for the first 2 weeks, until lactation is well established. Infants may be confused by a rubber nipple, which actually requires a different tongue and jaw motion. Furthermore, if the appetite is partially satiated by water or formula, the infant will take less from the breast, which will lead to a diminished milk production. In the breast-fed infant, water supplements may contribute to lactation failure in the mother and little or no weight gain in the infant. Water supplements for either breast or bottle-fed infants have not been shown to prevent or cure hyperbilirubinemia in the neonatal period.

Monitoring the Breast-fed Infant

Ordinarily, an infant is adequately nourished in the first few weeks of life if he or she receives at least six feedings a day and sleeps well between feedings. However, it is important also to check the number of wet diapers a day (should be at least six), number and quantity of stools, and weight gain over a period of time. The infant may actually feed 12 to 14 times a day and be doing well. The breast-fed infant should be seen when 10 to 14 days old, especially if the mother is a primipara. Failure to regain birth weight by 3 weeks of age or continuing to lose weight after 10 days of life indicates failure to thrive. Infants with this condition should be evaluated, including observing the infant at the breast.

Milk from strict vegetarian mothers may lack vitamin B_{12}. There also are reports of rare instances of ostensibly well nourished mothers whose milk had an extremely low phosphorus, chloride, or zinc content. The results were clinical symptoms of deficiency in each instance.

In lactation failure, the lactation reflex may be reestablished by the use of a device (the "Lact-Aid")* which permits simultaneous suckling at the breast and delivery of formula through a small tube.[2,3]

Nutrition for the Lactating Mother

The mother's diet should include sufficient additional sources of energy, protein, minerals, and vitamins to provide for adequate milk production and composition. Fluid intake should be at least 2 qt (liters) a day.

Data on the composition of mature human milk are given in Appendix K. The mother's diet must be sufficient to provide for adequate milk production, both in quality and quantity, if her own body stores are not to be depleted. The Recommended Dietary Allowances (RDA) for lactating women are listed in Appendix H.

In some respects the quantity and composition of human milk can be influenced by the mother's diet. Poorly nourished mothers produce less milk than well nourished mothers, and there is some evidence that dietary supplements can increase milk production and total milk lipid in these women. For specific nutrients, the following constituents have been shown to be responsive to the respective intakes of the mother: unsaturated fats (particularly linoleic acid), vitamin A, vitamin E, thiamine, riboflavin, niacin, pyridoxine, vitamin B_{12}, manganese, and iodine.[4] Maternal supplements have not been shown to alter milk composition for other nutrients. These are ascorbic acid, vitamin K, folate, biotin, pantothenic acid, sodium, calcium, iron, zinc, copper, and fluoride. For a third group of nutrients, the effects of maternal supplements are not known. These are vitamin D and selenium. The foregoing statements about maternal supplements pertain to well nourished mothers; the quality of milk from poorly nourished mothers can be improved by supplements of all the water-soluble vitamins.

Despite recent claims to the contrary, human milk contains little vitamin D—too little to prevent rickets—nor does it contain enough thyroid hormone to mitigate the impact of congenital cretinism. In addition, the mother does not provide for the vitamin K requirements of her nursing infant. The breast-fed

*Lact-Aid International, Inc., P.O. Box 1066, Athens, Tennessee 37303.

infant must rely on a vitamin K supplement to correct the prolonged prothrombin time observed immediately after birth.

Breast Feeding After Cesarean Delivery

The mother who plans to breast feed after a cesarean delivery should be able to do so if the infant is healthy. The mother may feel alert enough to put the infant to the breast within the first 12 hours. Most mothers find that nursing the infant in a semi-sitting position in bed is the most comfortable position (see Figure 3). By positioning a standard pillow on the mother's abdomen with the infant lying on the pillow, the full weight of the infant is not on the mother's incision. A small pillow also can be placed under the infant's head to assist in positioning him or her at the breast.

Pain medication is best given immediately after breast feeding to permit the level to peak before the next feeding. The medication used should be limited to short-acting drugs (aspirin, codeine).

After discharge home, mothers who had a cesarean delivery may have pain when getting the infant ready for a feeding. If the pain is severe, it can impair the let-down reflex. The father or a helper should assist in preparing the infant for a feeding.

Weaning

Mothers should be reminded that, if they must stop breast feeding, they should use infant formula rather than cow's milk until the infant is at least 6 months old.

Advantages of Human Milk

Human milk is unquestionably the best source of nutrition for full-term infants during the first months of life. Recent publications[5-8] have emphasized the advantages of human milk's biochemical composition, and particularly of its immunochemical and cellular components. Renewed interest in also providing preterm infants with human milk stems partly from nutritional considerations and, more importantly, from evidence that it confers some protection against infections and allergy. The degree of protection against necrotizing enterocolitis is uncertain. This disease has been reported in infants fed sterilized human milk, and it can occur in neonates fed fresh human milk.

Human milk has come back into favor in intensive care nurseries; consequently, there has been a resurgence of interest in human milk banks,[9] which stopped operating in North America shortly after World War II. However, the milk bank tradition was never abandoned in certain British hospitals and in Scandinavia. The Helsinki Children's Hospital experience now spans a 50-year period. The collection, processing, and storage of human milk may be initiated to meet the needs of preterm infants, of full-term newborn infants who temporarily cannot breast feed, or of sick infants with intractable diarrhea, the short-gut syndrome, or intolerance to cow's milk or soy proteins who are not responsive to other measures.

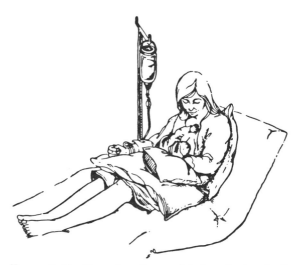

Figure 3. Position of mother and infant during feeding when mother has had a cesarean delivery. Pillows help position the infant to minimize pressure on the incision.

Contamination of Human Milk

An important property of breast feeding is the relative freedom from bacterial contamination of human milk. However, contamination can be a major problem with banked human milk. The precautions which need to be taken to make human milk microbiologically safe require careful attention, especially when human milk is collected and stored prior to feeding. Salmonella and group B streptococcal infections have occurred from infected breast milk. A variety of other bacteria, bacterial toxins, and viruses such as rubella, cytomegalovirus, and hepatitis B particles have been identified. Human milk also may be a vehicle for transmission of herpes simplex type I.

Composition of Human Milk

Human milk leukocytes are thought to constitute an important component of the anti-infective and immunologic properties of breast milk.[10] Colostrum and human milk phagocytes have a low-killing power but a considerable capacity for phagocytosis. They may sequester pathogens and prevent their attachment and subsequent colonization of the gut. In addition to the known enteromammary circulation of B lymphocytes, maternal T lymphocytes also may be absorbed intact through the gastrointestinal tract of newborn infants. This possibility raises theoretical questions about the safety of feeding "fresh" (unfrozen or unheated) human milk from a mother other than the infant's own. A syndrome resembling a graft versus host reaction has been observed in young animals fed milk leukocytes from a different species; this is not the case with human milk.

Doubts have been expressed regarding the adequacy of protein, sodium, chloride, phosphorus, and calcium in human milk for small preterm infants.[11,12] Nitrogen and mineral requirements of the small preterm infant are higher per unit weight than in the full-term infant. However, milk from mothers of young preterm infants generally has 10 to 30% more nitrogen, sodium, chloride, and magnesium than that of mothers who deliver at term.[13-15] But one recent study[16] disagrees. However, the calcium and phosphorus contents of "preterm" milk are, on the average, no higher than those of "term" milk, and most studies show that nitrogen and mineral contents are highly variable. Data on the benefits of the differences in composition of milk at term and preterm would be particularly important for extremely small preterm infants. Donated human milk is usually mature milk; therefore, it may not meet the protein and mineral needs of the extremely small preterm infant.[17] Years ago Hess and Lundeen[18] recommended the addition of skimmed cow's milk to human milk; and the possibility of adding human milk protein to human milk is now under study.

Collection and Treatment of Human Milk

Human milk can be made microbiologically safe if certain precautions are taken. Recent information suggests that bacterial contamination is minimized if the donor is properly selected and trained and if the first 10 ml of milk are rejected. Some authorities believe that manual expression is preferable to the suction breast pump. Milk samples identified by bacteriologic screening as unacceptable must be rejected. Healthy donors are generally recruited from mothers who nurse their infants but have extra milk. The screening of potential donors, their training, and facilities to carry out routine or spotcheck bacteriologic cultures are essential components of a human milk bank.

Heat treatment is a widely used method for reduction of bacterial contamination. However, it is important to restrict the extent and duration of heating to that required for the destruction of pathogens. Holder pasteurization (62.5°C for 30 minutes) appears to be adequate, although 6% of the samples may not be acceptable. Even this modest heat treatment has had significant adverse effects on the protective immunochemical constituents of human milk. At 80°C, the ability of human milk to inhibit the growth of added bacteria largely disappears. There is little information on the effect of heat treatment on the nutritional properties of human milk, and the results are conflicting.

The storage of milk by freezing is an alternative to heating for the preservation of optimal nutritional value and immunologic benefits. The use of stored frozen milk requires more attention to bacteriologic screening. Efforts should be made to collect clean milk with minimal bacterial contamination and to store it immediately in a freezer until it is gently thawed and fed.

There are at least three procedures for collecting human milk for infants who cannot be breast fed. These include: (1) collection of milk from a mother to be supplied to her infant, (2) collection of milk from healthy donors for feeding specific infants, and (3) pooling of milk from several donors.

Collection of Milk for a Woman's Own Infant

The collection of milk for a woman's own infant is the most physiologic method. As previously noted, the composition of milk from the mothers of preterm infants has a somewhat higher protein, nitrogen, and sodium content than that from mothers of full-term infants. Although milk from mothers of full-term infants may partly meet the needs of preterm infants, it lacks sufficient calcium and phosphorus. Furthermore, the mother who collects her milk for her infant usually is highly motivated and more likely to take antiseptic precautions in collecting, storing, and delivering the milk; she also is more likely to avoid exposing herself to toxic substances that might be secreted into the milk.

The greatest obstacle to the wider use of this method is a logistic one. A growing proportion of preterm infants are cared for in referral centers, which frequently are located at a considerable distance from the home. This makes it difficult for some mothers to deliver milk to the hospital on a regular basis, especially if they have other children and/or heavy family responsibilities. Because most donors cannot deliver fresh milk daily, human milk usually must be stored frozen, either in single donations or as pooled collections. Some mothers of preterm infants will experience lactation failure when they return home. This is not surprising because manual or mechanical expression is not as good as suckling for the stimulation of milk production and the let-down reflex.

The preservation of leukocytes in milk would be desirable when a woman's milk is fed to her infant, but there are practical obstacles to accomplishing this. Freezing is necessary when the interval between collection and feeding is longer than 24 hours; but this procedure destroys viable cells. Storage of human milk near body temperature is the most effective procedure to preserve viable cells; but this procedure carries an increased risk of unacceptable bacterial growth. Because of

these difficulties and unanswered questions regarding leukocytes from donor milk, a recent recommendation is that attempts to preserve the cells should not influence the processing
and storage conditions used for human milk.[19]

Collection of Milk for a Specific Infant

Providing milk from an individual donor for each infant has
been proposed as a means of decreasing the risk of infection
after a donor's milk has been shown to consistently meet the
criteria for numbers and types of bacteria. Disadvantages of
this system are that it complicates banking procedures, results
in some wastage of milk, and increases the risk of transmitting
undiluted toxic substances (e.g., drugs, nicotine, pesticides,
and environmental contaminants) which are secreted in milk.

Collection of Pooled Milk

Pooled milk from several donors simplifies routine procedures for ensuring microbiologic safety. The mixing of milk
from a group of donors also results in a more uniform nutrient
content and dilutes drugs or toxins which may be present in
the milk of an individual donor. A possible disadvantage of
pooled milk is the increased potential for the transmission of
viral infections, particularly if the milk is frozen only.

Conclusion

The experience of Finnish workers, as well as that of others,
shows that the banking of heat-treated and frozen human milk
is a practical and safe means of feeding preterm, newborn infants. The continuous and exclusive use of human milk is associated with a low incidence of infection and with a rate of
survival which is among the highest reported. The rate of
growth and weight gain also is considered satisfactory, although there is some controversy about whether weight gain is
quite as rapid as in formula-fed infants. Long-term studies
should be carried out to see if these infants grow and develop as
well, or better than, those on formula feedings.

It is still uncertain whether banked human milk will prove sufficiently superior to commercial infant formulas with respect to its nutritional and immunologic characteristics to compensate for the difficulties of maintaining bacteriologic control and to warrant the cost of setting up and running a milk bank for preterm infants.

References

1. Committee on Drugs: The transfer of drugs and other chemicals into human breast milk. PEDIATRICS, 72:375, 1983.
2. Weichert, C.E.: Lactational reflex recovery in breast-feeding failure. PEDIATRICS, 63:799, 1979.
3. Auerbach, K.G., and Avery, J.L.: Relactation: A study of 366 cases. PEDIATRICS, 65:236, 1980.
4. Committee on Nutrition: Nutrition and lactation. PEDIATRICS, 68:435, 1981.
5. Lawrence, R.A.: Breast-Feeding, A Guide for the Medical Profession, ed. 2. St. Louis: C. V. Mosby, 1985.
6. Nutrition Committee of the Canadian Paediatric Society and Committee on Nutrition: Breast-feeding. PEDIATRICS, 62:591, 1978.
7. Committee on Nutrition: Encouraging breast-feeding. PEDIATRICS, 65:657, 1980.
8. Committee on Nutrition: Human milk banking. PEDIATRICS, 65:854, 1980.
9. Human Milk Banking, Procedures and Protocols. San Jose, California (751 S. Bascom Avenue): Institute for Medical Research, 1983.
10. Pittard, W.B., III: Breast milk immunology: A frontier in infant nutrition. Amer. J. Dis. Child., 133:83, 1979.
11. Fomon, S.J., Ziegler, E.E., and Vazques, H.D.: Human milk and the small premature infant. Amer. J. Dis. Child., 131:463, 1977.
12. Forbes, G.B.: Nutritional adequacy of human breast milk for premature infants. In Lebenthal, E., ed.: Textbook of Gastroenterology and Nutrition in Infancy. New York: Raven Press, pp. 321-330, 1981.
13. Atkinson, S.A., Bryan, M.H., and Anderson, G.H.: Human milk: Difference in nitrogen concentration in milk from mothers of term and premature infants. J. Pediat., 93:67, 1978.
14. Gross, S.J., David, R.J., Bauman, L., and Tomarelli, R.M.: Nutritional composition of milk produced by mothers delivering preterm. J. Pediat., 96:641, 1980.
15. Lemons, J.A., Moye, L., Hall, D., and Simmons, M.: Differences in the composition of preterm and term human milk during early lactation. Pediat. Res., 16:113, 1982.

16. Anderson, D.M., Williams, F.H., Merkatz, R.B., Schulman, P.K., Kerr, D.S., and Pittard, W.B., III: Length of gestation and nutritional composition of human milk. Amer. J. Clin. Nutr., **37**:810, 1983.
17. Chance, G.W., Radde, I.C., Willis, D.M., Roy, R.N., Park, E., and Ackerman, I.: Postnatal growth of infants of <1.3 kg birth weight· Effects of metabolic acidosis, of caloric intake, and of calcium, sodium, and phosphate supplementation. J. Pediat., **91**:787, 1977.
18. Hess, J.H., and Lundeen, E.C.: The Premature Infant: Medical and Nursing Care, ed. 2. Philadelphia: J.B. Lippincott, 1949.
19. Widdowson, E.M.: Symposium report: Protective properties of human milk and the effects of processing on them. Arch. Dis. Child., **53**:684, 1978.

Chapter 2

FORMULA FEEDING OF INFANTS

The development of a substitute for maternal milk is an integral part of the history of pediatrics. The production of a safe, nutritious alternative to human milk remains one of the crowning achievements of pediatric medicine. This chapter will discuss the appropriate use of commercial infant formulas from a descriptive and a physiologic point of view.

Contemporary Formulas

The first year of the normal term infant can be divided into three biologic periods: a transition period of approximately 28 days; the first semester, from approximately 29 to 180 days; and the second semester, from 180 to 365 days. Maturation of organ function and changes in nutrient requirements which require pediatric supervision occur during the first year of the infant's life.

Approximately 60% of all infants born in the United States today begin breast feeding in the hospital. This is twice the frequency reported in 1970. Nevertheless, 48% of infants receive a commercially prepared formula in the hospital and are discharged home on this product (Fig. 4). By 2 months of age, 61% of all infants are receiving prepared formulas; usage peaks at about 67% by 3 to 4 months of age, then progressively falls to 14% at 12 months of age. The percentage of infants who are breast fed declines to 27% at 6 months of age, then to 9% by 12 months.

At the end of the first semester, many infants are placed on whole cow's milk or evaporated milk formulas prepared at home. The frequency of this type of milk feeding increases from 17% at 6 months of age to 85% at 1 year. When all types of milk feeding during the first year of life are considered, breast feeding accounts for 29%, commercial infant formulas for 45%, and cow's milk and evaporated milk for 26%.[1] Despite the increasing trend toward breast feeding in the United States, commercial infant formulas continue to play a substantial role in meeting the nutrient needs of infants.

Another component of the diet of infants in the United States is given in Figure 5. By 2 months of age, about 15% of the average infant's caloric intake is derived from prepared infant foods or puréed home foods, and this rises to 25% by 6 months of age. At 12 months of age, only 35% of the total energy intake is derived from milk; most of the remainder is derived from table foods. Figure 5 is designed so 100% equals the recommended energy intake of 115 kcal/kg per day at birth and 105 kcal/kg per day at the end of infancy.[2] The total energy intake does not equal the recommended energy intake between 4 and 8 months of age because evidence indicates an overestimate of energy needs by the National Research Council.

The data in Figures 4 and 5 show that infant feeding as currently practiced is not in complete agreement with the recommendations of the Committee on Nutrition.

Evolution of Infant Formulas

The composition of infant formulas has evolved over many years. Although most infants have thrived on modifications of cow's milk, a few have displayed signs and symptoms that suggest formula intolerance. Consequently, research to improve the acceptability and quality of infant formulas continues. In addition to formulas used for feeding normal term infants, there now are a number of special purpose formulas for infants with gastrointestinal or metabolic disturbances.[3] Cow's milk-based infant formulas comprise four fifths of the formulas used by term infants during the first semester of life.[1] These formulas are composed of reconstituted skimmed milk or a mixture of skimmed milk and electrolyte-depleted whey protein. Lactose is the carbohydrate in these formulas; and, because butter oil is less well digested and absorbed, a mixture of soy, coconut, corn, oleo, and safflower oils is used instead. The present milk-based formulas have been tested intensively under experimental and field conditions and are equal to human milk in providing adequate nutrition support to the normal infant. The Committee on Nutrition has prepared a recommended range of nutrient composition for these formulas (see Appendix I). These recommendations are followed by all the infant formula manufacturers. The composition of commercial infant formulas is shown in Appendix L.

Soy Formulas

Based on the hypothesis that cow's milk formula intolerances are a manifestation of either protein hypersensitivity or lactose intolerance, soy-protein-based formulas (which are lactose free) were developed in the late 1920's. Since then, these formulas have undergone a series of refinements and today represent a nutritionally sound and safe alternative to cow's milk-based formulas.[4] Soy-protein-based formulas now make up a fifth of the formulas produced and marketed in the United States.[1] The protein in soy-based formulas is an isolate treated to improve its biologic qualities. Methionine is added to upgrade the quality of the protein to equal that of casein in cow's milk. The carbohydrate is sucrose, corn syrup solids (smaller molecular weight corn starches), or a mixture of sucrose and corn syrup solids. The fat mixture consists of soy, oleo, coconut,

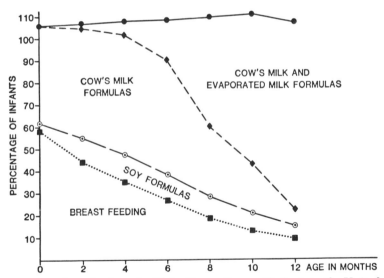

Figure 4. Distribution of milk feeding patterns of infants in the United States indicated by 2-month intervals. This information was based on a probability sample of 51,537 mothers surveyed on a quarterly basis by Martinez and Dodd.[1] The total percentage of infants either breast feeding or on formula exceeds 100% because a number of breast-feeding infants also received supplemental formula feedings.

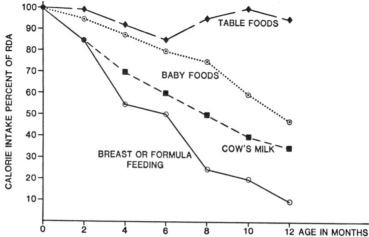

Figure 5. Average caloric intake of infants in 1979 divided according to human milk or formula feeding, cow's milk feeding, infant food intake, and table food intake. This information was obtained from a probability sample of 154 infants whose parents recorded food intake for a 4-day period during midweek. Human milk intake was indirectly estimated. The data are those of Johnson et al.[2] The total calories are compared to the Recommended Dietary Allowance of 115 kcal/kg and 105 kcal/kg at birth and 1 year of age. The deviation below 100% of recommended caloric intake is discussed in the text.

and safflower oils in various combinations chosen to mimic the digestibility of human milk fat.

As seen in Figure 4, the frequency of soy-formula use in the United States increases from 3% in the newborn period to a peak of 12% at 4 months of age. Forty percent of the infants who still receive formula at the end of the first year of life are receiving soy formulas.

Soy formulas have not proved to be completely hypoallergenic.[4] Early studies suggested that the use of soy protein instead of cow's milk protein could prevent the development of allergic disorders in later life, but others have failed to confirm this hypothesis. The best estimate, based on clinical rather than laboratory criteria, is that approximately 1 to 2% of infants develop an intolerance to cow's milk or soy protein.[5] Of the infants who develop clinical symptoms of cow's milk intolerance (estimated variously at 0.4 to 7.5%), 10 to 20% also develop soy-protein intolerance.[5,6] The data available to date have not revealed any relationship between serum milk-protein antibody levels and clinical symptoms of milk intolerance. Additional nonimmune and immune-mediated mechanisms must be explored before an explanation can be given for the clinical findings associated with formula intolerance. The benefits which have been attributed to the acute substitution of soy-protein formula for cow's milk were due, in part, to the replacement of lactose by sucrose or corn syrup, which probably accounts for the popularity of soy formulas in the post-diarrheal state. Lactase activity is diminished following acute viral gastroenteritis. Unfortunately, some investigations in this field have not discriminated between carbohydrate and protein intolerance in these infants.[5]

The development of a more refined soy-protein isolate has made the manufacture of high quality, soy-based formulas possible. Although the specific processing of soy proteins is kept confidential by the manufacturers, the primary objective is extraction of the major protein fraction. Heat treatment of soy protein reduces the activity of trypsin inhibitors and hemagglutinins and enhances protein digestibility and bioavailability of some minerals. For example, although iron absorption appears to be inhibited by soy products, absorption from soy-isolate formulas has been shown to be similar to that from cow's milk formula.[7] However, in the processing of isolates, the formation of tightly bound, protein-phytic acid-mineral complexes may reduce the availability of some minerals. Zinc in soy also appears to be less well absorbed; however, supplemental zinc absorption does not appear to be impaired. The amount of phytic acid in soy-based formulas and its effect on mineral and trace element availability needs to be more clearly delineated. Soy-based formulas contain minimal amounts of carnitine. However, there is insufficient evidence to conclude that carnitine should be added to formulas on a routine basis.

Use of Soy-based Formulas for Full-term Infants

Normal growth and development in full-term infants fed soy-protein formulas have been well documented in several studies. A recent review of this topic by Fomon and Ziegler[8] reported growth and nitrogen balance studies in infants fed soy-protein formula or cow's milk-protein formula. No significant differences were found between the two groups of infants in either weight or length. Furthermore, concentrations of serum urea nitrogen, total protein, and albumin did not differ significantly between the infants consuming cow's milk-based formulas and those consuming soy-protein formulas.

Use of Soy-based Formulas for Preterm Infants

In a comparative study of soy-protein and cow's milk-protein formulas in preterm infants, Naude et al.,[9] using a methionine-supplemented formula, found reduced weight and length growth and significantly lower serum albumin levels in infants fed soy-protein formula. However, Shenai et al.,[10] in a comparison of cow's milk-protein formula and soy-protein formula (methionine supplemented), found equal growth in length and weight and normal serum albumin levels in both groups.

Serum phosphorus levels were significantly lower, and alkaline phosphatase levels were higher in the soy-protein formula groups. Osteoporosis and rickets recently were reported in sick, very low-birth-weight infants fed soy-protein formulas for several months. (These conditions also can occur with standard formulas and human milk feedings.) The reason for the hypophosphatemia is not clear, but it may lie with the binding of some of the phosphorus with phytate in the formula, leading to its unavailability for intestinal absorption. The disadvantages of the soy-protein formula for very low-birth-weight infants, as discussed here, indicate that these formulas should not be used for feeding of these infants.

Prophylaxis of Allergic Disease in Newborn Infants

The role of soy-based formulas in the prevention of allergic disease in newborn infants remains controversial. Theoretically, any protein is a potential allergen, and examples of soy-protein allergy have been cited. Glaser and Johnstone's original paper[11] included a few infants fed meat-base formula and human milk as well as soy formulas; their main emphasis was on the exclusion of cow's milk from the moment of birth, and they dealt only with potentially allergic infants. More recent studies have failed to confirm their findings.

Current evidence suggests soy protein may be less allergenic than sterilized cow's milk protein and is probably a better source of nutrition in allergy-prone infants. However, whether or not soy protein represents the optimum form of prophylaxis for allergic disease is still controversial. The extent to which early exposure to antigen affects the subsequent development of allergic disease requires more sophisticated prospective studies.

Based on the information given here, soy-protein formulas can be recommended for use in (1) vegetarian families where animal-protein formulas are not desired; (2) the management of galactosemia, primary lactase deficiency, and secondary lactose intolerance; and (3) potentially allergic infants (with a family history of atopy) who have not shown clinical manifestations of allergy. However, these infants should be monitored closely for allergy to soy protein.

Other Formulas

Other formulas include Nutramigen (protein from hydrolyzed casein), Pregestimil (hydrolyzed casein, MCT oil), Portagen (casein, MCT oil), and Ross Carbohydrate-Free formula. All of these are lactose free; some contain modified starches, and some contain medium-chain triglycerides (MCT). All have been used in special situations, but none has been used extensively in the feeding of normal infants (see Appendix L for formula compositions).

Special formulas are available for use in preterm infants and in those with inborn errors of metabolism (see Appendix L).

Uses for Formulas

There are three general uses for infant formulas: (1) substitution for infants whose mothers do not choose to breast feed; (2) supplementation for infants whose mothers choose to omit a breast feeding; (3) if the mother's milk production is inadequate, complementation with a formula is indicated.

There are two major medical indications for substitution with formula feeding. (1) Infectious disease (such as neonatal listeriosis and maternal hepatitis B, chickenpox, and pertussis) is a contraindication to breast feeding, as is active cavitary tuberculosis and herpetic or syphilitic lesions of the breast. (2) Extreme caution is required in some women with metabolic disorders when breast feeding. If the mother has been heavily treated for toxemia at term, breast feeding should be delayed until the maternal phenobarbital dose is less than 160 mg per day. If the mother has thyrotoxicosis and is on antithyroid medication, care should be exercised in biochemical surveillance of the infant's thyroid status. A list of maternal medications which contraindicate breast feeding can be found in a recent statement by the Committee on Drugs.[12]

Formula Complementation

The indications for complementation with cow's milk formula in the first semester require individualized clinical judgments. Clinical assessment is required if growth has faltered or there are other signs of malnutrition. Complementation with infant formula is mandated if intake is inadequate. If the mother wishes to continue breast feeding, formula may be offered as a temporary complement; but, unless steps are taken to increase milk production, the mother's milk supply will decrease (see Chapter 1).

Complementation of the breast-fed infant's diet may become necessary near the end of the first semester because exclusive breast feeding eventually becomes inadequate for normal growth. If the mother is undernourished and/or socially disorganized, growth faltering of the exclusively breast-fed infant may occur before the age of 3 months. However, in a healthy environment, growth faltering is delayed until 6 months of age or later.

Infant formula is an appropriate complement to the diet of the growth faltering, breast-fed infant. The content and ratio of nutrients in infant formulas is adequate throughout infancy.[3]

The Use of Whole Cow's Milk in Infancy

The appropriate age at which pasteurized whole cow's milk (WCM) can be safely introduced into the infant's diet is unknown and remains controversial.[13] The consumption of excessive amounts of WCM has been associated with iron-deficiency anemia. Both the concentration and the bioavailability of iron are low in cow's milk, and some infants have occult bleeding from the gastrointestinal tract. The process by which the latter occurs is unknown.

There are some difficulties in using these findings as a basis for recommendations for feeding older infants because of the young age at which the infants studied were initially given

WCM. Fomon *et al.*[14] studied 81 normal infants between 112 and 196 days of age who had not previously consumed WCM: 39 infants were fed WCM; the remainder were fed either a commercial infant formula or sterilized cow's milk. All infants received daily supplements of 50 mg ascorbic acid and 12 mg of iron as ferrous sulfate. The proportion of infants between 112 and 140 days old who had guaiac-positive stools was significantly greater among the infants fed WCM than among those fed Enfamil or sterilized cow's milk. However, after 140 days of age, there was no difference between groups in the number of guaiac-positive stools. Furthermore, in these iron-supplemented infants, no significant differences were observed between feeding groups in mean hemoglobin, hematocrit, serum iron, total iron-binding capacity, or transferrin saturation. Hematologic values did not differ significantly between infants with and those without guaiac-positive stools. Although the study demonstrated no adverse effects from feeding WCM after 140 days of age, all infants under study were receiving a daily supplement of ferrous sulfate. However, a recent report by Sadowitz and Oski[15] has documented an appreciable number of iron-insufficient subjects fed WCM after 6 months of age, although the incidence was higher in those less than 6 months old.

Cow's Milk Allergy

Another area requiring further research is cow's milk-protein intolerance or "allergy," estimated at from 0.4 to 7.5% of the infant population in the first 2 years of life and manifested by a variety of symptoms and signs.[16] Of interest is the fact that many of the symptoms disappear by age 2 years.

Whether or not the percentage of infants with intolerance or "allergy" would decrease if cow's milk protein were withheld from the infant's diet for the first 4 to 6 months of life is debatable.

The Renal Solute Load

The increased renal solute load provided by WCM also needs to be considered. There is little direct evidence concerning this. The theoretic effect of substituting WCM for either human milk or commercial infant formula in infants 2 to 12 months old can be calculated by the method of Ziegler and Fomon.[17]

The substitution of WCM for commercial infant formula or human milk will result in an increase in urine osmolality at all ages. However, this increase was more dramatic during the first 6 months of life (49% increase) than during the second 6 months (18%). Hence, infants fed WCM-containing diets should have ready access to water, and water supplements are vital during hot weather or episodes of diarrhea.

Because WCM is a poor source of iron, linoleic acid, and vitamin C, these nutrients must be supplemented.

Fomon et al.[18] have observed that, although infants fed skimmed milk ad libitum continue to gain weight, they do so at a slower rate than infants fed formula or WCM. They also show a decrease in skinfold thickness, suggesting that body energy stores are being depleted. Of importance is the fact that skimmed milk has a much higher solute:energy ratio than WCM. Although a recent study suggests that the use of 2% cow's milk as part of a mixed second semester complementary diet can be satisfactory,[19] the Committee on Nutrition recommends that reduced-fat milks not be used for infants.

Evaporated milk is readily available and costs less than whole milk, although it is seldom used today. Other advantages of evaporated milk are that it can be kept for long periods without refrigeration if the can is not opened, and it is sterile. Past experience suggested that the heat used during the evaporation process renders the casein more digestible (smaller curd tension) and the product less allergenic than WCM. However, water must be added (54 parts water to 46 parts evaporated milk) to render it comparable to WCM, and instructions are necessary to avoid contamination. Evaporated milk is fortified with vitamin D but lacks a sufficient amount of vitamin C; and it contains more lead (34 μg/l reconstituted) than infant formulas (less than 10 μg/l).

Goat's milk is used in many parts of the world. It too does not contain enough iron, vitamin D, or vitamin C to meet the needs of infants, and it has the distinct disadvantage of a low folacin content (about one-tenth the level in WCM or human milk), so supplements of iron and all three vitamins are needed.

Mention should be made of some infant formulas based on indigenous foods in underdeveloped countries and used with success in those areas. These include a fortified soy-oats preparation[20] and Incaprina (an acronym derived from the Institute of Nutrition for Central America and Panama), which consists of whole ground sorghum (28%), ground corn (28%), cottonseed flour (38%), torula yeast (3%), dehydrated leaf meal (3%), plus calcium carbonate and vitamin A. A number of other plant protein mixtures also have been found to support the growth of several mammalian species and to cure infantile malnutrition.[21]

Although breast feeding is now strongly recommended for full-term infants, the experience of the past few decades has shown they can be satisfactorily nourished by formula.

References

1. Martinez, G.A., and Dodd, D.A.: 1981 milk feeding patterns in the United States during the first 12 months of life. PEDIATRICS, 71:166, 1983.
2. Johnson, G.H., Purvis, G.A., and Wallace, R.D.: What nutrients do our infants really get? Nutr. Today, July/August, 16:4, 1981.
3. Committee on Nutrition: Commentary on breast-feeding and infant formulas, including proposed standards for formulas. PEDIATRICS, 57:278, 1976.
4. Committee on Nutrition: Appraisal of nutritional adequacy of infant formulas used as cow milk substitutes. PEDIATRICS, 31:329, 1963.
5. Bock, S.A.: Food sensitivity. A critical review and practical approach. Amer. J. Dis. Child., 134:973, 1980.
6. Committee on Nutrition: Soy-protein formulas: Recommendations for use in infant feeding. PEDIATRICS, 72:359, 1983.
7. Rios, E., Hunter, R.E., Cook, J.D., Smith, N.J., and Finch, C.A.: The absorption of iron as supplements in infant cereal and infant formulas. PEDIATRICS, 55:686, 1975.
8. Fomon, S.J., and Ziegler, E.E.: Soy protein isolates in infant feeding. In Wilche, H.L., Hopkins, D.T., and Waggle, D.H., ed.: Soy Protein and Human Nutrition. New York: Academic Press, pp. 79-96, 1979.
9. Naudé, S.P.E., Prinsloo, J.G., and Haupt, C.E.: Comparison between humanized cow's milk and a soy product for premature infants. S. Afr. Med. J., 55:982, 1979.
10. Shenai, J.P., Jhaveri, B.M., Reynolds, J.W., Houston, R.K., and Babson, S.G.: Nutritional balance studies in very low-birth-weight infants: Role of soy formula. PEDIATRICS, 67:631, 1981.
11. Glaser, J., and Johnstone, D.E.: Prophylaxis of allergic disease in the newborn. J.A.M.A.. 153:620, 1953.
12. Committee on Drugs: The transfer of drugs and other chemicals into human breast milk. PEDIATRICS, 72:375, 1983.
13. Committee on Nutrition: The use of whole cow's milk in infancy. PEDIATRICS, 72:253, 1983.
14. Fomon, S.J., Ziegler, E.E., Nelson, S.E., and Edwards, B.B.: Cow

milk feeding in infancy: Gastrointestinal blood loss and iron nutritional status. J. Pediat., **98**:540, 1981.

15. Sadowitz, P.D., and Oski, F.A.: Iron status and infant feeding practices in an urban ambulatory center. PEDIATRICS, **72**:33, 1983.
16. Lo, C.W., and Walker, W.A.: Chronic protracted diarrhea of infancy: A nutritional disease. PEDIATRICS, **72**:786, 1983.
17. Ziegler, E.E., and Fomon, S.J.: Fluid intake, renal solute load, and water balance in infancy. J. Pediat., **78**:561, 1971.
18. Fomon, S.J., Filer, L.J., Jr., Anderson, T.A., and Ziegler, E.E.: Recommendations for feeding normal infants. PEDIATRICS, **63**:52, 1979.
19. Yeung, D.L., Pennell, M.D., Leung, M., and Hall, J.: The effects of 2% milk intake on infant nutrition. Nutr. Res., **2**:651, 1982.
20. Mermelstein, N.H.: Soy-oats infant formula helps fight malnutrition in Mexico. Food Technology, **37**:64, August, 1983.
21. Bressani, R., and Behar, M.: The use of plant protein foods in preventing malnutrition. Proceedings of the Sixth International Congress of Nutrition, August 9-15, 1963. Edinburgh: E. & S. Livingstone Ltd., p. 181, 1964.

Chapter 3

SUPPLEMENTAL FOODS FOR INFANTS

Recommendations and practices of feeding solid foods to infants are widely divergent in the United States[1] and other countries. Although few differences in health are noted from such divergent practices, the consequences may be subtle or may require long-term, careful observations.

Solid or supplemental foods seldom were recommended for infants before 1 year of age until about 1920. Human milk, for the most part, or modified cow's milk formulas supplied all or most of the nutritional needs of infants during the first year of life. The first supplements to the diet were cod liver oil to prevent rickets and orange juice to prevent scurvy.

Over the next 50 years, recommendations were made that some cereals and strained vegetables and fruits be introduced at about 6 months of age to: (1) supply energy, iron, vitamins, and possibly other factors; and (2) help prepare the infant for a more diversified diet. A wide variety of infant foods has since become available, and these have been introduced into the infant's diet earlier and earlier. Some reasons for the earlier introduction of solid foods were the desire of mothers to see their infants gain weight rapidly, the ready availability of convenient forms of solid foods, and the mistaken assumption that added solid foods help the infant sleep through the night.

Infant Feeding Periods

Infant feeding should be considered in three overlapping stages: the nursing period, during which human milk or an appropriate formula is the source of nutrients; a transitional period, during which specially prepared foods are introduced in addition to human milk or a formula; and a modified adult period, during which the majority of the nutrients come from the foods available from the table. The rate at which an infant progresses through these stages ideally should be determined by the rate of maturation of the nervous system, intestinal tract, and kidneys.

During the nursing period, the young infant is able to suck

and swallow only liquids. At this time the intestinal tract has not yet developed the defense mechanisms to cope with foreign proteins[2,3] and is best equipped to digest the protein, fat, and carbohydrate in human milk. The young infant's kidneys are not mature enough to handle large osmolar loads of protein and electrolytes.[4]

During the transitional period, the neuromuscular mechanisms needed for recognizing a spoon, masticating, and swallowing nonliquid foods are developing; and the infant can appreciate the variation in the taste and color of foods. At this time the intestine is developing defense mechanisms to protect the infant from foreign proteins; the ability to digest and absorb proteins, fats, and carbohydrates is increasing rapidly; and the kidneys are developing the ability to handle osmolar loads with less water.

With the onset of the modified adult period, the physiologic mechanisms have matured to near adult proficiency, and the infant is learning to feed himself or herself. At this time table food requires only minimal alteration, such as cutting into small pieces; and taste ability and preferences are becoming established.

Recommendations for the introduction of solid foods to infants should be based on current concepts of the infant's developmental processes.

The nursing period lasts for at least 4 to 6 months and is followed by the transitional period. The timing of this dietary change is in part related to the neuromuscular development of the infant. By 4 to 5 months of age, the extrusion reflex of early infancy has disappeared, and the ability to swallow nonliquid foods has become established. By 5 to 6 months of age, the infant will be able to indicate a desire for food by opening his or her mouth and leaning forward, and to indicate disinterest or satiety by leaning back and turning away. Until the infant can react in this manner, feeding of solid food supplements may represent a type of forced feeding.

The onset of the modified adult period is more a matter of individual preference, but it usually begins after 1 year of age.

Adequate intakes of human milk or a commercial infant formula[5] meet all the known nutritional requirements of infants for the first 6 months of life, with the possible exception of vitamin D and fluoride in breast-fed infants. Rickets has been reported in breast-fed infants. When climatic and social conditions interfere with radiation of vitamin D precursors in the skin, breast-fed infants should be given a supplement of 400 IU of vitamin D daily.

Although all known essential nutrients (except fluoride) are contained in presently available commercial infant formulas based on cow's milk, unrecognized deficits may be avoided by introducing supplemental foods at 4 to 6 months of age.

Introduction of Solid Foods

When solid foods are introduced, single-ingredient foods should be chosen and started one at a time at weekly intervals to permit the identification of food intolerance.

Infant cereals, which provide additional energy and iron, are a good choice for the first supplemental food given the infant. Single-grain cereals, particularly rice, are usually well tolerated. Four level tablespoons of dry infant cereal fortified with electrolytic iron and diluted with milk or formula provide about 7 mg of iron. Other solid foods include vegetables, egg yolk, fruits, and meats; the order of introduction is not critical. Most infant foods are high in carbohydrate and provide a balance to the high protein content of the diet when cow's milk is the major source of calories. Higher protein foods (e.g., meat or chicken) are appropriate choices in the breast-fed infant because of the lower protein content of human milk.

Combination foods of cereal and fruit provide about 5 mg of iron per 4½ oz jar and may be given to older infants after the tolerance for individual components has been established. Combination foods generally are more expensive than single foods. Juices should be introduced when the infant can drink from a cup. Juices provide carbohydrates and vitamin C. However, juice in bottles used as a pacifier predisposes to nursing-bottle caries.

The gradual introduction of a variety of foods contributes to a nutritionally balanced diet and helps promote good eating habits. Strained foods prepared at home are nutritionally equivalent to those obtained commercially. Care must be taken to avoid spoilage of both home-prepared foods and commercial foods after the jars have been opened. Home-prepared spinach, beets, turnips, carrots, or collard greens are not good choices for feeding during early infancy because they may contain sufficient nitrate to cause methemoglobinemia.

Salt and sugar are not added to most commercially prepared infant foods, but many of the combined dinners or desserts have added sugar. Similarly, there is no need to add salt or sugar to fresh or frozen foods when they are used for home preparation of infant foods. Canned foods which contain large amounts of salt and sugar are unsuitable for the home preparation of infant foods.

Texture and Form

Solid foods offered to infants less than 1 year old should require a minimum of chewing. Unfortunately, a number of deaths from choking and aspiration have occurred in infants and toddlers in recent years, including such foods as hot dogs, nuts (especially peanuts), grapes, carrots, and round candies.[6]

Water

During the nursing period, the amount of water needed by infants to replace water loss from the skin and lungs, feces, and urine, and to provide for growth, is available in human milk or infant formula. Healthy infants usually require little or no supplemental water, except in hot weather.

When solid foods are introduced, additional water frequently is required because the renal osmolar load is high in foods with a higher protein or electrolyte content such as strained meats, egg yolk, and "high-meat dinners." Fruit juices, fruits, puddings, vegetables, and desserts have a low renal solute load. Infants should be offered water as part of a feeding to allow them an opportunity to fulfill fluid needs without an obligatory intake of extra calories. Additional water should be provided when fluid intake is low or extrarenal losses are increased, such as during an illness. Table 1 lists the renal solute load provided by a number of foods commonly consumed by infants.

Sodium

The suggestion that salt intake is an etiologic factor in the development of hypertension in adults comes mainly from epidemiologic evidence and animal studies. Additional factors of genetic and nutritional origin play a role in pathogenesis of hypertension.[7] The hypotheses that the sodium content of infant foods contributes to hypertension in later life has not been confirmed in two areas: (1) Infant foods, even with salt added, have not been shown to contribute as much sodium to the diet as whole milk or table foods. (2) Studies of infants fed diets either high or low in sodium (9.2 mEq/100 kcal versus 1.9 mEq/100 kcal) from ages 3 to 8 months showed no correlation between salt intake during infancy and blood pressure at 1 and 8 years of age (see Chapter 32).

Concern about this possible problem led the manufacturers of infant foods to reduce and finally omit the addition of salt to their products. A series of infant dietary surveys reflect the changes in sodium intake by infants in the United States.[8,9] Their results are summarized in Tables 2 and 3.

The sodium intake is relatively high when table foods and cow's milk are consumed, and sodium intake is relatively low

Table 1
Renal Solute Load for Various Infant
Feeds

Product	Solute Load (mosmol/100 kcal)
Human milk	12
Whole cow's milk	33
Cow's milk (2% fat)	40
Skimmed cow's milk	66
Evaporated cow's milk with water 1:1 + 5 gm carbohydrates/dl	24
Infant formula*	16
Strained foods:	
Pears	5
Applesauce	5
Chicken with vegetables	30
Vegetables and beef	18

*Representative of the major commercial infant formulas.

Table 2
Sodium Concentration (mEq/100 kcal) in Infant Diets

Age (mo)	1969	1972	1974	1977	1977*	1979*	1983*
2	2.4	2.0	2.3	1.7	1.6	1.2	1.1
4	3.9	2.8	2.9	3.3	2.6	1.5	1.2
6	4.7	3.5	3.5	3.8	3.1	1.5	1.3
8	5.3†	4.3	5.0	4.7	3.6	2.3	2.7
10	5.5†	5.1	5.3	5.1	4.3	3.1	2.9
12	5.7†	5.8	6.0	6.2	6.2	3.9	5.0

*No added salt.
†No table food used.

when human milk or commercial infant formula and infant foods are the principle sources of calories. Only 6 to 28% of the total sodium intake comes from the salt in infant foods. Virtually every source of sodium in infant diets has been involved in the decrease in intake between 1972 and 1979, including an increase in breast feeding, a decrease in cow's milk intake (particularly during the early months of life), and a change in the selection of infant food with an increased use of fruits, vegetables, and juices. Selection of table foods containing less sodium accounts for the lower sodium intake of older infants.[10]

Sodium requirement for healthy infants is the sum of the needs for growth and obligatory losses (e.g., skin, stool, and urine). The need for growth approximates 0.5 mEq/kg per day between birth and 3 months of age and decreases to 0.1 mEq/kg per day after 6 months of age. Dermal losses range from 0.4 to 0.7 mEq/kg per day, depending on the environmental temperature. Human milk has a much lower sodium content than cow's milk. However, on the average, there is sufficient sodium to meet the infant's needs under usual environmental circumstances. The amount of sodium in individual samples of human milk is variable, with a range of 3 to 19 mEq per liter. With regard to higher intakes, there is evidence that uptakes up to 9 mEq/kg per day are tolerated by infants with only a minimal increase in extracellular space and changes in compensatory mechanisms. However, healthy infants can tolerate a range of sodium intakes without aberrations in their sodium homeostasis.[11]

At present, the recommended feedings for infants contribute less sodium to their diets than the table foods they frequently receive in the latter half of the first year of life. Further efforts at reducing the sodium concentration in foods designed primarily for infants would be unwise.[12]

Food Sensitivity

The gastrointestinal tract is permeable to macromolecules during early infancy. In addition, the production of IgA antibody is low in the neonate and does not reach appreciable levels until the infant is about 7 months old. IgA antibody secreted from the intestinal mucosa on stimulation of food protein is specifically directed against that food protein; and this antibody could decrease the amount of antigenic material passing through the mucosa. These considerations provide an argument for breast feeding alone during the nursing period and for using only hypoallergenic foods during the transitional period, especially in infants with a family history of allergy.[2]

An estimated 0.3 to 7% of infants are sensitive to cow's milk and other foods such as soy protein. However, these estimates are tentative because of the lack of simple, reliable, and objective means to verify the diagnosis of food allergy. There is a tendency to ascribe a variety of symptoms to food allergy; this may lead to the unjustified elimination of valuable foods from the diet (see Chapter 29).

Obesity

The use of infant formulas and the age of introduction of supplementary foods may be factors in the development of obesity. There is some evidence that artificially fed infants develop and gain weight more rapidly than breast-fed infants; the tendency to encourage infants to finish a bottle feeding may be a predisposing factor. In addition, solid foods do not appear to displace calories from bottle feedings; rather, they tend to constitute an additional supply of calories. There is a need for further studies on this issue.

Caloric density of commercially prepared foods varies considerably and is a factor in caloric intake. For example, strained fruits contain 45 to 70 calories per 100 gm (135 gm per jar); strained vegetables, 25 to 65 calories per 100 gm (128 gm

Table 3
Sources of Calories in Diets with Increasing Sodium Content

Sodium (mEq/100 kcal)	Average Age (mo)	Formula (%)	Infant Food (%)	Milk (%)	Table Food (%)
0.99-1.99	4.4	72.4	21.3	1.4	4.7
2.00-2.99	7.4	22.4	36.7	25.5	15.3
3.00-3.99	7.6	6.1	27.0	42.8	24.0
4.00-4.99	9.2	12.9	11.5	29.5	46.2
5.00-5.99	10.5	3.9	10.9	25.9	61.4

per jar); meats, 90 to 140 calories per 100 gm jar; and egg yolks, 195 calories per 100 gm jar.

Composition of Supplementary Foods

Most commercially prepared foods are labeled to indicate calorie and nutrient content. Physicians and parents should be familiar with the nutrition information on product labels. The renal solute load for representative foods is given in Table 1. Protein content is variable.

References

1. Committee on Nutrition: On the feeding of solid foods to infants. PEDIATRICS, 21:685, 1958.
2. Eastham, E.J., Lichauco, T., Grady, M.I., and Walker, W.A.: Antigenicity of infant formulas: Role of immature intestine on protein permeability. J. Pediat., 93:561, 1978.
3. Walker, W.A.: Antigen penetration across the immature gut: Effect of immunologic and maturational factors in colostrum. In Ogra, P.L., and Dayton, D.H., ed.: Immunology of Breast Milk. A Monograph of the National Institute of Child Health and Human Development. New York: Raven Press, pp. 227-235, 1979.
4. Ziegler, E.E., and Fomon, S.J.: Fluid intake, renal solute load, and water balance in infancy. J. Pediat., 78:561, 1971.
5. Committee on Nutrition: Commentary on breast-feeding and in-

fant formulas, including proposed standards for formulas. PEDIATRICS, **57**:278, 1976.

6. Foods and Choking in Children. (A report to the Food and Drug Administration on a conference held in Elkridge, Maryland, August 4-5, 1983.) Evanston, Illinois: American Academy of Pediatrics, December 1983.

7. Committee on Nutrition: Salt intake and eating patterns of infants and children in relation to blood pressure. PEDIATRICS, **53**:115, 1974.

8. Purvis, G.A.: What nutrients do our infants really get? Nutr. Today, **8**:28, September-October, 1973.

9. Johnson, G., and Purvis, G.A.: Unpublished data.

10. Council on Scientific Affairs, AMA: Sodium in processed foods. J.A.M.A., **249**:784, 1983.

11. Committee on Nutrition: Commentary on breast-feeding and infant formulas, including proposed standards for formulas. PEDIATRICS, **57**:278, 1976.

12. Nichols, B.L., Jr.: Sodium intake of infants in the United States. *In* Bond, J.T., Filer, L.J., Jr., Leveille, G.A., Thomson, A.M., and Weil, W.B., Jr., ed.: Infant and Child Feeding. New York: Academic Press, pp. 317-332, 1981.

Chapter 4

VITAMIN AND MINERAL SUPPLEMENT NEEDS OF NORMAL CHILDREN IN THE UNITED STATES

The last 50 years have witnessed a steadily increasing understanding of the biochemistry of vitamins and trace minerals and their role in human nutrition and intermediary metabolism. There also has been a growing public awareness of the sometimes dramatic clinical impact of vitamin and mineral administration in deficiency states. Indeed, the addition of vitamin D to milk almost has eliminated deficiency rickets in children in the United States.

As nutritional needs became more clearly defined, vitamins and minerals were incorporated into processed formulas to help provide an essentially complete diet for infants; specific nutrients likely to be lacking in the diet of older infants and children also were used to fortify certain foods, such as infant cereal. Supplemental vitamin and mineral drops or tablets continued to be used, probably to a greater extent than necessary considering the more extensive fortification of food.

Vitamin and/or mineral supplements are relatively inexpensive and available without prescription; therefore, they are used by a substantial proportion of the population. The widespread consumption of these supplemental products also is fostered by a combination of advertising pressure and concern about dietary adequacy. Many individuals regard vitamin and/or mineral supplements as a reliable method of ensuring that real or imagined dietary shortcomings are corrected. Others, on far less rational grounds, have come to regard supplements in a wide range of doses as the philosopher's stone for good health or as treatment for a wide array of ailments from mental retardation to the common cold. As a result, vitamin and mineral supplements are widely abused by the general public, occasionally to the point of toxicity.

This chapter will review the usual need for vitamin and mineral supplements in normal infants and children in the United States. In addition, the special needs of preterm and low-birth-weight infants and those of infants whose mothers are malnourished will be mentioned. The special requirements of infants and children with overt nutritional deficiencies, malabsorptive and other chronic diseases, rare vitamin-dependency conditions, inborn errors of vitamin or mineral metabolism, or deficiencies related to the intake of drugs will not be discussed. Many children with these disorders may require pharmacologic doses of vitamins, which should be individually prescribed by the physician.

Government Regulations and Commercial Practice

Vitamin and mineral preparations currently available in the United States for infants and children less than 4 years old are in accord with Food and Drug Administration (FDA) regulations.[1,2] Preparations for older children and adults are not subject to FDA regulations, and this may increase the likelihood of toxicity from these preparations. The FDA regulations, designed to minimize misuse, cover the specific vitamins and minerals and the minimum and maximum levels allowed and/or required in multivitamin and/or multimineral supplements for infants and children less than 4 years old and pregnant or lactating women.

The distinctions between the Recommended Dietary Allowances (RDA) and the US RDA follow. RDA's are established for numerous age groups and according to sex, and they are periodically published by the Food and Nutrition Board of the National Academy of Sciences, National Research Council. Using the RDA's as a basis, the FDA established US RDA's as reference figures for the nutrition labeling of foods and supplements. US RDA's are established for only three groups: infants, children from 1 to 4 years old, and adults and children 4 or more years old. The scientific basis for the types of supplements considered proper for infants and children has not changed substantially.

The FDA regulations were intended to require multivitamin and multimineral supplements to contain appropriate combinations of vitamins and/or minerals at levels which ranged from lower limits (considered sufficient to minimize the risk of deficiency) to upper limits (estimated to fully meet nutritional needs without undue excess). In almost all instances, the lower limits for individual nutrients were about 25 to 50% of the RDA, and the upper limits were 100 to 150% of the RDA. This type of regulation is useful because some previously available preparations called multivitamin or multimineral supplements omitted important nutrients considered conducive to good health. In addition, many preparations contained insignificant amounts of certain nutrients, and some contained levels of nutrients deemed excessive and possibly harmful if taken over a long period of time.

The products on the market for infants and children consist primarily of:

1. Liquid drop preparations for infants (a) vitamins A, D, and C, with or without iron; (b) vitamins A, D, C, and E, thiamin, riboflavin, and niacin; (c) vitamins A, D, E, and C, thiamin, riboflavin, niacin, and vitamin B_6, with or without iron.

2. Chewable tablets for young children (a) vitamins A, D, and C, with or without iron; (b) vitamins A, D, E, and C, thiamin, folic acid, riboflavin, niacin, vitamin B_6, and vitamin B_{12}, with or without iron.

Folic acid is omitted from liquid dietary supplements because it is relatively unstable in liquid preparations. No liquid multivitamin supplements containing folate are commercially available for this reason.

The foregoing combinations also are available with fluoride for infants and children residing in areas where the water is not fluoridated. However, because of their fluoride content, these preparations are only available on prescription. Supplements containing 0.25, 0.5, or 1.0 mg fluoride per dose enable physicians to prescribe the appropriate amount of fluoride supplements, when necessary, and the vitamins or vitamins and iron recommended for an individual child or age group.

Individual vitamin supplements rarely are used for infants, except for specific indications. Examples are the administration of vitamin K at birth to prevent hemorrhagic disease and vitamin E to prevent hemolytic anemia in small preterm infants.[3,4] Iron is the only mineral supplement commonly used for infants, either alone or in combination with vitamins.

Guidelines for Supplementation

Table 4 summarizes the following guidelines for the use of supplements in healthy infants and children. The indications for vitamin K and fluoride are discussed in the text. The normal infants and children indicated by Table 4 are assumed to be receiving an adequate milk intake, and those who are more than 6 months old are assumed to be receiving a variety of solid foods.

Newborn Infants

Vitamin K is an effective prophylaxis against hemorrhagic disease of the newborn because it prevents or minimizes the postnatal decline of the vitamin K-dependent coagulation factors (II, VII, IX, and X).

Vitamin K_1 should be given as a single, intramuscular dose of 0.5 to 1 mg or an oral dose of 1.0 to 2.0 mg. In rare instances, the dose may have to be repeated after about 4 to 7 days.

Vitamin K prophylaxis for newborn infants is now mandated by law in many states. Large doses of water-soluble vitamin K analogs can produce hyperbilirubinemia.

Table 4
Guidelines for the Use of Vitamin and Mineral Supplements in Healthy Infants and Children[*,†]

Child	Multi-vitamin	Vitamins			Minerals	
		D	E	Folate	Iron	Fluoride[‡]
Term infants (0-6 mo)						
Breast-fed	0	+	0	0	0	±
Formula-fed	0	0	0	0	0	±
Preterm infants						
Breast-fed[∥]	+	+	±	±	+	±
Formula-fed	+	+	±	±	+	±
Older infants (>6 mo)	0	+	0	0	±[§]	±
Children	0	0	0	0	0	±
Pregnant woman	±	0	0	±	+	0
Lactating woman	±	0	0	0	±	0

*Vitamin K for newborn infants is not shown.
†Extra calcium for pregnant and lactating women not shown.
‡Depending on local drinking water supply.
§Iron-fortified commercial infant formula and/or infant cereal is a convenient and reliable source.
∥Sodium content of human milk is marginal for these infants.

Breast-fed Infants

The renewed emphasis on human milk as an ideal food has raised questions about whether breast-fed infants require any vitamin or mineral supplements prior to the introduction of solid foods. This subject bears further discussion, particularly concerning the most widely used supplements: vitamins A, C, D, and E, iron, and fluoride. Multivitamin supplements should be given to breast-fed infants of mothers who are malnourished (a condition which is rare in the United States).

Because the vitamin D content of human milk is extremely low (about 22 IU/l), rickets can occur in breast-fed infants who do not have adequate exposure to sunlight. The results of studies purporting to show that human milk contains adequate quantities of vitamin D sulfate analogs have not been confirmed, and rickets is known to occur in breast-fed infants.[5,6]

Vitamin A deficiency rarely occurs in breast-fed infants. Historically, vitamin A supplementation was coupled with vitamin D supplementation because both were provided by cod liver oil. Currently there is little reason to provide vitamin A supplements; thus, there would be no harm in omitting vitamin A from supplements designed to provide vitamin D for breast-fed infants. Similarly, there is no evidence that supplementation with vitamin E is needed for the normal, breast-fed, term infant.

The maternal diet strongly influences the concentration of certain water-soluble vitamins in human milk. Vitamin B_{12} deficiency has been reported in breast-fed infants of strict vegetarian mothers. Thiamin deficiency also can occur in breast-fed infants of thiamin-deficient mothers, but this situation is virtually restricted to infants in countries where rice is a significant dietary staple.

Iron deficiency rarely develops before 4 to 6 months of age in breast-fed infants because neonatal iron stores can supply the major portion of iron needs during this period. Although human milk may contain little more than 0.3 mg iron per liter, about half of it is absorbed in contrast to the much smaller proportion assimilated from other foods.[7] This iron helps to delay the depletion of neonatal iron stores, but other sources of iron are required by 6 months of age. In normal, breast-fed, term infants, the addition of iron-fortified cereal after 6 months of age is desirable.[8]

The benefit of fluoride supplementation in the breast-fed infant is controversial. This is understandable because of the dearth of evidence that fluoride supplementation in the first 6 months of life alters the prevalence of dental caries in the secondary dentition. The view that fluoride supplementation is unnecessary during the first 6 months of life is tempered by the knowledge that unerupted teeth are being mineralized in early infancy; consequently, supplemental fluoride would be expected to have a beneficial effect during this period. In weighing these opposing views, the Committee on Nutrition favors initiating fluoride supplements shortly after birth in breast-fed infants but acknowledges that fluoride supplementation could be initiated at 6 months of age (see Chapter 17).

Fluoride supplements are available alone and in combination with vitamins, with or without iron. Thus, if iron or vitamin D supplements are indicated, it is acceptable to include 0.25 mg fluoride if the water supply contains less than 0.3 ppm of fluoride.

Formula-fed Term Infants

Infants consuming adequate amounts of commercial infant formulas which are in keeping with the recommendations of the Committee on Nutrition[9] do not need vitamin and mineral supplementation in the first 6 months of life. They also do not need supplements during the second 6 months of life if formula continues to be used in appropriate combination with solid foods. After 4 months of age, iron-fortified formula and/or iron-fortified cereal are convenient sources of iron and are preferable to the use of iron supplements. If powdered or concentrated formula is used, fluoride supplements should be administered only if the community water contains less than 0.3 ppm of fluoride. Ready-to-use formulas are now manufactured with water low in fluoride, and recommendations for fluoride supplementation should be similar to those for breast-fed infants.

Mothers who insist on using pasteurized cow's milk or evaporated milk formulas should be told to give their infant supplemental vitamin C as well as vitamin D if the milk is not fortified.

Vitamin K deficiency is seen occasionally in infants. It usually is associated with diarrhea and, especially with the administration of antibiotics, through a decrease in the synthesis of vitamin K by the intestinal microflora. The feeding of soy or other nonmilk-based, commercial infant formulas was associated with vitamin K deficiency, which was related in part to the type of oil used in the formula. In 1976, the Committee on Nutrition recommended that all infant formulas, particularly nonmilk-based, commercial infant formulas, be required to contain an appropriate level of vitamin K.[9]

Preterm Infants

The needs of preterm infants for certain nutrients are proportionately greater than those of term infants because of the increased demands of a more rapid rate of growth and less complete intestinal absorption.[10]

During the first weeks of life (prior to consumption of about 300 kcal per day, or reaching a body weight of 2.5 kg), a multivitamin supplement that contains the equivalent of the RDA's for term infants should be supplied. The components of this supplement ideally should include vitamin E in a form well absorbed by preterm infants, such as d-α-tocopheryl polyethylene glycol succinate. Folic acid deficiency has been reported in preterm infants, and folic acid supplementation should be included in the regimen. Folic acid is not present in liquid multivitamin-multimineral combinations because of its lack of stability. However, because the period of administration will generally be in a hospital, folate can be added to a multivitamin preparation in the hospital pharmacy in a concentration to provide 0.1 mg (the US RDA) per day. The shelf life of folate should be limited to 1 month, and the label should read "shake well" because folate will gradually precipitate. Iron supplementation is best delayed until after the first few weeks of life because extra iron may predispose to anemia when there is insufficient absorption of vitamin E.[11] Neonatal iron stores are abundant for several weeks, and iron needs for erythropoiesis are relatively small during the physiologic postnatal decline in hemoglobin concentration.

After several weeks of age, when the infant is consuming more than 300 kcal per day, or when the body weight exceeds 2.5 kg, a multivitamin supplement is no longer needed; but it is a convenient method for providing the few specific nutrients that still may be required. These include vitamin D in amounts sufficient to bring the total daily intake (from milk plus supplement) to at least 400 IU, iron (2 mg elemental iron per kilogram per day), and possibly folic acid.

There have been reports of rickets and osteoporosis in breast-fed, preterm infants, and photon densitometry of the radius and ulna shows that bone density is less than in infants fed formulas.[12] The problem is the low calcium and phosphorus content of human milk, the former at only one-third the level in cow's milk, the latter at only one-sixth. Commercial infant formulas (see Appendix L) supply two to three times as much calcium and phosphorus as human milk. Preterm milk is no richer in calcium and phosphorus than milk from mothers who deliver at term.

Preterm milk from some mothers can supply sufficient sodium to meet the needs of rapidly growing preterm infants. But mature milk has too little sodium; in fact, hyponatremia has occurred when mature milk is fed.

The need of preterm infants for other minerals (zinc, copper, and selenium) is now under study.

Home-prepared Evaporated Milk or Cow's Milk Formulas

Although home-prepared formulas are not used frequently in the United States, they are used extensively in other countries. Home-prepared formulas lack sufficient vitamin C, so this must be supplemented (also, some milks are not fortified with vitamin D). Pasteurized cow's milk may promote fecal blood loss in some infants, and it is a poor source of iron; so supplemental iron (1 mg elemental iron per kilogram per day) should be started no later than 4 months in term infants. Preterm infants will also need a daily multivitamin preparation that includes a well absorbed form of vitamin E, and they will require folacin.

Older Infants

During the second 6 months of life, the normal infant may be on a diet of milk or formula, mixed feedings, and increased amounts of table food. Cereal should be fortified with iron. Other vitamin and mineral supplements usually are not required, although it is important that the diet include an adequate source of vitamin C. Infants at special nutritional risk as a result of lifestyle, economic disadvantage, or intercurrent illness may require multivitamin and mineral supplements.

After Infancy

Recent national dietary and health surveys[13] have shown little evidence of vitamin or mineral inadequacies, with the exception of iron. The most prevalent nutritional lack in preschool-aged children of lower socioeconomic status was simply an insufficiency of food. Thus, there is little basis for routine vitamin and mineral supplementation in normal children, especially because the growth rate decreases after infancy. An exception is the need for fluoride if there is insufficient fluoride in the drinking water.

When evidence of significant nutritional inadequacy arises, as with iron, the fortification of foods seems to be the most effective means of dealing with the problem. Among the disadvantages of relying on vitamin and/or mineral supplements to supply essential nutrients is the fact that some of the children most at risk do not have ready access to the supplements or may not comply with long-term medication. However, supplements may be indicated in some situations and should be composed of the multivitamins and minerals that provide these nutrients at approximately RDA levels. Groups at particular nutritional risk include:

1. Children and adolescents from deprived families, or those who suffer from parental neglect or abuse.

2. Children and adolescents who have anorexia, or those who have poor and capricious appetites, or those who consume fad diets.

3. Children who are on dietary regimens to manage their obesity.

4. Pregnant teen-agers—iron and probably folic acid are needed by these young women, but uncertainty about overall nutritional status in those considered at special nutritional risk warrants use of a multivitamin-multimineral supplement. The nutritional needs of the pregnant and lactating woman are discussed more fully in the recommendations of an ad hoc committee on nutrition of the American College of Obstetricians and Gynecologists.[14]

5. Children and adolescents consuming vegetarian diets without adequate dairy products may need supplementation, particularly with vitamin B_{12}, which is absent from vegetable foods. Vitamin B_{12} and vitamin D deficiencies have been described.

Providing Vitamin and Mineral Needs with Available Preparations

Recommendations for the use of supplements can be conveniently met with currently available preparations. But it is difficult to supply trace minerals other than iron to infants and children who are considered to be in high-nutritional-risk categories because multimineral preparations have required the inclusion of calcium, phosphorus, and magnesium in relatively large quantities that would be difficult to supply in a liquid or small tablet form. However, there may be a clinical role for a multivitamin-trace mineral supplement that would include iron, zinc, copper, and possibly other trace minerals which probably could be prepared more easily in liquid or small tablet form.

There is sufficient evidence to support the inclusion of zinc[15] and copper in multivitamin-multimineral preparations in tablet form.[16] The requirements for other trace minerals (such as selenium,[17] chromium, manganese, and molybdenum) are under investigation; figures for these nutrients are included in the 1980 RDA's. These trace minerals eventually might be considered for inclusion in supplements for infants and children because evidence to warrant their use may be forthcoming. However, there currently is insufficient information on which to base detailed recommendations for dose and appropriate ages for administration.

The combination of vitamins A, C, and D for infants (with vitamin E and/or iron as optional ingredients) was originally designed to complement home-prepared formulas. Now that most infants in the United States are fed commercial infant formulas or human milk, these needs have shifted somewhat. There seem to be roles in infant feeding for combinations of vitamin D with iron, vitamin D with vitamin E and possibly folate, and vitamins D, E, folate, and iron (Table 4).

Conclusion

Although some comments in this chapter are relevant to future developments in supplementation, currently available supplements and foods can be used to meet all recognized nutritional needs of infants and children. Even though deficiencies have been recorded in the infant of a malnourished mother,[18] the normal, breast-fed, term infant of the well nourished mother has not been shown conclusively to need any specific vitamin and mineral supplement—**provided** the infant has **adequate** exposure to sunlight. Similarly, there is no evidence that supplementation is necessary for the full-term infant fed commercial infant formula and for the properly nourished, normal child.

References

1. Food and Drug Administration: Label statements concerning dietary properties of food purporting to be or represented for special dietary uses. Definitions and interpretation of terms. Code of Federal Regulations, **21**:125.1, 1973.
2. Food and Drug Administration: Foods for special dietary use. Dietary supplements of vitamins and minerals. Code of Federal Regulations, **21**:105.85, 1977.
3. Committee on Nutrition: Vitamin K compounds and the water-soluble analogues: Use in therapy and prophylaxis in pediatrics. PEDIATRICS, **28**:501, 1961.
4. Committee on Nutrition: Vitamin K supplementation for infants receiving milk substitute infant formulas and for those with fat malabsorption. PEDIATRICS, **48**:483, 1971.
5. von Sydow, G.: A study of the development of rickets in premature infants. Acta Paediat. Scand. (Suppl. 2), **33**:3, 1946.
6. Harrison, H.E., and Harrison, H.C.: Disorders of Calcium and Phosphate Metabolism in Childhood and Adolescence. (Schaffer, A.J., and Markowitz, M., ed.: Volume XX in the Series Major Problems in Clinical Pediatrics.) Philadelphia: W.B. Saunders, 1979.
7. Saarinen, U.M., Siimes, M.A., and Dallman, P.R.: Iron absorption in infants: High bioavailability of breast milk iron as indicated by the extrinsic tag method of iron absorption and by the concentration of serum ferritin. J. Pediat., **91**:36, 1977.
8. Committee on Nutrition: Iron supplementation for infants. PEDIATRICS, **58**:765, 1976.
9. Committee on Nutrition: Commentary on breast feeding and infant formulas, including proposed standards for formulas. PEDIATRICS, **57**:278, 1976.
10. Committee on Nutrition: Nutritional needs of low-birth-weight infants. PEDIATRICS, **60**:519, 1977.
11. Williams, M.L., Shott, R.J., O'Neal, P.L., and Oski, F.A.: Role of dietary iron and fat on vitamin E deficiency anemia of infancy. New Engl. J. Med., **292**:887, 1975.

12. Steichen, J.J., Gratton, T.L., and Tsang, R.C.: Osteopenia of prematurity: The cause and possible treatment. J. Pediat., **96**:528, 1980.

13. Dietary Intake Findings, United States, 1971-74. National Health Survey. DHEW Publication No. (HRA) 77-1647. Vital and Health Statistics, Series 11, No. 202. Hyattsville, Maryland: National Center for Health Statistics, 1977.

14. Pitkin, R.M., Kaminetzky, H.A., Newton, M., and Pritchard, J.A.: Maternal nutrition: A selective review of clinical topics. Obstet. Gynecol., **40**:773, 1972.

15. Committee on Nutrition: Zinc. PEDIATRICS, **62**:408, 1978.

16. Alexander, F.W.: Copper metabolism in children. Arch. Dis. Child., **49**:589, 1974.

17. Lombeck, I., Kasperek, K., Bonnermann, B., Feinendegen, L.E., and Bremer, H.J.: Selenium content of human milk, cow's milk and cow's milk infant formulas. Eur. J. Pediat., **129**:139, 1978.

18. Fomon, S.J., and Strauss, R.G.: Nutrient deficiencies in breast-fed infants. New Engl. J. Med., **299**:355, 1978.

Chapter 5

FEEDING FROM AGE 1 YEAR TO ADOLESCENCE

The period from the first birthday until adolescence is one of transition from the child who is a passive recipient of food, through an exploratory phase of eating, through needing consistent limits from the parents, and finally to total control of the diet. During this period the child learns the importance of good nutrition for physical growth and mental development and the role of food in social interactions. Food should never be used inappropriately to discipline or as the primary form of affection.

The Second Year of Life

By the age of 1 year, infants who have put everything and anything into their mouth and have to be protected from ingesting dangerous materials are well on the way to taking some initiative in their selection of foods and the way in which the foods will get into their mouth. Finger foods, use of a spoon, and drinking from a cup involve the child's increasing dexterity and coordination. Children of this age do best if offered three meals and two snacks of an appropriate size each day. However, their food intake may be rather large on occasion and almost negligible at other times. Actual food intake may increase little compared to the first year of life, which may lead to a perception of a poor appetite. Unpredictable whims may make today's favorite meal unacceptable tomorrow. Or only one type of food may be acceptable for many days. Studies have shown that children will, over time, select a balanced diet if presented with a variety of foods. An increasing variety in taste, color, consistency, and temperature will help to maintain an adequate nutritional intake. Dependence on a single food, such as milk, or the consumption of large volumes of liquid will lead to nutritional imbalance. The use of added salt should be discouraged. Sugar in the form of soft drinks and candy, whether the items are purchased or home made, should be minimized.

The types of foods chosen must be appropriate for the child's ability to chew and swallow. Foods which are likely to be aspirated such as hot dogs, nuts (especially peanuts), grapes, carrots, and round candies should be avoided.[1] Young children are extremely curious, have limited patience, and have limited dexterity; these factors should be considered if young children eat with the rest of the family. Early nutritional guidance is based on consistent limit setting to mold the child's mobility, curiosity, and hunger drive. This molding will be in the family pattern. Demands for food or for drink frequently become attention-getting devices which may lead to an inappropriate intake if not recognized for what they are.

During this period, as well as in the later years, variety can be perceived in terms of what nutritionists have labeled the "basic four" food groups:

1. meat, fish, poultry, eggs;
2. dairy products—milk, cheese, and milk products;
3. fruits and vegetables;
4. cereal grains, potatoes, rice.

In assessing a child's nutrient intake, the physician or dietitian should take the occasion to survey the eating habits and patterns of the family because these play a significant role.

The Preschool Years

The years from age 2 to 5 are characterized by an increasingly active participation in family life. There also is increasing maturity in language and social skills appropriate to eating. Meals should become important social as well as nutritional functions and separated as much as possible from the stresses of the day and the tribulations of family life. A regular meal schedule to meet the increasing needs for energy use is important. During this period of life, the child is subjected to pressure from the media (especially television) concerning food selection. It is a challenge for the family to cope with these outside pressures so they do not dictate entirely the child's eating habits.

The School Years

Many changes occur in the child's life when formal education begins. He or she has to maintain a schedule which reinforces the limit setting in the preschool years. The noon meal frequently is at school, and there may be added choices to make. The child needs to learn to eat foods offered under conditions which may be considerably different from those at home. Meeting school bus schedules may supersede breakfast if time is short. The energy used at school needs to be replenished when the child comes home in the afternoon; but this snack should only "tide" the child over until the evening meal, not replace it. Parental control over the amount and type of these snacks is necessary.

During the later elementary school years, the child's need for energy increases and the pressures and temptations to replace the school lunch with other purchases may be great. This can take the form of foods high in energy but low in other nutrients or involve skipping a meal. These assertions of independence may appear to negate the nutrition lessons learned earlier. The older child is more likely to respond to reasoning to please parents or other caretakers.

Early involvement in competitive sports may be another influence on the child's eating behavior. The need to please a coach as well as parents may lead to discrepancies in advice which may be difficult to reconcile. Regimens designed for older children or professional athletes should not be applied to young amateurs.[2]

Summary

Adequate nutrition of the preschool and school-age child is based on a variety of foods of basic nutritional value. Eating patterns learned at home must compete with food selection choices promoted by the media and the children and adults with whom the child works and plays. The family will establish basic eating patterns which will be particularly important in the eating behavior learned by the child. This behavior is increasingly subject to outside influences as the child matures, yet the child's ability to make choices grows in scope and depth with age.

References

1. Foods and Choking in Children (a report to the Food and Drug Administration on a conference held in Elkridge, Maryland, August 4-5, 1983). Evanston, Illinois: American Academy of Pediatrics, December 1983.
2. Committee on Sports Medicine: Sports Medicine: Health Care for Young Athletes. Evanston, Illinois: American Academy of Pediatrics, pp. 161-175, 1983.

Bibliography

The following books are recommended for parents and older children:

Jane Brody's Nutrition Book. New York: W.W. Norton & Company, 1981

Winick, M.: Growing up Healthy. New York: William Morrow & Company, 1982.

Lambert-Lagacé, L.: Feeding Your Child from Infancy to Six Years Old. New York: Beaufort Books, Inc., 1982.

Chapter 6

ADOLESCENT NUTRITION

Approximately 39 million people, or 17% of the population in the United States, are aged 10 to 19 years. Based on dietary histories, some adolescents have been reported to have insufficient intakes of calcium, iron, and vitamin A. There are special situations, such as pregnancy and physical conditioning, during which the adolescent will have increased nutrition requirements.

Pediatricians and other health professionals should be aware of the health hazards associated with undernutrition and overnutrition during adolescence and be able and willing to provide nutrition counseling.

In this chapter, normal nutrition needs, food habits, and general nutrition concerns of adolescents will be discussed. Approaches for providing adequate nutrition support to pregnant adolescents and adolescents who are involved in athletic activities will be included. The Nutrition Committee of the Canadian Paediatric Society recently published a statement on adolescent nutrition,[1] and the American Academy of Pediatrics has published a handbook, *Sports Medicine: Health Care for Young Athletes*, which includes nutrition information for adolescent athletes.[2]

Factors Influencing Nutrition Needs of Adolescents

The onset of puberty—with its associated increased growth rate, change in body composition, physical activity, and onset of menstruation in girls—affects normal nutrition needs during adolescence. Increased growth rates occur in girls between 10 and 12 years of age, and in boys about 2 years later. Growth in girls is accompanied by a greater increase in the proportion of body fat than in boys, and in boys it is accompanied by a greater increase in the proportion of lean body mass and blood volume than in girls. Total body calcium shows a male:female ratio similar to that of lean body mass.

Recommended Dietary Allowances

The *Recommended Dietary Allowances*, from the National Research Council, provides guidelines for normal nutrition of adolescent males and females in two age categories, 11 to 14 years and 15 to 18 years (see Appendix H; also see Appendix H for the Canadian recommendations for age groups 10 to 12, 13 to 15, 16 to 18, and 19 to 24 years). A distinction must be made between energy allowances and allowances for protein, vitamins, and minerals. Energy allowances are based on median energy intakes of children doing light activities. Among teenagers, there is individual variability in the rates of physical growth, timing of the growth spurt, and physiologic maturation. In addition, individual physical activity patterns vary widely. For these reasons, it is recommended that assessment of energy needs of adolescents should be arrived at from observations of appetite, growth, activity, and weight gain in relation to deposition of subcutaneous fat. When food intake is restricted in the physically active adolescent, the sequence of events that follow will be a restriction of growth, a reduction of physical activity, then a drop in basal metabolic rate. For protein, vitamins, and minerals, the RDA's are designed to meet the needs of practically all healthy adolescents; hence, they exceed the requirements for the average person. However, the experimental evidence to justify the RDA's for adolescents (and young children) is extremely limited.

During adolescence, increases in the requirement for energy and such nutrients as calcium, nitrogen, and iron which reside in lean body mass depend on an increase in lean body mass (LBM) rather than an increase in body weight, with its variable fat content. Based on data collected for 570 males and 450 females 8 to 25 years old, Forbes showed that, between the ages of 10 and 20, the male LBM increases by an average 35 kg from 27 to 62 kg and the female LBM increases by 19 kg from 24 to 43 kg.[3] Assuming that the lean body contents of calcium, iron, nitrogen, zinc, and magnesium of adolescents are the same as those of adults, the daily increments of body nutrients for the growing adolescent can be estimated (Table 5). If maintenance needs (at present unknown for adolescents) were to be added to growth needs, appropriate daily requirements could be derived. Inherent in this method is the limitation that the increments in body content of these nutrients, hence the increased nutrient needs, are not constant throughout adolescence but are associated with the growth rate rather than chronologic age *per se*.

Table 5
Daily Increments in Body Content of Minerals and Nitrogen During Adolescent Growth*

Mineral	Sex	Average for Period 10-20 yr (mg)	At Peak of Growth Support (mg)
Calcium	M	210.0	400.0
	F	110.0	240.0
Iron	M	0.57	1.1
	F	0.23	0.9
Nitrogen†	M	320.0	610.0
	F	160.0	360.0
Zinc	M	0.27	0.50
	F	0.18	0.31
Magnesium	M	4.4	8.4
	F	2.3	5.0

*Adapted from Forbes.[3]
†Multiply by 0.00625 to obtain grams of protein.

Nutrition Concerns During Adolescence

The National Health and Nutrition Examination Survey (1971-1974) found that, of all age groups, adolescents had the highest prevalence of "unsatisfactory" nutritional status.[4] Based on dietary recall, adolescents' intake of calcium, vitamin A, vitamin C, and iron tended to fall below the RDA levels, with iron deficiency being more common in males than in females during adolescence.* The nutrient intakes of boys tended to come closer to RDA levels simply because they ate relatively greater amounts of food, whereas girls frequently dieted. Soft drinks, coffee, tea, and alcoholic beverages frequently replaced milk and juice. Milk intake was diminished in nonwhite adolescents, possibly because of lactose intolerance.

Food habits of adolescents differ from those of other age groups. They are characterized by an increased tendency to skip meals (especially breakfast and lunch), snacking (especially candies), inappropriate consumption of fast foods, and dieting. Some adhere to vegetarianism or to extremely restric-

*In this connection, it should be remembered that the RDA's are designed to meet the estimated needs of 95% of the population and thus clearly exceed average requirements.

tive dietary regimens such as Zen macrobiotic diets. These behavioral patterns are explained by the teen-ager's newly found independence, difficulty in accepting existing values, dissatisfaction with body image, search for self-identity, peer acceptance, and conformity of lifestyle. Diet counselors should have a complete understanding of these behavioral patterns. As a result of typical adolescent food behaviors, the following aspects related to the adolescent's diet deserve special mention.

1. Energy—The low energy intake by many adolescents creates difficulties in planning diets which contain adequate levels of nutrients, especially iron.

2. Calcium—A low calcium intake associated with a high protein intake may unfavorably affect the teen-ager's calcium balance.

3. Iron—The need for iron for both boys and girls is increased from 11 to 18 years, in the former to sustain the rapidly enlarging LBM and hemoglobin mass, in the latter to offset menstrual losses. Iron-deficiency anemia is one of the most common nutritional disorders in this age group, and it is more frequently found in adolescent boys than girls.

4. Zinc—Zinc is an essential element for adolescent growth. Some observers feel that the intake of this element is marginal in certain segments of the population in the United States. A zinc-deficiency syndrome characterized by growth failure, hypogonadism, and decreased taste acuity has been described in children in the Middle East.

5. Vegetarianism—Vegetarian teen-agers who do not eat eggs and meat or drink milk are vulnerable to deficiencies of several nutrients, particularly vitamins D and B_{12}, calcium, iron, zinc, and perhaps other trace elements.

6. Dental caries—Although dental caries begin in early childhood, this condition may be the most prevalent nutrition-related problem of teen-agers. Low fluoride intake and a high consumption of sugared foods are the major nutritional factors implicated in the widespread occurrence of dental caries. A complete discussion of this all-too-common problem is to be found in Chapter 17.

7. Obesity and anorexia nervosa—These two major nutrition-related health problems of adolescents are discussed elsewhere (see Chapters 28 and 21).

8. Conditioned deficiencies—A number of drug-nutrient interactions have been described.[5] Anticonvulsant drugs, especially phenytoin and phenobarbital, interfere with the metabolism of vitamin D. Protracted use of these drugs can

lead to rickets and/or osteomalacia; hence, supplementation with vitamin D is desirable. Isoniazid interferes with pyriodoxine metabolism. The possible influence of oral contraceptives is currently being studied; there is evidence to suggest that serum lipid values are increased.[6,7]

Nutritional Considerations During Pregnancy

The Impact of Pregnancy on the Teen-ager

About 600,000 live births per year are reported for girls in their teens; more than a tenth of these infants are born to mothers 15 years old or younger.

Pregnancy is believed to put additional stress on the nutrition status of the growing and maturing teen-ager. Because the adolescent growth spurt is not complete until a few years after menarche, fetal demand for nutrients could place maternal growth in jeopardy. This is especially true in the early maturing girl and in those whose prepregnancy nutrition status is unsatisfactory. Although it is widely recognized that the fetus may be protected from the vagaries of maternal diet, except in extreme malnutrition, supplementation of poor maternal diets with calories and nutrients results in improved maternal weight gain during pregnancy and a reduction in the prevalence of low-birth-weight infants.[8] However, an extensive study of normal pregnant women showed no effect on birth weight from protein and energy supplements.[9]

The concept that pregnancy may have a significant impact on the growth of the teen-ager has been challenged.[10] Citing nitrogen and calcium as examples, Forbes showed that the nutrient requirements for the adolescent growth spurt, which is waning by the time pregnancy is possible, represent only a small amount above what is considered the requirement for a nongrowing, pregnant adult. However, nutritional considerations may become extremely important in the teen-ager who is undergrown, undernourished, or chooses to nurse her infant.

There also is some difficulty in accepting the widely held belief that the incidence of low-birth-weight infants is higher in teen-age pregnancies than in others. Garn and Petzold[11] recently showed that the birth weight of infants born to teen-age mothers is similar to those born to older women, when race and maternal stature are considered.

Recommended Dietary Allowances

Regardless of whether or not an adverse biologic outcome is likely to occur in a teen-age pregnancy, the pregnant teen-ager should receive sound nutritional advice and support. Recommended dietary allowances for teen-agers who are pregnant and lactating may be derived by adding the allowances for these conditions to those for the nonpregnant age groups (Appendix H). A total weight gain of 11 to 13 kg during pregnancy is considered optimal for adequate fetal development. Too little weight gain has been associated with the delivery of low-birth-weight infants. Too rapid a weight gain has been associated with toxemia, a condition most prevalent in low-income, nonwhite women who enter pregnancy with decreased nutritional reserves and poor medical attention.

The studies of Hytten and Leitch[12] have provided information on the composition of the weight gain during pregnancy and of the theoretic energy and protein needs. Of a total weight gain of 12.5 kg, the fetus, placenta, and amniotic fluid accounts for about 4.8 kg; the remaining 7.7 kg is maternal lean tissue (3.7 kg) and body fat (4 kg).

The total increment in protein is 900 gm, in calcium it is 27 gm, and in iron it is 800 mg; these amount to 5.0 gm, 150 gm, and 4.4 mg per day, respectively, for the second and third trimesters, when most of the weight gain is occurring. The additional need for protein represents only a small increment (about 10%) over the requirement for the nonpregnant woman. Furthermore, calcium and iron absorption are increased during pregnancy, and the additional need for iron is lessened by cessation of menstruation.

An estimated total of 80,000 additional kilocalories are required to sustain a normal pregnancy; averaged over the entire pregnancy, this amounts to 290 extra kilocalories per day, or about 13% more than is recommended in the nonpregnant woman.

The energy allowance for the pregnant teen-ager, as for other teen-agers, should be tailored to individual needs. Energy consumption over and above requirements will lead to accumulation of fat, which may persist after childbirth and become a factor in the development of adult obesity. An energy intake below requirements could lead to suboptimal pregnancy weight gain. The pregnant adolescent, in denying the pregnancy, may diet for several months in the hope she will not become heavier.

Lactation

In many respects lactation is a greater nutritional burden than pregnancy. Each 850 ml of human milk contains 600 kcal, 9.5 gm protein, and 250 mg calcium, plus, of course, trace elements and most of the vitamins; and the concentration of the latter group can be influenced by the mother's diet (see Chapter 1). Assuming 80% efficiency, the lactating woman requires an additional 750 kcal per day to produce 850 ml milk and an additional 18 gm protein and 500 mg calcium (the latter two values are based on 50% absorption).

Counseling the Pregnant Teen-ager

Pregnant teen-agers are just as likely as other teen-age girls to have patterns of meal skipping, poor quality snacks, eating away from home, overconcern about weight, and limited food choices. Deficiencies of calcium, vitamin A, and iron—most frequently reported in the diets of adolescents—may have deleterious effects on the outcome of the pregnancy. Folate deficiency also has been reported in the pregnant teen-ager's diet. The pregnant teen-ager who is a strict vegetarian may have additional deficiencies such as protein, riboflavin, vitamin B_{12}, vitamin D, and trace minerals. The pregnant adolescent also may be particularly vulnerable to zinc deficiency. Appropriate vitamin and mineral supplementation is indicated for those who habitually consume inadequate diets. Recommendations for folate and iron supplementation should be made routinely (see Chapter 23).

The counselor should realize that, in addition to nutritional risks, the teen-age mother may experience a host of social disabilities such as disrupted schooling, disrupted family life, decreased earning capacity, and dependency on public assistance.

There is concern for adolescents who are pregnant. They need early and continuous medical, emotional, and nutritional support. A comprehensive health care program for the pregnant adolescent should include proper prenatal care, monitoring weight gain, nutritional assessment, counseling and support, psychologic counseling, family planning, and continued schooling. The counselor should gain the pregnant teen-ager's trust and confidence and should include, whenever possible, the parents or other caregiver in the counseling sessions. Many teen-agers · are responsive to suggestions that incorporate ethnic foods into their eating patterns. Pregnancy may provide the educator with a unique opportunity to make the teen-ager understand and improve her eating habits.

Nonnutritional factors also can influence pregnancy outcome; the influence of cigarette smoking is the best documented.[13] Pregnant women should be informed of the adverse effects of smoking and of the use of narcotic drugs.

Nutrition and the Adolescent Athlete

Adequate nutrition is essential for the peak performance of athletes.[2] In the highly competitive world of sports, it is easy for the athlete, coach, trainer, and/or parent to fall victim to nutrition misinformation or quackery.

Energy Intake and Distribution

Caloric intake must satisfy the need for basal metabolism, physical activity, and growth. Energy expenditure for basal metabolism depends on sex and body size. Because energy and nutrient needs for basal metabolism and physical activity take priority over those for growth, insufficient food intake can lead to suboptimal growth, which, in itself, can reduce physical performance. Attempts by athletes to gain or lose weight rapidly should be discouraged because these practices are associated with changes in body composition which may lead to reduced ability to perform.

Energy intake is the principal dietary determinant of athletic performance. The RDA's for energy of adolescents include energy cost of light physical activity. Energy costs of a variety of physical activities are known (Table 6). To obtain a rough estimate of the energy needs, the athlete may simply add 600 to 1,200 kcal, depending on the nature of the sport, to the RDA for weight. An optimum distribution of calories in the diet of an adolescent athlete is: protein, 15%; fat, 30%; and carbohydrate, 55%.

Protein

Contrary to the widely held belief, physical training does not call for an excessively large intake of protein. A small increase in daily protein intake may be justified to meet the need for building muscle mass and blood volume during training. If a balanced diet is consumed, the additional 600 to 1,200 kcal will add 22 to 45 gm protein per day. This would raise the daily protein intake to levels that are more than adequate.

Table 6
Energy Cost of Physical Activities

Activity	Men	Women
	kcal per hour	
In bed, asleep or resting	65	54
Sitting quietly	83	69
Standing quietly	105	82
Walking 3 mph	222	180
Recreation:		
Light activity (billiards, bowling, golf, sailing, and so forth)	150-300	120-240
Moderate activity (canoeing, dancing, horseback riding, swimming, tennis, and so forth)	300-450	240-360
Heavy activity (basketball, football, rowing, and so forth)	450+	360+

*Adapted from Durnin and Passmore.[14]

Vitamins, Minerals, and Water

If the diet has the prescribed calories and is structured from a variety of nutritious foods, the requirements of vitamins and minerals will ordinarily be met. However, there are circumstances in which supplementation with certain minerals and water becomes desirable.

Profuse sweating during heavy exercise may cause depletion of body sodium, potassium, and iron. Sodium chloride lost through sweating amounts to about 22 mM per liter of water loss. Because sweat is hypotonic, the problem with sweating is not so much the loss of electrolytes as dehydration which can lead to anorexia, inability to work, and lassitude. Under no circumstances should fluid intake be restricted as a means of weight control. Satisfaction of thirst alone is not an adequate means of ascertaining fluid replacement. Replacement of lost electrolytes with salt tablets may become necessary under conditions of profuse sweating, but this should be combined with fluid intake. Dilute glucose-electrolyte drinks may be ingested during prolonged periods of training and competition. In extreme salt loss, rehydration without adequate electrolyte replacement can lead to symptoms similar to those encountered in heat exhaustion.

Iron deficiency is a common problem in female athletes, and it also can occur in boys undergoing the adolescent growth spurt. During training and competition, iron-deficiency anemia can lead to loss of strength and endurance and to easy fatigability.

Fuel for Exercise and "Carbohydrate Loading"

Energy for exercise is derived from the phosphocreatine-ATP system. For sustained muscular activity, ATP should be replenished constantly. In the muscle cell, energy for the enzymatic synthesis of ATP is derived from the metabolic breakdown of carbohydrate, fat, or protein. With a normal diet adequate in calories, carbohydrate and fat are the prime sources of energy for muscle contraction. The relative efficiencies with which these energy sources are used depend on the level of oxygen consumption and the duration of activity.

In short-term activities such as sprinting, which involve maximal muscular effort, glycogen appears to be used preferably over fat for ATP synthesis. In endurance-type activities such as distance running and cycling, although fat provides a sizable amount of energy, muscle and liver glycogen are essential for repeated muscular contractions. When the muscle glycogen supply is nearly exhausted, the muscle fibers will fail to contract properly and lead to weakness. The total glycogen content of the body is only about 500 gm, which is equivalent to 2,000 kcal. The athlete can increase the muscle glycogen content well above normal levels by a procedure known as "carbohydrate loading;" this procedure consists of several days of carbohydrate deprivation followed by several days of high carbohydrate intake. The athlete should continue exercise programs during this procedure. Any diet rich in carbohydrate will promote glycogen storage and thus help to improve the athlete's endurance.

In other sports such as football and basketball, where repeated strenuous training is involved, the muscle glycogen level gradually drops and the athlete's performance level deteriorates. This condition can be reversed only by proper nutrition and rest.

A precompetition meal containing large amounts of protein and fat may interfere with respiration and place excessive stress on circulation when eaten within 2 hours of strenuous exercise.

Consumption of candy and sugar drinks before exercise to obtain a "quick energy lift" may actually impair performance endurance activities. These feedings stimulate the release of insulin, which with exercise causes mild hypoglycemia. However, after exercise is initiated, the ingestion of sugar does not produce hyperinsulinemia. Sugar taken during exercise tends to maintain blood glucose at a normal level and reduces the need to break down liver glycogen.

Weight Control

Many young male athletes may want to improve their sports performance by increasing body weight. They should realize that what is needed is an increase in LBM and not excess body fat. This can be achieved only through muscle work and an appropriate increase in the intake of calories and nutrients. Drugs, hormones, and supplements of protein, vitamins, or other nutrients are not recommended. Serial measurements of skin-fold thickness will detect any undesirable increase in body fat.

Some athletes, particularly female athletes involved in

gymnastics and ballet and male wrestlers, may want to reduce their body weight. The athlete should attempt to reduce body weight by reducing body fat. This is done not by ingesting hypocaloric diets, which will reduce the athletic performance, but by working harder. The fat content of the body may be reduced to approximately 5 to 7% of the body weight. If further effort is made to reduce weight, it also will result in the loss of muscle tissue, which will reduce the physical performance of the athlete.

Although not every youngster can be an accomplished athlete, all should be encouraged to participate in physical exercise, which can serve to counterbalance the sedentary influence of the ubiquitous automobile. Physically active adults tend to have low blood cholesterol levels, and participation in physical fitness programs might even divert the adolescents' attention from such undesirable behaviors as substance abuse and overeating. A clear-cut benefit of physical activity is that it requires more intake of energy but no increase in specific nutrients, so it serves to prevent nutrient deficiencies.

Summary

Typical adolescent food habits include increased meal skipping, snacking, consumption of fast foods, and dieting. These habits make adolescents highly vulnerable to such nutritional deficiencies as calcium, vitamin A, iron, and ascorbic acid. Diet counselors should have a full understanding of adolescent behavioral patterns.

Special nutritional concerns among adolescents are vegetarianism, dental caries, oral contraceptives, pregnancy, obesity, anorexia nervosa, and athletic activities.

References

1. Canadian Paediatric Society Nutrition Committee: Adolescent nutrition. 1. Introduction and summary (first of a six-part series). Canad. Med. Assn. J., 129:419, 1983.
2. Committee on Sports Medicine: Sports Medicine: Health Care for Young Athletes. Evanston, Illinois: American Academy of Pediatrics, 1983.

3. Forbes, G.B.: Nutritional requirements in adolescence. *In* Suskind, R.M., ed.: Textbook of Pediatric Nutrition. New York: Raven Press, pp. 381-391, 1981.
4. Caloric and Selected Nutrient Values of Persons 1-74 Years of Age. DHEW Publication No. (PHS) 79-1657. Washington, D.C.: National Center for Health Statistics.
5. Roe, D.A.: Diet-drug interactions and incompatibilities. *In* Hathcock, J.N., and Coon, J., ed.: Nutrition and Drug Interrelations. New York: Academic Press, pp. 319-345, 1978.
6. Committee on Nutrition of the Mother and Preschool Child: Oral contraceptives and nutrition. Food and Nutrition Board of the National Research Council. Washington, D.C., 1975.
7. Wahl, P., Walden, C., Knopp, R., Hoover, J., Wallace, R., Heiss, G., and Rifkind, B.: Effect of estrogen/progestin potency on lipid/lipoprotein cholesterol. New Engl. J. Med., **308**:862, 1983.
8. Osofsky, H.J., and O'Connell, E.J.: Nutritional factors in pregnancy affecting fetal growth and subsequent infant development. *In* Suskind, R.M., ed.: Textbook of Pediatric Nutrition. New York: Raven Press, pp. 1-19, 1981.
9. Rush, D., Stein, Z., and Susser, M.: A randomized controlled trial of prenatal nutritional supplementation in New York city. PEDIATRICS, **65**:683, 1980.
10. Forbes, G.B.: Pregnancy in the teenager: Biological aspects. *In* McAnarney, E.R., and Stickle, G., ed.: Pregnancy and Childbearing During Adolescence: Research Priorities for the 1980s. New York: Alan R. Liss, pp. 85-90, 1981.
11. Garn, S.M., and Petzold, A.S.: Characteristics of the mother and child in teenage pregnancy. Amer. J. Dis Child., **127**:365, 1983.
12. Hytten, F.E., and Leitch, I.: The Physiology of Human Pregnancy. Oxford: Blackwell Scientific, 1964.
13. The Collaborative Perinatal Study: The Women and Their Pregnancies. DHEW Publication No. (NIH) 73-379. Washington, D.C.: U.S. Government Printing Office, pp. 72-80, 1972.
14. Durnin, J.V.G.A., and Passmore, R.: Energy, Work and Leisure. London: Heinemann Educational Books Ltd., 1967.

Chapter 7

NUTRITIONAL NEEDS OF PRETERM INFANTS

Optimal nutrition is critical in the management of the ever-increasing number of surviving, small preterm infants. Although the goal of nutrition for preterm infants is not known definitely, achieving a postnatal growth which approximates the growth *in utero* of a normal fetus at the same post-conception age appears to be the most logical approach at present.[1,2] The growth should begin by the second week after birth, after the initial changes in body water distribution have taken place and the infant has accommodated in a nonstressful way to the provision of enteral feeds and parenteral supplements. The fetal standards of growth to be considered in this chapter include not only weight and length but also values for rate of retention of individual nutrients and minerals (Table 7).[2] The quality of postnatal growth may differ from the quality of fetal growth, depending on the type of milk consumed, e.g., *ex utero* weight gain of a preterm infant taking an artificial formula includes more fat than the weight gain of a fetus of the same maturity.[3]

Caloric Requirement

The energy expenditures for maintenance and the energy costs of growth are the determinants of the caloric requirements of the growing infant. The energy expenditure for growth includes both the energy value of the new tissue stores and the energy cost of the tissue synthesis. The estimated "basal" or maintenance metabolic rate of preterm infants, including an irreducible amount of physical activity, is lower in the first week after birth than later; and, in a thermoneutral environment, it is approximately 50 kcal/kg per day by 2 to 3 weeks of age. Each gram of weight gain, including the stored energy and the energy cost of synthesis, requires 5 to 6 kcal. Thus a daily weight gain of 15 gm/kg requires a caloric expenditure of approximately 75 kcal/kg above the 50 kcal/kg

Table 7
Estimated Requirements and Advisable Intakes for Protein and Major Minerals
as Derived by the Factorial Approach*

Requirement	Tissue Increment (per day)	Dermal Loss (per day)	Urine Loss (per day)	Intestinal Absorption (% intake)	Estimated Requirement (per day)	Advisable Intake		
						per day	per kg†	per 100 kcal‡
Body weight 800 to 1,200 gm (26-28 weeks gestational age)								
Protein (gm)	2.32	0.17	0.68	87‡	3.64	4.0	4.0	3.1
Sodium (mEq)	1.63	0.06	1.21	90	3.22	3.5	3.5	2.7
Chloride (mEq)	1.23	0.10	1.18	90	2.79	3.1	3.1	2.4
Potassium (mEq)	0.87	0.12	1.11	83	2.52	2.5	2.5	1.9
Calcium (mg)	116.0	2.0	4.0	65	188.0	210.0	210.0	160.0
Phosphorus (mg)	75.0	1.0	25.0	80	126.0	140.0	140.0	108.0
Magnesium (mg)	3.2	–	2.0	60	8.7	10.0	10.0	7.5
Body weight 1,200 to 1,800 gm (29-31 weeks gestational age)								
Protein (gm)	3.01	0.25	0.90	87	4.78	5.2	3.5	2.7
Sodium (mEq)	1.77	0.09	1.81	90	4.08	4.5	3.0	2.3
Chloride (mEq)	1.30	0.15	1.77	90	3.47	3.8	2.5	2.0
Potassium (mEq)	1.03	0.18	1.66	83	3.45	3.4	2.3	1.8
Calcium (mg)	154.0	3.0	6.0	65	251.0	280.0	185.0	140.0
Phosphorus (mg)	98.0	2.0	37.0	80	171.0	185.0	123.0	95.0
Magnesium (mg)	4.0	–	3.0	60	11.7	13.0	8.5	6.5

*Adapted from Ziegler and co-workers.[2]
†Assuming body weight of 1,000 and 1,500 gm, respectively, for the 800 to 1,200 and 1,200 to 1,800 gm infants.
‡Assuming calorie intake of 130 kcal/kg per day.

maintenance expenditure. Estimated mean caloric requirements of preterm infants during the neonatal period are shown in Table 8.

There are individual variations among infants in activity, their ease of achievement of basal energy expenditure at thermoneutrality, and the efficiency of their nutrient absorption. In practice, intake by the enteral route of approximately 120 kcal/kg per day enables most preterm infants to achieve satisfactory rates of growth. More calories may be given if growth is unsatisfactory at these intakes. Newborn infants who are growth retarded frequently require an increased energy intake for growth because of both higher maintenance needs and higher energy costs of new tissue synthesis.

Protein Amount and Type

Up to the 1940's, preterm infants were usually fed human milk. However, at that time Gordon and co-workers[4] found that preterm infants would gain weight better when fed various artificial formulas than when fed the pooled, banked human milk then available. Weight gain of the infants appeared to correlate more with the electrolyte or ash intake than with the protein intake.[1] Intakes between 2.25 and 5.0 gm protein per kilogram per day were adequate but not toxic. The estimated requirements based on the fetal accretion rate of protein are 3.5 to 4 gm/kg per day[2] (Table 7).

The type of protein most suitable for preterm infants was studied by Gaull, Räihä, and co-workers.[5,6] They compared whey-predominant (60:40 ratio of whey:casein proteins) to casein-predominant (18:82 ratio of whey:casein proteins) formulas, each at two concentrations—1.5 gm/dl and 3 gm/dl. The metabolic effects and resultant growth following feeding of each of the four formulas were compared to the effects of feeding pooled milk from mothers of term infants. The BUN was higher in infants fed both of the 3 gm/dl formulas and the 1.5 gm/dl 18:82 formula than with the 1.5 gm/dl 60:40 formula. Metabolic acidosis and elevated plasma tyrosine and phenylalanine levels were found with the 3 gm/dl 18:82 formula, and plasma taurine levels were maintained longer with the 60:40 formulas. Gaull and co-workers[5,6] concluded there were no advantages, and some metabolic disadvantages, to the 3 gm/dl over the 1.5 gm/dl formulas, and that infants fed the whey-predominant (60:40) formulas, with whey:casein protein ratios similar to human milk, had metabolic indices and plasma amino acid levels closer to those of infants fed pooled, mature human milk.

Fats

Fat provides the major source of energy for growing preterm infants. In human milk, about 50% of the energy is from fat; and, in commercial formulas, fat provides 40 to 50% of the energy. The preterm infant digests and absorbs the predominantly saturated triglycerides of cow's milk poorly. The recognition of the magnitude of this fat malabsorption led to the use of low-fat formulas for preterm infant feeding in the 1940's and 1950's.[1] By 1960, after unsaturated, long-chain triglycerides from vegetable oils were recognized as being better absorbed than cow's milk fats, vegetable fats were used in commercial infant formulas for feeding of preterm infants. However, medium-chain triglycerides (MCT) are even better absorbed,[1] presumably because their digestion and absorption are not dependent on duodenal intraluminal bile salt levels, which are low in the preterm infant. Thus, the recently developed special formulas for preterm infants contain a mixture of MCT and predominantly unsaturated, long-chain triglycerides. The essential fatty acid requirement of at least 3% of total calories in the form of linoleic acid is amply met by this fat mixture. However, the gain in energy through improved absorption of

Table 8
Estimated Requirement for Calories in a
Typical, Growing, Preterm Infant*

Item	Kilocalories (per kilogram per day)
Resting caloric expenditure	50
Intermittent activity	15
Occasional cold stress	10
Specific dynamic action	8
Fecal loss of calories	12
Growth allowance	25
Total	120

*Adapted from Committee on Nutrition.[1]

MCT may be offset by an increased frequency of intestinal disturbances (abdominal distension, loose stools, vomiting) attributable to the MCT lipid.

The fat of human milk is well absorbed by the preterm infant. One reason for the relatively efficient absorption of human milk fat is the distribution of fatty acids in the triglyceride molecule. Palmitic acid in the beta position, as in human milk fat, leads to better absorption than seen with cow's milk fat, which has stearic acid in the beta position. Lingual lipase acting in the stomach starts the digestion, and bile salt-activated lipase in the milk continues digestion in the duodenum. These lipase activities substitute for the low pancreatic lipase of preterm infants and appear to proceed well in the low intraluminal bile salt concentrations of these infants.

Carbohydrates

The ability of the preterm infant to digest lactose may be poor in the first days of life because of a low intestinal mucosal lactase activity.[1] In the absence of adequate lactase activity, undigested lactose may be present in high concentrations in the lower intestinal tract and serve as a substrate for proliferation of potentially pathogenic bacteria. Additionally, the lactose may cause intestinal distension by its osmotic effect. However, glycosidase enzymes for glucose polymers are active in small preterm infants, and these polymers are well tolerated clinically by preterm infants. Also, glucose polymers add fewer osmotic particles to the formula per unit weight than lactose. On the basis of these advantages, the carbohydrate portions of the various special formulas for preterm infants contain approximately 50% lactose and 50% glucose polymers.

Minerals

Sodium and Potassium

Preterm infants, particularly those with a birth weight of less than 1,500 gm, do not have well developed renal sodium conservation mechanisms. The fractional excretion of sodium is high for the first 10 to 14 days after birth. Thus, the low sodium concentrations of human milk or of some commercial infant formulas designed for the feeding of term infants lead to hyponatremia when these milks are used as the sole source of sodium for a small preterm infant. Special formulas for preterm infants should provide 2.5 to 3.5 mEq of sodium per kilogram per day at full feeding levels.[7] However, small preterm infants (<1.5 kg) may require 4 to 8 mEq of sodium per kilogram per day to prevent hyponatremia. The potassium requirement for preterm infants appears to be similar to that of term infants, which is 2 to 3 mEq of potassium per kilogram per day.

Calcium and Phosphorus

Adequate amounts of calcium and phosphorus for normal bone growth and mineralization are difficult to supply to small preterm infants. As a result, osteopenia is a frequent feature in these infants, and some develop rickets. The commercial infant formulas designed for term infants and human milk are more discrepant in calcium and phosphorus content, relative to fetal accretion rates, than in other nutrient or mineral content.[1] The advisable intake for an 800 to 1,200 gm preterm infant is 210 mg calcium per kilogram per day to meet the fetal retention rate, which takes into account limited intestinal absorption.[2] The formulas commonly used for term infants contain 44 to 52 mg/dl calcium, and the bone mineral content (BMC) by photon absorptiometry in preterm infants consuming these formulas is far below the normal fetal values.[8] But with calcium intakes of 200 to 250 mg/kg per day and phosphorus intakes of 110 to 125 mg/kg per day, the BMC of preterm infants increases at the fetal rate. The role of vitamin D and its active metabolites in the genesis of the bone disease of small preterm infants will be discussed.

There is evidence that the special commercial infant formulas with added calcium and phosphorus now available for preterm infants can lead to postnatal bone growth and mineralization at fetal rates.[9] Overall growth and clinical status of the infants fed these formulas have been normal, and serum calcium and phosphorus concentrations are in the normal range.

Zinc and Manganese

Zinc metabolism in the preterm infant is complex. Theoretically, the fetal retention rate of 250 μg/kg per day[10] could be met by preterm infants who are fed their mothers' milk. However, when these infants are fed heat-treated human milk, they are in negative zinc balance until about 70 days of age, apparently because of limitations in intestinal absorption of zinc.[11] Recent evidence indicates that zinc absorption in preterm infants may be highly correlated with fat and nitrogen absorption. A positive zinc balance may appear earlier in the postnatal period when fat absorption is improved by having 40 to 50% of the fat as MCT.[12]

The Committee on Nutrition has proposed that infant formulas for full-term infants supply at least 0.5 mg of zinc and 5 μg of manganese per 100 kcal. There is no reason to modify these recommended levels for preterm infants.

Copper

Copper retention by the fetus is 51 μg/kg per day.[13] This amount of copper is available from the milk of mothers of preterm infants, with a copper content ranging from 58 to 72 μg/dl during the first month after birth. However, copper balances are negative in preterm infants until the fifth week of life.

Evaluation of copper nutrition in the neonatal period is complicated by the primary correlation of the serum copper level with the serum ceruloplasmin level, which rises after birth. The serum copper level may increase while the copper balance is negative. Increases in copper concentration in formulas from 50 μg/dl to 160 μg/dl did not lead to higher serum copper levels,[14] although huge doses of 1,500 μg/dl per day increase serum levels.[15]

Because clinical neonatal copper deficiency can occur with low copper intakes, close attention to the copper intake of preterm infants is important. The Committee's recommended copper intake of 90 μg per 100 kcal continues to be appropriate.[1]

Iron

On a weight basis, the iron content at birth of preterm infants is lower than the content of full-term infants. Much of the iron is in the circulating hemoglobin, and the frequent blood sampling the preterm infant may be subjected to further depletes the amount of iron available for erythropoiesis. The early physiologic anemia of prematurity is not benefited by iron therapy,[1] and there are frequent clinical indications for maintaining the preterm infant's hematocrit above 40% by transfusions of red blood cells (apnea of prematurity, long-term requirement for supplemental oxygen, patent ductus arteriosus). In addition, high levels of oral iron supplements can interfere with vitamin E metabolism in small preterm infants. Thus, there is no clear indication for iron supplementation during the first 1 to 2 months of life, although it has been suggested[2] that oral iron supplements be started at about 2 weeks of age, or when enteral feedings are tolerated, at a dose of 2 to 3 mg/kg per day. Vitamin E supplements should be given if iron is administered.

When preterm infants reach about 2 kg in weight and/or go home, iron supplementation is needed. Human milk-fed infants should receive 2 to 3 mg iron per kilogram per day as ferrous sulfate, and formulas with iron usually contain sufficient supplemental iron (see Chapter 23). A somewhat higher total daily dose of iron (supplement plus iron in the formula) is recommended for preterm infants by Siimes[16] to be started by 2 months of age and continued to 12 to 15 months of age (birth weight 1,500 to 2,000 gm, 2 mg/kg per day; 1,000 to 1,500 gm, 3 mg/kg per day; less than 1,000 gm, 4 mg/kg per day).

Iodine

The recommended minimum requirement of iodine in normal infants (5 μg/100 kcal) is based on the iodine content of human milk. The uptake of radioiodine by the thyroid gland of preterm infants has been found to be in the normal range for children and adults; therefore, 5 μg iodine per 100 kcal also is assumed to be adequate for preterm infants.

Other Trace Minerals

Although other minerals (such as cobalt, molybdenum, selenium, and chromium) are probably essential in trace amounts for infants, there is no information at this time on which to base recommendations.

Vitamins

The recommended oral intake of vitamins A, K, thiamin, riboflavin, niacin, pyridoxine, pantothenic acid, vitamin B_{12}, and biotin by preterm infants is the same as that recommended for full-term infants. All preterm, as well as term, infants should receive at least 1 mg vitamin K at birth. The Committee on Nutrition recommends that daily multivitamin supplements be given when enteral feedings are established. The most appropriate supplements are those that contain the National Research Council's Recommended Dietary Allowance (NRC-RDA) of vitamins A, C, D, E, and B complex (see Appendix H). Be aware that liquid multivitamin drops for infants do not contain folic acid. The Committee on Nutrition suggests that the NRC-RDA of folate can be added to the multivitamin preparation in the hospital pharmacy.

Vitamin C

There have been conflicting reports on the need for high ascorbic acid intakes in preterm infants to enhance the activity of hepatic p-hydroxyphenylpyruvic acid oxidase and to lower blood tyrosine and urinary tyrosine metabolite levels. Some investigators have reported no detrimental effects of transient neonatal tyrosinemia,[17,18] but one study reported a lowering of I.Q. values at 7 to 8 years of age in affected children.[19]

Because of the uncertainties, there have not been consistent recommendations regarding vitamin C supplementation. Although the Nutrition Committee of the Canadian Paediatric Society recommended vitamin C supplements for preterm infants in 1976, it did not do so in 1981.[20] Ziegler and co-workers[2] recommended an intake of 60 mg vitamin C per day by preterm infants. Because of the absence of compelling evidence for a high vitamin C requirement in preterm infants, the Academy's Committee on Nutrition does not recommend a supplement in addition to the 35 mg in the daily oral multivitamin mixture.

Vitamin D

The role of vitamin D deficiency in the development of the osteopenia and rickets of small preterm infants is uncertain.

Although some investigators have suggested that some small preterm infants have a high vitamin D requirement because of a relative insensitivity to active vitamin D metabolites, others have found that preterm infants given a high calcium formula plus 600 to 700 IU vitamin D per day did show normal serum 25-OH-vitamin D levels and calcium retentions similar to the fetal retention rate.[21]

The prevention of severe bone disease in preterm infants appears to rely on both supplemental oral calcium and phosphorus and at least 500 IU vitamin D per day. The latter can be achieved by giving 400 IU per day in a multivitamin supplement, in addition to the vitamin D in the formula. There is no evidence that administration of the active vitamin D metabolites, 25-OH-vitamin D or 1,25-diOH-vitamin D, is necessary or advisable.

Vitamin E

The requirement for vitamin E, alpha-tocopherol, in the small preterm infant is higher than that of the term infant because fat absorption is limited. The signs of vitamin E deficiency in the preterm infant include a mild hemolytic anemia[22] and mild generalized edema.[23] Vitamin E deficiency is exacerbated by a high iron intake which interferes with vitamin E absorption and vitamin E-mediated stabilization of the erythrocyte cell membrane, as well as by a high intake of polyunsaturated fatty acids which leads to a higher vitamin E requirement.[1]

The recommended intake of vitamin E is 0.7 IU vitamin E (0.5 mg d-alpha-tocopherol) per 100 kcal and at least 1.0 IU vitamin E per gram of linoleic acid.[1] In addition, it has been suggested that the preterm infant receive 5 to 25 IU of supplemental vitamin E per day because of concerns about the adequacy of its intestinal absorption.[1]

Folic Acid

Although clinical deficiency of folic acid is unusual, many preterm infants show laboratory evidence of folate deficiency by hypersegmentation of their neutrophils. Although a dose of 20 μg folate per day to preterm infants does not prevent low serum folate levels after 2 weeks, 50 μg is effective, and

Dallman[24] has suggested that preterm infants weighing less than 2,000 gm receive this amount. Be aware that the usual liquid multivitamin preparations for infants do not contain folic acid.

Caloric Density and Water Requirements

The caloric density of both preterm and term human milk is about 67 kcal/dl at 21 days of lactation. More detailed data are given in Appendix K. Formulas of this caloric density have been used for feeding preterm infants. However, more concentrated milks, 81 kcal/dl (24 kcal/oz), are preferred by many when commercial infant formulas are used. The increased concentration allows feeding volumes to be smaller, an advantage when gastric capacity may be limited. The volume given when formulas of this concentration are fed at the rate of 120 kcal per kilogram per day, 150 ml per kilogram per day, provides sufficient water for most preterm infants for the excretion of protein metabolic products and electrolytes derived from the formula. However, if lower volumes of formula are given, insufficient water may be provided for renal excretion when relatively constant extrarenal losses occur.

Human Milk

Preterm infants fed with their mother's milk have a more rapid rate of growth in weight, length, and head circumference, as well as a shorter time to regain birth weight, than those fed milk from the mothers of term infants.[25] Pooled human milk from mothers of term infants does not meet all nutritional requirements of preterm infants and results in a slower rate of growth than is found with consumption of milk from mothers of preterm infants or commercial infant formulas.[26-28] The low protein concentration of pooled, term human milk is probably the major cause of the poor growth; metabolic complications include hyponatremia at 4 to 5 weeks,[29] hypoproteinemia at 8 to 12 weeks,[1,30] and rickets at 4 to 5 months.[31]

Milk from mothers of preterm infants, especially during the first 2 weeks after delivery, contains more calories; higher concentrations of fat, protein, and sodium; but slightly lower concentrations of lactose, calcium, and phosphorus than milk from mothers of term infants.[32-35] These differences in composition may be mainly a result of the lower daily volume of milk produced by the mothers of preterm compared to mothers of term infants. The higher fat content leads to the higher caloric density of preterm milk, which may be advantageous for the small infant with limited gastric capacity. The higher protein content of preterm milk is sufficient to meet the fetal growth requirement for nitrogen[2] when the milk is consumed at 180 to 200 ml per kilogram per day.

Human milk contains taurine, a sulfur-containing amino acid not present in cow's milk.[1] The role of this amino acid in the human infant is not clear, and its essential nature has not been established. Recent studies of preterm infants receiving taurine-supplemented whey protein-predominant commercial formula have shown that the added taurine did not enhance growth,[36] the production of tauro-conjugated bile acids,[37] or fat absorption.[38]

The anti-infectious qualities of human milk are important attributes. The secretory IgA in the milk inhibits adherence and proliferation of bacteria at epithelial surfaces, and it is important in controlling the microbial environment of the intestinal tract. The secretory IgA is present in higher concentration in milk from mothers of preterm infants than in milk from mothers of term infants.[39]

Chessex and co-workers[40] have shown that the nitrogen and fat composition of the weight gain in preterm infants fed their mother's milk was similar to that reported for fetuses of similar postconceptional age. However, a note of caution regarding the feeding of mother's milk to their preterm infant has been raised by Forbes,[41] who is concerned about the variability in composition of human milk aliquots and the difficulty of assuring an adequate nutrient intake for the infant, especially calcium and phosphorus.

Mixtures of whey-predominant protein, carbohydrate, calcium, phosphate, trace minerals, and vitamins for addition to milk from the mothers of preterm infants have been developed by commercial infant formula manufacturers. When these supplements are added to milk from mothers in the first postpartum month, the resultant nutrient, mineral, and vitamin concentrations approach those of the formulas developed for feeding preterm infants. However, there have been no published studies on the nutritional effects of human milk fortified in this manner.

Commercial Formulas for Preterm Infants

Many results of studies on nutrient, electrolyte, mineral, and vitamin needs and tolerances of preterm infants, which were discussed earlier in this chapter, have been applied to the development of formulas specifically designed to meet the needs of small preterm infants. The common features of these commercial infant formulas are the use of whey-predominant proteins, carbohydrate mixtures of lactose and glucose polymers, and fat mixtures containing combinations of MCT and relatively unsaturated long-chain triglycerides. The formulas differ in content of sodium, calcium, phosphorus, vitamins, and minerals (see Appendix L). Each of the special formulas has been shown to be associated with adequate growth and metabolic stability.[25,42]

Methods of Enteral Feeding

The method of enteral feeding chosen for each infant should be based on gestational age, birth weight, clinical state, and experience of nursing personnel. Coordination of sucking, swallowing, and respiration appears at approximately 32 to 34 weeks' gestation. Preterm infants of this gestational age who are alert and vigorous may be fed by nipple. Infants who are less mature, are weak, or are critically ill will require alternate modes of feeding by vein or tube to avoid the risk of aspiration and to conserve energy.

Gastric feeding of boluses of milk can lead to disturbances of respiratory function in infants with respiratory problems; thus, in some infants, continuous transpyloric feedings by nasal or oral tubes have become popular.[1] Clinical results of this feeding mode have been excellent in many nurseries, but there have been some criticisms that bypassing the stomach and duodenum by a jejunal tube may cause inefficient utilization of the nutrients in the formula.[43] Continuous gastric feedings may be tolerated by many small infants better than bolus gastric feedings, and they are satisfactory if gastric emptying is not limiting in the infant. Bolus feedings into the stomach via gavage tube or by nipple, every 2 to 3 hours, is the goal after the preterm infant shows a clearing of the respiratory distress and gastric emptying is not a problem. Whatever the mode of feeding, the formula volume should be advanced slowly—over at least 10 to 14 days in infants who weigh less than 1,000 gm and 6 to 8 days in infants who weigh more than 1,500 gm.

Parenteral Nutrition

Parenteral administration of glucose, fat, and amino acids is frequently an essential part of the nutritional care of preterm infants, particularly those who weigh less than 1,500 gm. The high incidence of respiratory problems, limited gastric capacity, and intestinal hypomotility in small preterm infants dictates the need to advance the volume of enteral feedings slowly. The availability of parenteral nutrition components enables the supplementation of the slowly enlarging enteral feedings so the total daily intake by both routes meets the infant's nutrition needs. When required, full nutrition requirements can be met for considerable periods by the parenteral route alone.

A positive nitrogen balance, and thus the achieving of an anabolic state, can occur with parenteral lipid and/or glucose caloric intakes of 60 kcal per kilograms per day and amino acid intakes of 2.5 to 3.0 gm per kilogram per day.[44,45] With higher nonprotein caloric intakes of 80 to 85 kcal per kilogram per day and amino acid intakes of 2.7 to 3.5 gm per kilogram per day, nitrogen retention occurs at the fetal rate.[46,47] Growth requires a minimum parenteral nonprotein caloric intake of 70 kcal per kilogram per day.

The nonprotein caloric sources are glucose and lipid. Glucose presents several problems as the sole nonprotein caloric source. Concentrations of glucose higher than 13 gm/dl cause undue local irritation of peripheral veins. In addition, small preterm infants have a poor glucose tolerance in the first days of life, with hyperglycemia (>125 mg/dl) appearing frequently at glucose infusion rates exceeding 6 mg per minute.[48] Thus, to avoid the potentially damaging effects of widely varying serum osmolality and to avoid the dehydrating effects of an osmotic diuresis from significant glycosuria, glucose infusion rates should start at a rate less than 6 mg/kg per minute (8.6 gm/kg per day). Usually a steady increase of the glucose infusion rate stimulates endogenous insulin secretion and an infusion rate of 11 to 12 mg/kg per minute (130 to 140 ml/kg per day of a 13 gm/dl solution) is tolerated after 5 to 7 days of feeding. If not, insulin may have to be administered to achieve a caloric intake sufficient for growth. Care must be exercised in the use of insulin because the very low-birth-weight infant may experience wide swings of blood glucose with resulting periods of hypoglycemia. Blood glucose levels also may be augmented by intravenous lipid supplements through effects of serum free fatty acids on glucose and insulin metabolism.

The availability of intravenous lipid preparations has allowed the provision of calories adequate for growth via peripheral veins. The lipids have a high concentration of calories (1.1 kcal/ml in the 10% preparations) but are isosmolar with plasma and thus are not irritating to the veins. The tolerance for parenteral fat is less in newborn infants than in older children and is further diminished in the small preterm infant.[49,50] In addition, intra-uterine growth-retarded infants have even less parenteral fat tolerance than would be predicted from their gestational ages. Thus, in preterm infants, lipids should be administered continuously 24 hours a day, should be started at a dose of 0.5 to 1.0 gm/kg per day, and should be slowly increased by 0.5 gm/kg per day to a maximum of 2.0 to 3.0 gm/kg per day. To avoid hyperlipemia, the rate of lipid infusion should not exceed 0.25 gm/kg per hour. Fat tolerance cannot be reliably assessed by visual estimation of plasma lactescence in a spun hematocrit tube. Such monitoring should be supplemented by periodic estimations of the serum triglyceride level, which should be kept under 150 mg/dl.

Hyperlipemia should be avoided because it can interfere with pulmonary gas diffusion.[51] Additional possible pulmonary complications of parenteral lipid in preterm infants include deposition of fat globules in capillaries or alveolar macrophages and fat in pulmonary arteriolar lining calls.[52,53] However, these changes also can occur in preterm infants who have not received parenteral lipids.[54] The role of carnitine deficiency in causing the poor lipid tolerance of the parenterally fed preterm infant is uncertain. These infants usually do not receive carnitine in the parenteral solutions, and their blood and tissue carnitine levels are low.[55] However, there is no evidence that providing carnitine would be beneficial.

The use of intravenous lipids should be restricted in the presence of hyperbilirubinemia.

The nitrogen in parenteral nutrition solutions is most commonly provided as a mixture of crystalline amino acids. These mixtures have generally replaced the protein hydrolysates used previously. The nitrogen of the amino acid solutions is utilized better than the nitrogen of protein hydrolysates.[46] There also is a lower incidence of hyperammonemia. However, hyperammonemia, as well as metabolic acidosis, can be seen when parenteral amino acids are given at a rate exceeding 3.5 gm/kg per day.

None of the amino acid mixtures available for parenteral use in the United States is specifically designed for use in small preterm infants. Moreover, the appropriate protein model for the amino acid composition of this type of parenteral solution is not known. In addition, it is not clear whether newborn infant amino acid requirements are the same as those for infants given parenteral amino acids. Cysteine has been considered an essential amino acid for newborn infants because of low activities of cystathionase, the enzyme which converts methionine to cysteine in hepatic tissue.[1] However, cysteine supplementation of cysteine-free parenteral amino acid solutions did not improve nitrogen balance or growth of preterm and term newborn infants.[56]

The intravenous requirements of calcium and phosphorus each are at least 30 to 40 mg/kg per day. The estimated intravenous requirement of magnesium is 15 to 25 mg per day.

The parenteral trace metal requirements for infants have been estimated by Shils and co-workers[57] to be zinc, 300 μg/kg per day; copper, 20 μg/kg per day; chromium, 0.14 to 0.2 μg/kg per day; and manganese, 2 to 10 μg/kg per day. Approximate amounts of trace metals, based on these estimates, should be added to each daily fluid volume. However, more recent studies by Zlotkin and Buchanan[58] suggest that higher intakes, 438 μg/kg of zinc per day and 63 μg/kg of copper per day, are needed for preterm infants to duplicate intra-uterine accretion rates of these metals.

Other trace elements, the need for which is based on animal experiments or presence in human enzyme systems, include selenium, vanadium, molybdenum, nickel, tin, silicon, and arsenic. Specific recommendations for the use of these elements await further studies.

Recommended vitamin requirements for infants can now be met by giving the daily amount recommended for children,[59] now available commercially in a lyophilized preparation (MVI-Pediatric). The amounts of the vitamins per day are: A, 1,495 IU; D, 260 IU; C, 52 mg; K, 130 mg; E, 4.55 IU; thiamin, 0.78 mg; riboflavin, 0.91 mg; pyridoxine, 0.65 mg; niacin, 11 mg; B_{12}, 0.65 μg; folic acid, 91 μg; pantothenic acid, 3.25 mg; and biotin, 13 μg. Evidence that fat-soluble vitamins are lost to the intravenous tubing has been presented.[60]

Conclusion

Nutrition plays a major role in the ultimate well-being of the ever-increasing number of preterm infants who survive. Recognizing the potential damage from inadequate nutrition during the early neonatal period, the dilemma of feeding the preterm infant is that of attempting to provide sufficient nutrition to assure optimal development without additional morbidity or mortality associated with feeding. Nutrition needs can be provided by the enteral or parenteral routes, or a combination of both methods. Current research has focused on the use of the preterm infant's mother's milk and on special formulas for infants needing substitutes for human milk. The use of parenteral supplements and, indeed, long-term, total parenteral feeding has improved the ability to provide adequate nutrition for these vulnerable infants.

References

1. Committee on Nutrition: Nutritional needs of low-birth-weight infants. PEDIATRICS, 60:519, 1977.
2. Ziegler, E.E., Biga, R.L., and Fomon, S.J.: Nutritional requirements of the premature infant. In Suskind, R.M., ed.: Textbook of Pediatric Nutrition. New York: Raven Press, pp. 29-39, Textbook of Pediatric Nutrition. New York: Raven Press, pp. 29-39, 1981.
3. Reichman, B., Chessex, P., Putet, G., Verellen, G., Smith, J.M., Heim, T., and Swyer, P.R.: Diet, fat accretion, and growth in premature infants. New Engl. J. Med., 305:1495, 1981.
4. Gordon, H.H., Levine, S.Z., and McNamara, H.: Feeding of premature infants. A comparison of human and cow's milk. Amer. J. Dis. Child., 73:442, 1947.
5. Gaull, G.E., Rassin, D.K., Räihä, N.C.R., and Heinonen, K.: Milk protein quantity and quality in low-birth-weight infants. III. Effects on sulfur amino acids in plasma and urine. J. Pediat., 90:348, 1977.
6. Räihä, N.C.R., Heinonen, K., Rassin, D.K., and Gaull, G.E.: Milk protein quantity and quality of low-birthweight infants. I. Metabolic responses and effects on growth. PEDIATRICS, 57:659, 1976.
7. Fomon, S.J., Ziegler, E.E., and Vázquez, H.D.: Human milk and the small premature infant. Amer. J. Dis. Child., 131:463, 1977.
8. Minton, S.D., Steichen, J.J., and Tsang, R.C.: Bone mineral con-

tent in term and preterm appropriate-for-gestational-age infants. J. Pediat., 95:1037, 1979.

9. Greer, F.R., Steichen, J.J., and Tsang, R.C.: Effects of increased calcium, phosphorus, and vitamin D intake on bone mineralization in very low-birth-weight infants fed formulas with Polycose and medium-chain triglycerides. J. Pediat., 100:951, 1982.
10. Shaw, J.C.L.: Trace elements in the fetus and young infant. I. Zinc. Amer. J. Dis. Child., 133:1260, 1979.
11. Dauncey, M.J., Shaw, J.C.L., and Urman, J.: The absorption and retention of magnesium, zinc, and copper by low-birth-weight infants fed pasteurized human breast milk. Pediat. Res., 11:1033, 1977.
12. Voyer, M., Davakis, M., Antener, I., and Valleur, D.: Zinc balances in preterm infants. Biol. Neonate, 42:87, 1982.
13. Shaw, J.C.L.: Trace elements in the fetus and young infant. II. Copper, manganese, selenium, and chromium. Amer. J. Dis. Child., 134:74, 1980.
14. Hillman, L.S., Martin, L., and Fiore, B.: Effect of oral copper supplementation on serum copper and ceruloplasmin concentrations in premature infants. J. Pediat., 98:311, 1981.
15. Manser, J.I., Crawford, C.S., Tyrala, E.E., Brodsky, N.L., and Grover, W.D.: Serum copper concentrations in sick and well preterm infants. J. Pediat., 97:795, 1980.
16. Siimes, M.A.: Iron requirement in low birthweight infants. Acta Paediat. Scand. (Suppl. 296), p.101, 1982.
17. Avery, M.E., Clow, C.L., Menkes, J.H., Ramos, A., Scriver, C.R., Stern, L., and Wasserman, B.P.: Transient tyrosinemia of the newborn: Dietary and clinical aspects. PEDIATRICS, 39:378, 1967.
18. Light, I.J., Sutherland, J.M., and Berry, H.K.: Clinical significance of tyrosinemia of prematurity. Amer. J. Dis. Child., 125:243, 1973.
19. Menkes, J.H., Welcher, D.W., Levi, H.S., Dallas, J., and Gretsky, N.E.: Relationship of elevated blood tyrosine to the ultimate intellectual performance of premature infants. PEDIATRICS, 49:218, 1972.
20. Nutrition Committee: Feeding the low-birthweight infant. Canad. Med. Assn. J., 124:1301, 1981.
21. Huston, R.K., Reynolds, J.W., Jensen, C., and Buist, N.R.M.: Nutrient and mineral retention and vitamin D absorption in low-birth-weight infants: The effect of medium-chain triglycerides. PEDIATRICS, 72:44, 1983.
22. Oski, F.A., and Barness, L.A.: Vitamin E deficiency: A previously unrecognized cause of hemolytic anemia in the premature infant. J. Pediat., 70:211, 1967.
23. Ritchie, J.H., Fish, M.B., McMasters, V., and Grossman, M.: Edema and hemolytic anemia in premature infants: A vitamin E deficiency syndrome. New Engl. J. Med., 279:1185, 1968.
24. Dallman, P.R.: Iron, vitamin E, and folate in the preterm infant. J. Pediat., 85:742, 1974.

25. Gross, S.J.: Growth and biochemical response of preterm infants fed human milk or modified infant formula. New Engl. J. Med., **308**:237, 1983.
26. Davies, D.P.: Adequacy of expressed breast milk for early growth of preterm infants. Arch. Dis. Child., **52**:296, 1977.
27. Fomon, S.J., and Ziegler, E.E.: Protein intake of premature infants: Interpretation of data. J. Pediat., **90**:504, 1977.
28. Atkinson, S.A., Bryan, M.H., and Anderson, G.H. Human milk feeding in premature infants: Protein, fat, and carbohydrate balances in the first two weeks of life. J. Pediat., **99**:617, 1981.
29. Engelke, S.C., Shah, B.L., Vasan, U., and Raye, J.R.: Sodium balance in very low-birth-weight infants. J. Pediat., **93**:837, 1978.
30. Rönnholm, K.A.R., Sipilä, I., and Siimes, M.A.: Human milk protein supplementation for the prevention of hypoproteinemia without metabolic imbalance in breast milk-fed, very low-birth-weight infants. J. Pediat., **101**:243, 1982.
31. Greer, F.R., Steichen, J.J., and Tsang, R.C.: Calcium and phosphate supplements in breast milk-related rickets: Results in a very-low-birth-weight infant. Amer. J. Dis. Child., **136**:581, 1982.
32. Atkinson, S.A., Anderson, G.H., and Bryan, M.H.: Human milk: Comparison of the nitrogen composition in milk from mothers of premature and full-term infants. Amer. J. Clin. Nutr., **33**:811, 1980.
33. Gross, S.J., David, R.J., Bauman, L., and Tomarelli, R.M.: Nutritional composition of milk produced by mothers delivering preterm. J. Pediat., **96**:641, 1980.
34. Anderson, G.H., Atkinson, S.A., and Bryan, M.H.: Energy and macronutrient content of human milk during early lactation from mothers giving birth prematurely and at term. Amer. J. Clin. Nutr., **34**:258, 1981.
35. Lemons, J.A., Moye, L., Hall, D., and Simmons, M.: Differences in the composition of preterm and term human milk during early lactation. Pediat. Res., **16**:113, 1982.
36. Järvenpää, A.-L., Räihä, N.C.R., Rassin, D.K., and Gaull, G.E.: Feeding the low-birth-weight infant: I. Taurine and cholesterol supplementation of formula does not affect growth metabolism. PEDIATRICS, **71**:171, 1983.
37. Järvenpää, A.-L., Rassin, D.K., Kuitunen, P., Gaull, G.E., and Räihä, N.C.R.: Feeding the low-birth-weight infant. III. Diet influences bile acid metabolism. PEDIATRICS, **72**:677, 1983.
38. Järvenpää, A.-L.: Feeding the low-birth-weight infant. IV. Fat absorption as a function of diet and duodenal bile acids. PEDIATRICS, **72**:684, 1983.
39. Gross, S.J., Buckley, R.H., Wakil, S.S., McAllister, D.C., David, R.J., and Faix, R.G.: Elevated IgA concentration in milk produced by mothers delivered of preterm infants. J. Pediat., **99**:389, 1981.
40. Chessex, P., Reichman, B., Verellen, G., Putet, G., Smith, J.M., Heim, T., and Swyer, P.R.: Quality of growth in premature infants fed their own mothers' milk. J. Pediat., **102**:107, 1983.

41. Forbes, G.B.: Human milk and the small baby. Amer. J. Dis. Child., 136:577, 1982.
42. Curran, J.S., Barness, L.A., Brown, D.R., Holzman, I.R., Rathi, M.L., Silverio, J., and Tomarelli, R.: Results of feeding a special formula to very low birth weight infants. J. Pediat. Gastroenterol. Nutr., 1:327, 1982.
43. Roy, R.N., Pollnitz, R.P., Hamilton, J.R., and Chance, G.W.: Impaired assimilation of nasojejunal feeds in healthy low-birth-weight newborn infants. J. Pediat., 90:431, 1977.
44. Anderson, T.L., Muttart, C.R., Bieber, M.A., Nicholson, J.F., and Heird, W.C.: A controlled trial of glucose versus glucose and amino acids in premature infants. J. Pediat., 94:947, 1979.
45. Rubecz, I., Mestyán, J., Varga, P., and Klujber, L.: Energy metabolism, substrate utilization, and nitrogen balance in parenterally fed postoperative neonates and infants. J. Pediat., 98:42, 1981.
46. Duffy, B., Gunn, T., Collinge, J., and Pencharz, P.: The effect of varying protein quality and energy intake on the nitrogen metabolism of parenterally fed very low birth weight (<1600 g) infants. Pediat. Res., 15:1040, 1981.
47. Zlotkin, S.H., Bryan, M.H., and Anderson, G.H.: Intravenous nitrogen and energy intakes required to duplicate in utero nitrogen accretion in prematurely born human infants. J. Pediat., 99:115, 1981.
48. Dweck, H.S., and Cassady, G.: Glucose intolerance in infants of very low birth weight. I. Incidence of hyperglycemia in infants of birth weight 1,100 grams or less. PEDIATRICS, 53:189, 1974.
49. Andrew, G., Chan, G., and Schiff, D.: Lipid metabolism in the neonate. I. The effects of Intralipid infusion on plasma triglyceride and free fatty acid concentrations in the neonate. J. Pediat., 88:273, 1976.
50. Shennan, A.T., Bryan, M.H., and Angel, A.: The effect of gestational age on Intralipid tolerance in newborn infants. J. Pediat., 91:134, 1977.
51. Greene, H.L., Hazlett, D., and Demaree, R.: Relationship between Intralipid-induced hyperlipemia and pulmonary function. Amer. J. Clin. Nutr., 29:127, 1976.
52. Friedman, Z., Marks, K.H., Maisels, M.J., Thorson, R., and Naeye, R.: Effect of parenteral fat emulsion on the pulmonary and reticuloendothelial systems in the newborn infant. PEDIATRICS, 61:694, 1978.
53. Dahms, B.B., and Halpin, T.C., Jr.: Pulmonary arterial lipid deposit in newborn infants receiving intravenous lipid infusion. J. Pediat., 97:800, 1980.
54. Hertel, J., Tygstrup, I., and Andersen, G.E.: Intravascular fat accumulation after Intralipid infusion in the very low-birth-weight infant. J. Pediat., 100:975, 1982.
55. Penn, D., Schmidt-Sommerfeld, E., and Pascu, F.: Decreased tissue carnitine concentrations in newborn infants receiving total parenteral nutrition. J. Pediat., 98:976, 1981.

56. Zlotkin, S.H., Bryan, M.H., and Anderson, G.H.: Cysteine supplementation to cysteine-free intravenous feeding regimens in newborn infants. Amer. J. Clin. Nutr., **34**:914, 1981.

57. AMA Department of Foods and Nutrition: Guidelines for essential trace element preparations for parenteral use. A statement by an expert panel. J.A.M.A., **241**:2051, 1979.

58. Zlotkin, S.H., and Buchanan, B.E.: Meeting zinc and copper intake requirements in the parenterally fed preterm and full-term infant. J. Pediat., **103**:441, 1983.

59. American Medical Association, Department of Foods and Nutrition. Multivitamin preparations for parenteral use—A statement by the Nutrition Advisory Group. J. Parent. Enter. Nutr., **3**:258, 1979.

60. Gillis, J., Jones, G., and Penchaz, P.: Delivery of vitamins A, D, and E in total parenteral nutrition solutions. J. Parenter. Enter. Nutr., **7**:11, 1983.

Basic Nutrition Information

Chapter 8

ENERGY

The body needs energy* for various metabolic functions (digestion, circulation, tissue synthesis, maintenance of electrochemical gradient across the cell membrane, and so forth), for maintenance of body temperature, and for external work. No nutrient can satisfy nutritional needs if energy intake is inadequate. Hence, adequate energy intake is a prime factor in health; and, in evaluating the adequacy of an individual's diet, an estimate of energy intake is essential. Several components of total energy expenditure have been identified. Basal metabolic rate (BMR) refers to expenditure at rest after an overnight fast. The thermogenic effect of food is the increment in energy expenditure which follows food intake ("specific dynamic action"). This effect persists for several hours. In the adult it accounts for about 10% of total daily energy expenditure, but it probably is more in infants because their food intake is proportionately larger. Physical activity also is a component of the energy requirement, which will vary with body size and the vigor and duration of the activity. Estimates of energy expenditure for various adolescent activities are given in Chapter 6; there are no reliable estimates of energy expenditures for infants and younger children.

Relative organ size also is a determinant of energy expenditure. Brain and liver, both of which have high metabolic rates compared to muscle, make up a larger proportion of body weight in the infant; the adult body has a larger proportion of muscle.[1] For example, brain accounts for 60% of the total BMR in the young infant but only 25% in the adult; values for muscle are 8 and 30%, respectively. Adipose tissue has a relatively low metabolic rate.

The process of growth demands additional energy. In the young infant this amounts to about one third of the total energy requirement; however, in the normal child and adolescent, the relative growth rate is so slow (less than 0.1% per day) that this aspect of the energy requirement is negligible. However, during "catch-up" growth, infants and children have

---

*The unit employed in this handbook is the kilocalorie, defined as the amount of heat required to raise 1 kg of water 1°C, from 15 to 16°C. For those who wish to use the Joule (see Appendix U), 1 kcal = 4.184 kJ, or conversely, 1 kJ = 0.239 kcal.

been observed to consume one and one-half to two times the usual intake. Some interrelationship must exist between the growth requirement, small as it is, and the other components of energy because growth falters if there is caloric deprivation and accelerates if there is caloric excess.[2]

Studies of children and adolescents recovering from malnutrition and growing preterm infants show that the energy cost of tissue synthesis and storage averages about 5 kcal per gram of weight gain.[3-5] This value depends on the relative amounts of protein and fat in the tissue gained. The former requires 8.7 kcal/gm (or 1.3 to 1.8 kcal/gm lean body mass, depending on age), the latter requires 12 kcal/gm.[3] Note that these values are higher than the metabolizable energy provided by ingested protein (4 kcal/gm) and fat (9 kcal/gm); that for carbohydrate is 4 kcal/gm.

Pregnancy and lactation both require additional energy; estimates can be found in Chapter 6. Energy expenditure is increased by fever and infection, and it is altered by thyroid function.

The importance of energy as the prime nutrient of the diet is illustrated by several studies. The speed of recovery from severe infantile malnutrition is more closely related to energy than to protein intake.[6] Pregnancy outcomes in malnourished women can be improved as much by additional "empty" calories as by protein supplements.[7] The minimal protein requirement of healthy young adults is inversely related to energy intake.[8]

Energy intake is regulated, and with a fair degree of precision; this is evident from the fact that many infants and children grow in regular fashion, and that many adults maintain stable body weight for long periods. Hence, energy intake is nicely balanced against energy expenditure. Young infants have been determined to "eat for calories,"[9] as do animals.[10] Observations on young children fed *ad libitum* while recovering from malnutrition showed that their voracious appetites abated as they approached normal weight for height.[11] The seat of appetite control is not known, although evidence suggests it lies somewhere within the central nervous system, with assistance perhaps from various gastrointestinal hormones. When, for one reason or another, the regulatory process(es) fail, the result is overeating or anorexia.

The average diet of individuals in the United States supplies 12 to 15% of calories from protein. The balance of calories is derived from carbohydrate, fat, and alcohol; the latter accounts for as much as 10% of the total calories in adults. Total energy requirement depends on body size; the values listed in Appendix G are estimates of average requirements for various age groups. Although these estimates can be used to judge the adequacy of intake, there is some variation among normal individuals. Growth rate serves as a good "bioassay" for the adequacy of energy intake.

References

1. Holliday, M.A.: Body composition and energy needs during growth. *In* Falkner, F., and Tanner, J.M., ed.: Human Growth: 2. Postnatal Growth. New York: Plenum Press, pp. 117-139, 1978.
2. Forbes, G.B.: Nutrition and growth. J. Pediat., **91**:40, 1977.
3. Spady, D.W., Payne, P.R., Picou, D., and Waterlow, J.C.: Energy balance during recovery from malnutrition. Amer. J. Clin. Nutr., **29**:1073, 1976.
4. Reichman, B., Chessex, P., Putet, G., Verellen, G., Smith, J.M., Heim, T., and Swyer, P.R.: Diet, fat accretion, and growth in premature infants. New Engl. J. Med., **305**:1495, 1982.
5. Whyte, R.K., Haslam, R., Vlainic, C., Shannon, S., Samulski, K., Campbell, O., Bayley, H.S., and Sinclair, J.C.: Energy balance and nitrogen balance in growing low birthweight infants fed human milk or formula. Pediat. Res., **17**:891, 1983.
6. Waterlow, J.C.L.: The rate of recovery of malnourished infants in relation to the protein and calorie levels of the diet. J. Trop. Pediat. African Child Health, **7**:16, 1961.
7. Lechtig, A., Delgado, H., Lasky, R., Yarbrough, C., Klein, R.E., Habicht, J.-P., and Béhar, M.: Maternal nutrition and fetal growth in developing countries. Amer. J. Dis. Child., **129**:553, 1975.
8. Garza, C., Scrimshaw, N.S., and Young, V.R.: Human protein requirements: A long-term metabolic nitrogen balance study in young men to evaluate the 1973 FAO/WHO safe level of egg protein intake. J. Nutr., **107**:335, 1977.
9. Fomon, S.J.: Infant Nutrition, ed. 2. Philadelphia: W.B. Saunders, 1974.
10. Adolph, E.F.: Urges to eat and drink in rats. Amer. J. Physiol., **151**:110, 1947.
11. Ashworth, A.: Growth rates in children recovering from protein-calorie malnutrition. Brit. J. Nutr., **23**:835, 1969.

Chapter 9

PROTEINS

Dietary protein provides amino acids for the continuous synthesis of body proteins and other important tissue constituents. This turnover of protein can be rapid, as it is in bone marrow and in gastrointestinal mucosa, or it can be slow as it is in collagen. Some of the amino acids released during the degradation of tissue are reutilized. Other amino acids are metabolized or lost in urine, feces, sweat, desquamated skin, hair, and nails. Dietary amino acids are needed to replace these losses, even after growth has ceased. There is little, if any, capacity for the storage of amino acids and proteins.

The amino acids which cannot be synthesized by adults are referred to as essential: leucine, isoleucine, valine, threonine, methionine, phenylalanine, tryptophan, lysine, and probably histidine. Cystine and tyrosine are partially essential in that the intake of these amino acids reduces, but does not obviate, requirements for methionine and phenylalanine. The rates of synthesis of cystine and tyrosine, and perhaps taurine, are insufficient during early development to meet all of the needs of the term or preterm infant. After the requirements for essential amino acids have been met, the additional dietary nitrogen required can be provided as nonessential amino acids or, to a limited extent, as simple nitrogenous compounds. The synthesis of nonessential amino acids may require energy and stress the immature organism.

Factors Affecting Dietary Protein Requirements

Dietary requirements for protein are affected by a variety of factors including: sex, age, growth, pregnancy, lactation, and possibly genetic variation. The protein requirements of men per unit of body weight are greater than those of women because of their greater relative lean body mass; and the requirements of the young are greater than those of the aged.

Dietary factors may alter requirements for protein; there are two important examples of this kind of interaction:

1. On a fixed, adequate protein intake, caloric intake is the major determinant of nitrogen utilization; whereas, on a fixed,

adequate caloric intake, protein is the crucial determinant.

2. Animal proteins contain essential amino acids in amounts which more closely meet human needs than plant proteins. However, mixtures of different plant proteins can be nutritionally equivalent to animal proteins such as milk and egg proteins.

Infections and stressful stimuli, such as those associated with severe thermal or physical injury, are among environmental factors which increase individual protein needs. Athletic activity and heavy physical work increase caloric needs but probably do not increase the need for protein.

Methods for Determining Protein Requirements

Protein Quantity

The minimal needs for protein have been estimated using various approaches.[1] In the factorial method, "obligatory" losses of nitrogen via urine and feces (i.e., excretion on extremely low protein intakes) are measured with corrections for skin and miscellaneous nitrogen losses. In growth, pregnancy, and lactation, further calculations are made for body nitrogen gains, nitrogen content of the fetus and placenta, and the output of milk protein and nonprotein nitrogen. These total obligatory nitrogen losses have been determined under conditions of low protein intake. However, the utilization of dietary protein is less efficient at requirement levels of intake than at low levels of protein intake; and the obligatory nitrogen losses lead to an underestimation of the amount of dietary nitrogen required to maintain body nitrogen. Thus, a correction factor, usually 30% in all age groups, is used, although the correct figure is not known. This factorial method is convenient but of limited reliability.

The nitrogen balance method involves determination of the intake and excretion of nitrogen during a short period, usually at least 3 days. The apparent retention is calculated. This method is subject to systematic errors[2] and is not appropriate for the estimation of body composition. But this method is useful for comparing two sources of protein at nearly equal levels of protein intake. Requirements based on nitrogen balance studies overestimate the protein requirement.

In infants with rapid growth rate, weight gain and linear

growth can be used for estimating protein requirements when energy requirements are met. The addition of estimates of body composition makes this approach more reliable.

Stable isotopes such as ^{15}N can be used to label amino acids. The isotopes can be administered as a single dose, permitting calculation of the rates of protein synthesis, degradation, and the size of several body amino acid pools. The application of these techniques to the determination of protein requirements is still in the process of development.[3]

Protein Quality

The quality of proteins is determined mainly by the essential amino acid content and pattern. Generally speaking, vegetable proteins are of lower quality than animal proteins (soy protein is an exception). Except in neonates, and possibly young infants, there is no definitive evidence that the pattern of intake of essential amino acids required is different among the age groups. The available data on the oral and parenteral requirements for individual essential amino acids are limited.

The relative requirements for each of the essential amino acids are thought to decrease more rapidly with age than those for total nitrogen. The quality of proteins is more critical in infants and small children. Because it is difficult to measure directly the nutritive value of proteins in humans, various chemical and biological assays of protein quality have been developed. These values must be applied with reservation.[1]

Clinical and laboratory methods for the evaluation of protein quality in humans are based on the same principles as those used in animals, but they require considerable modification for application to humans. Despite its limitation, the most useful criterion currently available is nitrogen balance. The determination of plasma amino acids and their turnover rates as measured by stable isotopes may offer an additional means of evaluating the nutritional significance of dietary protein quality in humans.

Protein Allowances

Because of the factors and methodologic limitations, it is difficult to be entirely confident about recommendations for protein and amino acid intakes for either individuals or populations. But recommendations are needed to guide the design of diets and the content of educational programs in nutrition and for planning specific intervention programs. Recommended allowances for protein intake are intended to apply only to healthy individuals whose energy intake is adequate. Nitrogen balance cannot be achieved on low energy intakes.

Infants

One nutritional statement which can be made with confidence is that the ideal food for full-term infants is human milk. It is the lowest in protein content of any species and contains only 0.8 to 0.9 gm/dl of pure protein and 0.2 to 0.3 gm protein equivalents per deciliter of nonprotein nitrogen compounds. The protein composition of human milk, in which the whey proteins rather than the caseins are the dominant protein constituents, is exceptional because of its high cystine content, high cystine:methionine ratio, and low content of tyrosine and phenylalanine (see Appendix K).

The low protein content of human milk implies that these proteins have a high nutritional quality and are digested and absorbed efficiently. The same increments of growth are obtained with the low protein intake of human milk as are observed with the higher protein intake of various commercial infant formulas. The total protein equivalent of 1.5 gm/dl in the commercial infant formulas (see Appendix L) available in the United States, and derived from bovine milk proteins, provides a margin of safety for the lower sulfur-containing proteins. Even though commercial infant formulas have a whey-protein:casein ratio similar to that of human milk, the specific proteins of bovine whey differ considerably from those of human whey. The long-term health consequences of protein intakes greater than those of human milk are not known.

A 4 kg, full-term infant taking 800 ml of human milk per day receives about 7.2 gm protein, plus 1.6 gm of protein equivalents (gm of nitrogen × 6.25) of nonprotein nitrogen compounds per day. This is about 1.8 gm/kg per day of high-quality protein and 0.4 gm protein equivalents per day. This protein intake will satisfy the infant's requirements for both maintenance and growth without an amino acid or solute excess.

The protein content of human milk decreases during lactation, and the infant's growth rate decreases as he or she becomes older; therefore, the protein requirement per unit of body weight decreases with age. However, the accurate determination of the protein requirement after weaning is subject to the caveats previously cited. The protein requirement of older infants fed proteins other than those of human milk have been estimated at about 1.5 to 2.0 gm/kg per day (see Appendix H). The essential amino acids in pooled human milk constitute about 45% of the total amino acids. The requirements for essential amino acids probably do not remain that high later in childhood. The protein requirements of preterm infants are reviewed in Chapter 7.

Children

There is a continuing but slow decline in protein needs relative to weight during the preschool and school-age years. Current protein allowances have been derived by estimating the average requirements by the factorial method, and by assuming that the variability of protein needs among the individual children is the same as that for other age groups. Recent recommendation will be found in Appendix H. Appropriate corrections must be made for dietary proteins which are of lower quality than any acceptable reference proteins.

Adolescents

Few data are available on the protein requirements of adolescents. Recommendations for this group have been extrapolated from studies in infants and adult men. At one time the "adolescent growth spurt" was believed to result in a substantial increase in protein requirements; but more recent recommendations have not emphasized the growth spurt because it is small relative to actual body size.

Effects of Too Little and Too Much Protein

There are two classic syndromes of infantile malnutrition: (1) kwashiorkor, which is the result of a greater deficiency of protein than of calories; and (2) marasmus, which is the result of deficiencies of both protein and calories (see also Chapter 21).

The effects of too much dietary protein have not been studied extensively. Multination studies have shown a correlation between protein intake and the prevalence of atherosclerosis, but a casual relationship has not been established. The concentration of blood urea nitrogen is a function of protein intake in both infants and adults. High intakes in small infants also can result in acidosis, aminoacidemia,[4] and cylinduria.[5] Studies in adults show that high protein intakes lead to hypercalcuria and even a negative calcium balance.[6] More studies are needed to determine the upper limits of protein intake consistent with the maintenance of good health. Note that the average diet of individuals in the United States provides 12 to 15% of calories from protein, a protein:calorie ratio clearly in excess of both the Recommended Dietary Allowance for the United States and the Recommended Nutrient Intakes for Canadians, which are 6 to 9% of calories from protein.

References

1. Committee on Dietary Allowances and Food and Nutrition Board: Recommended Dietary Allowance, ed. 9, revised. Washington, D.C.: National Academy of Sciences, pp. 39-41, 1980.
2. Wallace, W.M.: Nitrogen content of the body and its relation to retention and loss of nitrogen. Fed. Proc., 18:1125, 1959.
3. Heine, W., Richter, I., Plath, C., Wutzke, K., Oswald, F., and Töwe, J.: Evaluation of different ^{15}N-tracer substances for calculation of whole body protein parameters in infants. J. Pediat. Gastroenterol. Nutr., 2:599, 1983.
4. Gaull, G.E., Rassin, D.K., Räihä, N.C.R., and Heinonen, K.: Milk protein quantity and quality in low-birth-weight infants. III. Effects on sulfur amino acids in plasma and urine. J. Pediat., 90:348, 1977.
5. McCann, M.L., and Schwartz, R.: The effects of milk solute on urinary cast excretion in premature infants. PEDIATRICS, 38:555, 1966.
6. Linkswiler, H.M.: Calcium. In Hegsted, H.M., Chichester, C.O., Darby, W.J., McNutt, K.W., Stalvey, R.M., and Stotz, E.H., ed.: Nutrition Reviews': Present Knowledge in Nutrition, ed. 4. New York: The Nutrition Foundation, pp. 232-240, 1976.

Chapter 10

CARBOHYDRATE AND DIETARY FIBER

Carbohydrate

Although there is an obligatory, metabolic requirement for carbohydrate, relatively little carbohydrate is needed in the diet; however, low carbohydrate diets demand excessive intakes of protein and/or fat. During periods of fasting, the adult liver and kidney synthesize about 180 gm of glucose daily for use by tissues incapable of using fatty acids mobilized from adipose tissue; about 80% of this glucose is required by the central nervous system (small amounts of energy for this organ can be supplied by ketones). The total glycogen reserves in the adult amount to about 500 gm, one fifth of which is in liver. Obviously, much of the glucose supplied by the liver (muscle glycogen does not contribute directly) is the result of gluconeogenesis.

The newborn infant contains about 34 gm of glycogen. Only 6 gm of this is in the liver, and most of it is accumulated during the last weeks of fetal life.

Carbohydrate-free diets lead to ketosis, as does fasting; indeed, ketosis will occur when carbohydrate intake drops below about 10% of total calories. Ketosis occurs more readily in children than adults when they are fasted or given extremely low carbohydrate diets, and low carbohydrate-high fat diets (the ketogenic diet) have been used in the treatment of epilepsy and as a diagnostic test for ketotic hypoglycemia.

In addition to glycogen stores in the liver and skeletal muscle, the body contains carbohydrate in many different forms: mucopolysaccharides; structural carbohydrates which are important constituents of connective and collagenous tissues; and as components of nucleic acids, glycoproteins, glycolipids, and various hormones and enzymes.

Lactose is the major dietary carbohydrate normally consumed by young infants; however, at an early age, infants in the United States are fed a variety of other carbohydrates, including sucrose, natural and modified starches, starch hydrolysates, and small amounts of monosaccharides and indigestible carbohydrate (e.g., fiber). Absorption of carbohydrate into the portal circulation is mainly in the form of the monosaccharides glucose, fructose, and galactose. Fructose and galactose are rapidly converted to glucose by the liver. Maintenance of an adequate, but not excessive, concentration of glucose in the blood is controlled through complex hormonal interactions involving insulin, glucagon, and pituitary and adrenal hormones.

The consumption of large amounts of sucrose increases the likelihood of dental caries, especially when the sucrose-containing foods are of a texture which permits them to adhere to the tooth surfaces (see Chapter 17). Xylitol, a pentose alcohol, has been used with some success in trials in Scandinavia.[1] It has a sweet taste and is noncariogenic because it cannot be metabolized by oral microorganisms. However, xylitol is expensive to manufacture; this as well as concern about possible carcinogenic potential has forestalled clinical trials in the United States.

Approximately 20% of infants fed commercial infant formulas in the United States receive lactose-free soy isolate formulas containing sucrose or corn syrup solids, or a combination of both as the carbohydrate source(s). Corn syrup is a generic term for products derived from cornstarch by hydrolysis with acid or enzymes. These products are classified according to their chemical-reducing power relative to glucose, which has a dextrose equivalent (D.E.) of 100%. The D.E. of corn syrups ranges from less than 20% to more than 95%. A low D.E. corn syrup is lightly hydrolyzed, thus more starch-like than a corn syrup of high D.E. containing large amounts of glucose.

Many special formulas (e.g., Nutramigen, Pregestimil) and strained foods contain modified corn or tapioca starches. These formulas may provide approximately 15% of the total calories in the form of modified starch, which is used to facilitate suspension of insoluble nutrients during feeding. The amount of modified starch added to a few commercial infant desserts may amount to as much as 45% of the total solids content. The glucose units in these starches are chemically cross-linked by phosphate and adipate or acetyl-attached groups. Modified food starches also possess certain technical properties such as altered viscosity and "mouth feel," freeze-thaw stability, gel clarity, and stability in acid products. Animal studies have shown that caloric availability of modified food starches is similar to unmodified starches. No well controlled studies to evaluate digestibility of modified food starches by human infants have been conducted. Only 1 in 100 to 200 anhydroglucose units within the starch molecule may be chemically cross-linked;

therefore, it is unlikely that a major reduction in digestibility would occur.[2]

Fiber

Dietary fiber has been defined as the part of material in foods impervious to the degradative enzymes of the human digestive tract. The dietary fiber of plants consists of carbohydrate compounds, including cellulose, hemicellulose, pectin, gums, mucilages, and a noncarbohydrate polymer of phenylpropane, lignin. These substances, are present in the cell walls of all parts of the plant, including the leaf, stem, root, and seed.

Crude fiber and dietary fiber are not the same. Crude fiber refers to the residue left after strong acid and base hydrolysis of plant material. This process dissolves pectin, gums, mucilages, and most of the hemicellulose; and it mainly is a measure of the cellulose and lignin content. Clearly, this method tends to underestimate the total amount of fiber in the food. Most food composition tables give only crude fiber values.

Current interest in fiber was stimulated by the suggestion that fiber might help to prevent certain diseases common in the United States, namely diverticular disease, cancer of the colon, irritable bowel syndrome, obesity, and coronary heart disease.[3,4] African blacks in rural areas where the fiber intake was high rarely had these diseases; however, during the past 20 years as this population moved to the cities and adopted Western habits (including a Western diet), they began to suffer from the same "Western-type" diseases.

A high-fiber diet increases fecal bulk; produces softer, more frequent stools; and decreases transit time through the intestine. These factors may be responsible for the supposed beneficial effects of fiber. A decreased transit time implies less time for potential carcinogens to be in contact with the intestinal mucosa. The increased bulk would dilute potential carcinogens and produce less straining at stool.

Obesity is rare in populations which consume most carbohydrate as complex carbohydrate and have a high-fiber intake. The lower energy density of this type of diet could increase satiety; however, in many cultures where this type of diet is common, the total energy intake is low by Western standards.

Arteriosclerosis and coronary heart disease also may be inversely related to low-fiber intake. Subjects consuming from 12 to 36 gm of pectin daily for several weeks have shown a reduction of total serum cholesterol ranging from 8 to 30%.[5]

The different fractions of fiber have different physiologic effects. Pectin has a cholesterol-lowering effect, which may be caused by bile acid sequestration and increased stool-fat content. Lignin has bile acid-binding properties *in vitro*, but these have not yet been demonstrated *in vivo*. There are conflicting data about whether lignin lowers serum cholesterol. Cellulose and hemicellulose have been shown to increase output of fecal bile acid.

Most evidence for the beneficial effects of fiber is epidemiologic and refers almost entirely to adults; and the diseases mentioned (with the exception of obesity) require years to develop. In addition to fiber intake, there are many variables in the populations studied, such as intake of saturated fats and sucrose, exercise, and stress, all of which are implicated as causative factors in these diseases.

There are some indications that the current intake of fiber by children in the United States is low; possibly, 75% of children eat less than the recommended amounts of fruits and vegetables. A recommendation for an increased fiber intake in children would mean an increase in the consumption of fruits, vegetables, legumes, and whole grain cereals and breads; consequently, there would be a decrease in the intake of some highly processed foods. The dietary goals promulgated by the McGovern Committee of the U.S. Senate[6] include such a recommendation.

Objections have been made to an increased fiber intake for children. Children have a small stomach capacity, and the caloric density of high-fiber foods is low. Therefore, children would be unable to ingest adequate calories. This could be a problem in strict vegetarians, although it could be solved easily by including nuts and legumes (which are relatively high in both protein and fat) in the diet.

The second objection is that dietary fiber may influence adversely the absorption of certain essential minerals such as calcium, iron, copper, magnesium, phosphorus, and zinc. One advantage of white flour is that the removal of the husk (bran) means much of the phytate (inositol hexaphosphate) is removed. These minerals may form insoluble compounds with phytate that render them unavailable. If the intake of these minerals is low and the small amount consumed is chelated, a deficiency state may be produced. This may be a serious problem for children in developing countries if the main source of

Table 9
Edible Fiber of Foods (per serving)

Food	Serving Size	Moderate Fiber (2-4 gm)	High Fiber (5+ gm)
Breads	1 slice	whole wheat, cracked wheat, bran muffin	–
	4	rye wafers	–
Cereals	1 oz	Bran Flakes, Raisin Bran, Shredded Wheat, oatmeal	All Bran, Bran Buds, Corn Bran
Vegetables	½ cup	beets, broccoli, brussels sprouts, cabbage, carrots, corn, green beans, green peas	spinach
	1 med	baked potato with skin	corn on the cob
	½	avocado	–
Fruits	1 med	apple with peel, dates, fig, mango, nectarine, orange, pear	–
	½ cup	applesauce (unsweetened), raspberries, blackberries	cooked prunes
Meat substitutes	½ cup	–	baked beans, black beans, garbanzos, kidney beans, lentils, lima beans, pinto beans
	2 tbsp	peanut butter	–
	¼ cup	peanuts, roasted	–

zinc is bread. For example, in the rural populations in Iran where zinc deficiency occurs, unleavened whole grain bread accounts for approximately 75% of the energy intake.[7] However, it is not clear how relevant this observation is for children in the United States where bread and cereals account for approximately 20% of the zinc intake, and the intake of animal protein is high. Also, the phytate in whole wheat can be destroyed by yeast fermentation, and bread in this country is generally made with yeast. Although it is believed that mineral deficiencies are unlikely to develop in children on typical Western diets, even with a reasonable increase in their dietary fiber intake,[8] there is little direct evidence to support this belief.

Limited results from metabolic studies suggest that moderate amounts of dietary fiber do not significantly affect mineral status. A study was done in 1943 on children 4 to 12 years old who consumed from 4 to 6 gm of crude fiber (cellulose and hemicellulose) per day for periods ranging from 30 to 225 successive days.[9] All children enjoyed buoyant health and satisfactory bowel elimination, without any evidence of untoward effects. Unfortunately, because no nitrogen or mineral balance studies were actually conducted on the children, this conclusion may not be valid. Based on fecal analysis, the older children also seemed to have an increased ability to decompose cellulose and hemicellulose.

A more recent, rigorously conducted study investigated the effect of three fibers (hemicellulose, cellulose, and pectin) at a level of 14.2 gm per day on copper, zinc, and magnesium utilization by adolescent boys.[10] Some alteration in mineral utilization was found. Hemicellulose supplementation resulted in significantly increased fecal zinc, copper, and magnesium excretions and significantly lowered zinc, copper, and magnesium retentions. Cellulose had a directionally similar effect, but to a lesser degree. Pectin had the least influence on mineral utilization and retention, which corresponded primarily to smaller losses of these minerals in the feces. Serum levels of zinc, copper, and magnesium were resistant to change. However, each fiber was consumed for only 4 days, and longer periods may be required before serum changes are detected.

Other studies have shown that feces of individuals fed diets of increasing fiber content contain progressively greater amounts of nitrogen and fat.[11]

The effect of fiber on the efficiency of absorption of various nutrients may be of nutritional significance when diets marginal in nutrient content and high in fiber are consumed; however, the average diet consumed in the United States is so low in fiber content that a moderate increase in fiber intake would not measurably influence absorption of the nutrients present in adequate amounts.

More work needs to be done in this area before any firm recommendations can be made. It is not known whether an increased fiber intake during pregnancy would have any effect on the fetus and newborn infant in terms of vitamin and mineral status, nor is it known what effect the fiber intake of nursing mothers has on the mineral composition of their milk.

Nevertheless, a substantial amount of fiber probably should be eaten to ensure normal laxation. Fiber probably is not needed in infants less than 1 year old. For older infants and children, the diet should include whole grain cereals, breads, fruits, and vegetables. However, a diet that places emphasis on high-fiber, low-calorie foods, to the exclusion of the other common food groups, is not recommended for children.

Table 9 lists the various food groups of high and moderately high fiber content. Note that vegetables and fruits contain more fiber per calorie than other foods.

References

1. Scheinin, A., Mäkinen, K.K., and Ylitalo, K.: Turku sugar studies V: Final report on the effect of sucrose, fructose and xylitol diets on the caries incidence in man. Acta Odontol. Scand., 34:179, 1976.
2. Committee on Nutrition: Review of safety and suitability of modified food starches in infant foods. Unpublished report to the FDA, May 1978.
3. Burkitt, D.P., Walker, A.R.P., and Painter, N.S.: Dietary fiber and disease. J.A.M.A., 229:1068, 1974.
4. Huang, C.T.L., Gopalakrishna, G.S., and Nichols, B.L.: Fiber, intestinal sterols and colon cancer. Amer. J. Clin. Nutr., 31:516, 1978.
5. Mendeloff, A.I.: Current concepts: Dietary fiber and human health. New Engl. J. Med., 297:811, 1977.
6. Select Committee on Nutrition and Human Needs, U.S. Senate: Dietary Goals for the United States, ed. 2, December 1977.
7. Sandström, B., Arvidsson, B., Cederblad, Å., and Björn-Rasmussen, E.: Zinc absorption from composite meals: I. The significance of wheat extraction rate, zinc, calcium, and protein content in meals based on bread. Amer. J. Clin. Nutr., 33:739, 1980.
8. Saperstein, S., and Spiller, G.A.: Dietary fiber. Amer. J. Dis. Child., 132:657, 1978.

9. Hummel, F.C., Shepherd, M.L., and Macy, I.G.: Disappearance of cellulose and hemicellulose from the digestive tracts of children. J. Nutr., **25**:59, 1943.

10. Drews, L.M., Kies, C., and Fox, H.M.: Effect of dietary fiber on copper, zinc, and magnesium utilization by adolescent boys. Amer. J. Clin. Nutr., **32**:1893, 1979.

11. Southgate, D.A.T., and Durnin, J.V.G.A.: Calorie conversion factors. An experimental reassessment of the factors used in the calculation of the energy value of human diets. Brit. J. Nutr., **24**:517, 1970.

Chapter 11

FATS AND FATTY ACIDS

Fats provide a concentrated source of energy, and two of the fatty acids are essential because they cannot be synthetized by the body. Fats contribute to the taste and texture of foods, although, in the absence of antioxidants, they may produce derivatives with an unpleasant taste and odor. The observations of Hansen and co-workers[1] in the late 1950's proved that fat was essential in the human diet.

Vegetable oils usually contain substantial amounts of linoleic acid, one of the essential fatty acids. For example, corn and soy oils contain more than 50% of this acid, but coconut oil contains only 1.5% linoleic acid. In addition, the proportion of unsaturated fatty acids (containing one or more double bonds) to saturated fatty acids (containing no double bonds) in plant oils is higher than in most fats of domesticated animals. Arachidonic acid can be derived from linoleic acid and is essential for the body. Cow's milk fat contains much less essential fatty acid than human milk fat, which has led manufacturers of infant formulas to add vegetable oil (usually soy or corn, which are both rich in linoleic acid) to the skimmed cow's milk base of their preparations.

Under normal circumstances, it is difficult to design a diet deficient in essential fatty acids. Deficiencies in essential fatty acids most frequently are encountered in relation to parenteral alimentation or in patients who have cystic fibrosis or other causes of fat malabsorption.

Biochemistry

Fats may be regarded as the fatty acid esters of alcohols. The most common fat is triglyceride, the combination of glycerol with three fatty acids. Other lipids contain sugar, amino acid, phosphate, and choline moieties in varying proportions with fatty acids, including the fatty acid esters of sphingosine (sphingolipids), glycolipids, phospholipids, and sterol esters. Fatty acids are usually described in biochemical shorthand. The number of carbon atoms in the chain of fatty acids is written first, then the number of double bonds. The position of the

first double bond from the methyl end of the chain is written
with the prefix "ω".

An example of a short-chain length fatty acid is the following: $CH_3CH_2CH_2COOH$, or butyric acid written as (4:0).

A medium-chain fatty acid, such as decanoic, is $C_9H_{19}COOH$
(10:0).

A long-chain polyunsaturated fatty acid, such as linoleic

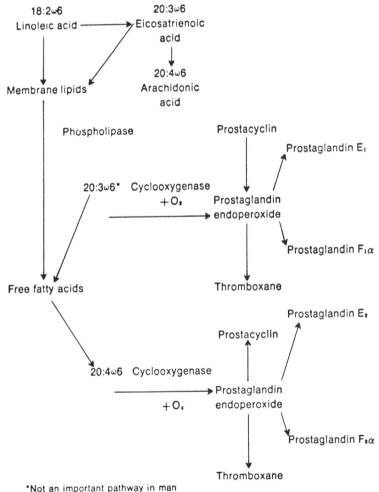

*Not an important pathway in man

*Figure 6. Essential fatty acids and prostaglandins. Linolenic acid
18:3ω3 is also thought to be essential.*

acid, is $CH_3(CH_2)_4CH = CHCH_2CH = CH(CH_2)_7COOH$ ($18:2\omega6$).

Most fatty acids have an even number of carbon atoms because they are synthesized or degraded two carbon units at a time.

Fatty acids essential for man are the derivatives of $18:2\omega6$ or linoleic acid. This acid cannot be made in mammalian tissues. Linoleic acid and its most important derivative, $20:4\omega6$, arachidonic acid, are components of cell membranes. An additional function is to serve as precursors for prostaglandins.

The fatty acid $18:3\omega3$, linolenic acid, is present in many structural lipids of the brain and nerves. There is now evidence which suggests that linolenic acid is essential for humans.[2] A 6-year-old child was given an intravenous fat emulsion deficient in linolenic acid. A syndrome of neurologic disease with both sensory and motor deficits resulted. These were reversed following infusion of a fatty acid emulsion rich in linolenic acid. Fortunately, elaborate fatty acid determinations were available to substantiate the deficiency and recovery on a biochemical basis.

The pathways of linoleic acid metabolism and related prostaglandin metabolism are shown in Figure 6.

Thromboxanes and prostacyclins are powerful but short-lived cellular regulatory agents derived from the precursor, prostaglandin endoperoxide. Not all tissues produce thromboxane, and the pattern of production of different prostaglandins varies in different tissues. Prostacyclin is one of the most potent physiologic anticoagulants known, whereas thromboxane stimulates coagulation. Prostacyclin also is a potent vasodilator. The various prostaglandins have a wide range of known physiologic and metabolic effects. The biologic antioxidant, vitamin E, appears to help regulate prostaglandin production and prevents oxidation of unsaturated fatty acids. A diet high in polyunsaturated fat should contain an appropriate amount of vitamin E (at least 0.5 mg tocopherol equivalents per gram linoleic acid) to ensure the normal metabolism of these fatty acids. Failure to do so has been associated with a hemolytic state, particularly when extra iron (a free-radical generator) is added to the diet.[3]

Absorption of Fats

The principal form of fat, triglyceride, is emulsified by the bile salts. The small emulsion particles or micelles provide a large surface area for the action of pancreatic lipase or human milk lipase, which mainly removes the two outer fatty acids from the glycerol and leaves an easily absorbable monoglyceride. The triglyceride is enzymatically reassembled from the monoglyceride and two fatty acids in the upper small bowel mucosa. In long-chain triglycerides, it is then coated with protein and extruded as chylomicrons into the lacteals. Medium- and short-chain fatty acids (with 2 to 10 carbon atoms) short circuit this complex system and are absorbed directly into the portal venous system. The longer the chain length of saturated fatty acids, the slower the rate of absorption. The introduction of double bonds into the longer fatty acids enhances absorption. Malabsorption of fatty acid may cause calcium wastage by the formation of insoluble soaps.

Deficiency

Deficiency symptoms in infants may result when less than 1% of the caloric intake is linoleic acid. This may be a consequence of feeding a skimmed milk diet or special fat-free diets for a variety of pathologic conditions, or of prolonged fat-free intravenous alimentation. Steatorrhea could possibly cause nonabsorption of essential fatty acids, but this does not seem to occur in celiac disease. However, it does occur in cystic fibrosis and hepatobiliary disease.

The clinical picture of isolated essential fatty acid deficiency in children is unclear because experimental depletion in otherwise healthy and calorically satisfied infants has been attempted only in one series of investigations.[1] A flaky skin condition appeared about 1 week after an essential fatty acid-deficient diet was instituted. This condition was present over the dorsal surfaces of the body. Hansen and co-workers[1] reported a "syrupy diarrhea" in the majority of subjects. The experiment was terminated after about 12 weeks. Poor hair growth, thrombocytopenia, failure to thrive, and increased susceptibility to infection also were found.

Human milk contains 7% or more of calories as linoleic acid, depending on the maternal diet, and most commercial infant formulas contain more than 10%. Unmodified cow's milk has only about 1%, which is less than the presumed daily requirement of 2.7%[4] (see Appendix I). However, there is no evidence that infants with unmodified cow's milk as their sole source of fat develop clinical evidence of fatty-acid deficiency.

Biochemical Markers of Essential Fatty-acid Depletion

Currently there is variation among laboratories about normal concentrations of linoleic and arachidonic acids, and there are limitations in providing generally agreed on figures (Appendix V) for plasma or red cell levels. The fatty acid eicosatrienoic acid (20:3ω9) can be synthesized by humans, but it is not normally present in serum. When depletion of the ω6 (linoleic) family of fatty acids occurs, the 20:3ω9 fatty acid becomes detectable in serum, indicating essential fatty acid deficiency. As the levels of fatty acids with three double bonds increase, the arachiodonic acid (with four double bonds) decreases. Thus the ratio of triene (three double bonds) to tetraene (four double bonds) increases. This ratio is normally less than 0.4.

The normal, full-term, newborn infant has lower serum levels of essential fatty acid than older children, and the level of eicosatrienoic acid (20:3ω9) is slightly higher. Normal levels in preterm infants and the requirements for essential fatty acid have not been accurately defined. However, the dietary requirements in preterm infants may be higher for essential fatty acids than in older children because of poor fat absorption and minimal depot stores. Both full-term and preterm infants can develop fatty-acid deficiency within 1 week when receiving intravenous alimentation without added lipids.[5]

The long-term effects of essential fatty-acid deficiency in infants are not clear. These acids are important constituents of cell membranes, brain lipids, and precursors of such potent bioregulators as the prostaglandins. Platelet dysfunction occurs in neonates with essential fatty-acid deficiency.[6] Research in experimental animals has shown a greater susceptibility to infection secondary to essential fatty-acid deficiency. Thus, it seems wise to avoid any degree of deficiency by ensuring that formulas contain at least 300 mg of linoleic acid per 100 kcal, even though this level may be significantly above the minimum need. This goal can be attained readily in infants by the use of human milk or formula with added soy or other vegetable oil. After solid foods are introduced into the diet, the use of vegetable oils (such as those found in margarine, peanut butter, and cereals) can be used as sources of essential fatty acids. Hydrogenated coconut oil does not furnish essential fatty acids.

In patients with steatorrhea, the provision of essential fatty acids either in the diet or by intravenous alimentation is useful in maintaining normal essential fatty acid intakes. Medium-chain length fatty acid triglyceride (MCT) also is a useful source of calories in malabsorptive states; but, of course, these do not provide essential fatty acids. However, formulas containing MCT are supplemented with oils high in linoleic acid. Altered prostaglandin levels have returned to normal in children with cystic fibrosis following linoleic acid supplementation.

There is still much controversy over the role of the dietary saturated:unsaturated fatty acid ratio in the genesis of coronary heart disease. Until this is resolved, it seems appropriate to recommend that essential fatty acids (i.e., linoleic acid) should provide at least 3% of the caloric intake of the normal diet. Ethnic differences exist for the intake of fat by children; but, in most Western societies, total fat intakes account for 30 to 40% of the total caloric intake. If about half this intake comes from plant sources, the essential fatty acid requirements will be met easily.

Disorders of fat metabolism are reviewed in Chapter 24.

References

1. Hansen, A.E., Haggard, M.E., Boelsche, A.N., Adams, D.J.D., and Wiese, H.F.: Essential fatty acids in infant nutrition. III. Clinical manifestations of linoleic acid deficiency. J. Nutr., 66:565, 1958.
2. Holman, R.T., Johnson, S.B., and Hatch, T.F.: A case of human linolenic acid deficiency involving neurological abnormalities. Amer. J. Clin. Nutr., 35:617, 1982.
3. Williams, M.L., Shott, R.J., O'Neal, P.L., and Oski, F.A.: Role of dietary iron and fat on vitamin E deficiency anemia of infancy. New Engl. J. Med., 292:887, 1975.
4. Naismith, D.J., Deeprose, S.P., Supramaniam, G., and Williams, M.J.H.: Reappraisal of linoleic acid requirement of the young infant, with particular regard to use of modified cows' milk formulae. Arch. Dis. Child., 53:845, 1978.
5. Friedman, Z., Danon, A., Stahlman, M.T., and Oates, J.A.: Rapid onset of essential fatty acid deficiency in the newborn. PEDIATRICS, 58:640, 1976.
6. Friedman, Z., Lamberth, E.L., Jr., Stahlman, M.T., and Oates, J.A.: Platelet dysfunction in the neonate with essential fatty acid deficiency. J. Pediat., 90:439, 1977.

Chapter 12

CALCIUM, PHOSPHORUS, AND MAGNESIUM

Calcium, phosphorus, and magnesium comprise about 98% of the total mineral in the body. Each mineral has an important role in the body economy, and regulatory mechanisms exist for stabilizing their concentrations in body fluids. Failure of these regulatory mechanisms, or the placing of a grossly excessive burden on them by dietary deficiency or excess, can result in clinical symptoms and signs. In the discussion to follow, all of the regulatory mechanisms are presumed to be in proper working order, with no malfunction of the kidney or gastrointestinal tract and no drugs which might lead to a "conditioned" deficiency having been administered.

Body Content

Chemical analyses have been made of a number of fetuses and several adults. Estimates of total body calcium and phosphorus also have been made in a large number of adults by neutron activation analysis.*

Estimates of total body calcium in children and adults have been developed through extrapolation of measurements of the metacarpal cortex thickness and of photon densitometry of the distal radius and ulna. Three important considerations have emerged from these analyses: (1) in fetal life the increase in body calcium content is most rapid during the final 2 months of gestation; (2) total body calcium increases rapidly during adolescence; and (3) in the adult, body calcium content appears to be a function of stature (tall individuals have a much larger burden than short ones). Therefore, in general, women's bodies contain considerably less calcium than men's. In adults body

---

*The subject is bombarded by a known flux of neutrons, and the induced radioactivity is measured in a whole body counter.[1] The reactions of interest here are ^{48}Ca, (n, γ) ^{49}Ca, and ^{31}P (n, α) ^{28}Al; both products are strong gamma emitters. The reaction ^{26}Mg (n, γ) ^{27}Mg is also known, but no data for man have been reported. This technique has been used only in adults, although the radiation dose is less than a roentgen.

calcium is calculated to increase an average of 20 gm for each centimeter increment in height, from 770 gm in short women to 1,290 gm[1,2] in tall men. Therefore, there is no single, adult value for total body calcium.

Table 10 gives data on total body calcium, phosphorus, and magnesium at various ages.† Bone accounts for 99% of the total body calcium, 80% of the phosphorus, and 60% of the magnesium. Bone crystal is hydroxyapatite, which has the formula $Ca_{10}(PO_4)_6(OH)_2$, and which has the property of accepting—either by substitution in the crystal lattice or by surface adsorption—a number of elements in trace amounts, including magnesium, fluorine, sodium, strontium, radium, and lead. Neuman and Neuman[8] have shown that certain elements also tend to concentrate in the hydration shell which surrounds the bone crystals. Young bone has a greater ability than old bone to accept such substitutions, a fact of obvious clinical importance as regards fluorine and lead, and perhaps the fallout product strontium[90] also.

Phosphate is the major anion of intracellular fluid, and magnesium is second only to potassium as a major cation.

The levels of calcium, phosphorus, and magnesium in serum are, respectively, 10, 3.5, and 2 mg/dl; infants and children have higher phosphorus levels (4 to 6 mg/dl). Of the total amount of calcium in serum (i.e., the value reported from routine analyses), about 33% is bound to protein and 12% is complexed with organic compounds; consequently, the level of ionized calcium is only 5.5 mg/dl. Most of the magnesium in serum is ultrafiltrable. The serum levels of each of these elements are maintained at fairly constant values by the combined action of a number of homeostatic mechanisms.

Functions

Calcium has a structural function because it is the major component of bone mineral. Trace amounts also are present in soft tissue, including bone cells, where calcium plays an important role in cellular metabolism: activation of synaptic transmitter substances, mitochondrial function, the formation

---

†Some prefer to express these values as mM: 1 mM of calcium is 40.08 mg; of phosphorus, 30.97 mg; and of magnesium, 24.30 mg.

Table 10
Mineral Content[1,3-7]
(in gm)

Sources	Total Body Content				Grams per Kilogram Fat-free Weight		
	1,000 gm Fetus	Full-term Newborn Infant	Adult Male*	Adult Female†	1,000 gm Fetus	Full-term Newborn Infant	Adult
Carcass analysis							
calcium, gm	6.2	27	1,030-1,230	860	6.4	11	22
phosphorus, gm	3.9	16	500-660	450	4.0	6.3	11
magnesium, gm	0.21	0.81	26-28	15	0.22	0.33	0.46
Neutron activation			Male‡	Female§			
calcium, gm	–	–	1,110±170	826±69	–	–	–
phosphorus, gm	–	–	510±86	398±41	–	–	–

*Four subjects[5-7] (only three subjects for magnesium).
†One subject.[4]
‡Nine subjects 30 to 39 years old (±S.D.).[1]
§Seventeen subjects 30 to 49 years old (±S.D.).[1]

of cyclic AMP, modulation of the excitatory threshold, and sodium permeability of cells.

Magnesium is a cofactor for a large number of enzyme systems, including ATP formation, phosphate transfer systems, and ribosomal protein synthesis; and, as mentioned previously, it is the major cation of intracellular fluid.

Phosphorus is essential to the cellular economy. Ribonucleic acids are polyphosphate polymers; ATP contains phosphate, as do phospholipids; and the various steps of glycolysis involve phosphorylated intermediates.

Alterations in serum calcium and magnesium lead to clinical symptoms and signs (the hypocalcemia secondary to hypoproteinemia is an exception), but changes in serum phosphorus are usually well tolerated. However, one study reported respiratory failure and severe muscle weakness in two patients who had severe hypophosphatemia (0.5 mg/dl); others have reported anemia, defective chemotaxis, decreased glucose utilization by erythrocytes, and a decrease in myocardial performance.[9,10] A low serum phosphorus may delay the return of consciousness in diabetic coma.

Regulation

Factors which regulate calcium metabolism include the mucosa of the upper small intestine, parathyroid hormone, thyrocalcitonin, vitamin D, the kidney, and bone. The gastrointestinal tract regulates calcium absorption; a portion of the calcium is absorbed by passive diffusion and a portion of it is actively transported. Indeed, much of the calcium ingested in food is rejected by the gastrointestinal tract and appears in the feces. Parathyroid hormone acts to enhance intestinal absorption (possibly by facilitating vitamin D metabolism in the kidney), the release of calcium from bone, and renal excretion. The concentration of ionized calcium in the fluid perfusing the parathyroid gland is a major determinant of the rate of synthesis and release of this hormone. Thyrocalcitonin, a hormone elaborated by the "C cells" of the thyroid and the ultimobranchial gland of lower vertebrates, acts to inhibit bone resorption. Vitamin D has two functions: (1) facilitation of intestinal absorption, and (2) release of calcium from bone. To achieve these effects, the vitamin—whether it is acquired from the diet or manufactured in the skin by the action of sunlight—must undergo sequential hydroxylation in the liver and kidney; the final product, 1,25-dihydroxycholecalciferol, is the active form. Anticonvulsant drugs, such as phenobarbital and dilantin, can interfere with vitamin D metabolism. The tremendous reservoir of calcium in bone also serves a regulatory function because a portion of bone calcium exchanges readily with the calcium of extracellular fluid.

The physical forces of muscle tension and gravity also play a role in preserving skeletal integrity because, in the absence of these forces, bone mass is lost.

The regulation of magnesium and phosphorus metabolism is less well understood. Parathyroid hormone seems to have some effect on magnesium absorption from the intestine and on renal tubular reabsorption; these effects are well established for phosphorus. The existence of an active transport system for magnesium in the intestine can be inferred from the fact that, although rare, there are patients who have a congenital defect in magnesium absorption. Vitamin D facilitates phosphorus absorption, but it apparently plays no role in magnesium absorption.

Calcium metabolism should be viewed from two areas, factors which (1) act to stabilize the serum concentration because this largely determines whether clinical symptoms occur, and (2) act to ensure preservation of total bone mass. If regulatory functions are intact, dietary deficiencies or excesses almost never lead to alterations in serum calcium. For example, fasting subjects maintain a normal serum level over long periods, as do breast-fed, newborn infants despite low calcium intakes during the first 2 to 3 days of life. Dietary excesses lead to prompt increases in fecal calcium excretion. Therefore, if serum calcium is elevated or depressed, one or more of the regulatory functions is at fault—lack or excess of vitamin D, hyper- or hypoparathyroidism, intestinal malfunction, and so forth.

Dietary deficiency in the growing organism can lead to osteoporosis, a term reserved for a diminished bone volume but normal bone composition. This condition is common in small preterm infants, for whom it is difficult, if not impossible, to provide an intake of calcium and phosphorus commensurate with their relatively high growth rate. Osteoporosis also may be seen in children suffering from malabsorption. Bone mineral also is lost whenever the normal physical forces acting on the skeleton are lessened: bed rest, muscle paralysis, immobilization, and true weightlessness such as that experienced by the astronauts.

Calcium absorption (variously reported at 21 to 70%)[11] is influenced by a number of factors in addition to parathyroid hormone and vitamin D. Young infants absorb more calcium than adults, and relative absorption is increased by dietary lactose, by a low calcium diet, and during pregnancy. Absorption is decreased by excessive dietary phosphate and alkali. Serum calcium levels are reduced in states of magnesium deficiency. Phosphorus absorption varies inversely with dietary calcium content, and it can be impaired by certain medications (e.g., antacids containing aluminum or magnesium). Magnesium deficiency has been described in patients with severe protein deficiency and in those suffering from alcoholism, but the responsible mechanisms involved are not known.

A certain amount of calcium in feces has its origin not in the diet but in the digestive secretions—the so-called endogenous fecal calcium. Endogenous fecal calcium has been estimated at anywhere from 32 to 290 mg per day in adults, but there are no data for children.

Calcium continues to be excreted in the urine of adults with low dietary intake; the amounts are between 100 and 200 mg per day.

The upper limits of normal urinary calcium for individuals in the United States on unselected diets is 4 mg/kg per day for children and adults.

An observation of considerable practical interest is that large amounts of dietary protein enhance urinary calcium excretion and may even lead to a negative calcium balance.[11] This observation and the fact that the typical diet of individuals in the United States is high in protein points up the need to revaluate this aspect of calcium nutrition.

Calcium-phosphorus Ratio

The calcium-phosphorus ratio varies widely in foods, from a high of 2.8 gm:1 gm in green vegetables to a low of 0.06:1 in meat. The ratio for human milk is 2:1, for cow's milk it is 1.2:1, and for commercial infant formulas it is 1.2-2:1. The high phosphorus content of cow's milk with its lower calcium-phosphorus ratio is one factor in the pathogenesis of neonatal tetany, a situation which is rarely encountered in the breast-fed infant.

In recent years processors have added polyphosphates to certain foods to the extent that the calcium-phosphorus ratio of the typical diet of individuals in the United States has been lowered somewhat. However, studies of primates and adult humans fed large amount of phosphorus have failed to show clear-cut adverse effects.

Requirements

Calcium requirements have been a matter of intense debate for many years. The reasons include:

1. "... the wide range of intakes with which people in various parts of the world maintain themselves without apparent signs of either calcium deficiency or calcium excess;"[11] obviously, the human organism can adapt to variations in intake;

2. the imprecision of the metabolic balance technique;

3. the difficulties in extrapolating animal data to humans;

4. the lack of an easily recognizable deficiency syndrome.

Calcium is needed for skeletal growth, to cover excessive losses (e.g., lactation), and for maintenance (endogenous fecal losses and the urinary excretion which continues with a low calcium diet). Of particular importance is the growth requirement.

Preterm Infants

The amount of calcium, phosphorus, and magnesium required for growth of the preterm infant can be estimated by determining the accretion rate of these minerals during fetal life. During the past century, a number of fetuses, ranging in weight from a few grams to 4,300 gm have been analyzed for various constituents. Plots of body content against body weight on double logarithmic coordinates showed straight line relationships for all three minerals. The increment in mineral content for a given body weight is, for practical purposes, a linear function of weight gain.

Figure 7 is based on these relationships. For example, a 1,000 gm infant gaining weight at the rate of 20 gm per day needs to retain 4.7 mg magnesium, 90 mg phosphorus, and 150 mg calcium for growth. The values for a 2,500 gm infant gaining at a similar rate would be 5.3 mg, 105 mg, and 190 mg, respectively.

The amount of mineral needed is a function of growth rate rather than of time alone. Figure 7 shows it also varies with body weight; large infants require more mineral per unit weight gain than small infants.

Human milk, even if it is taken in large amounts (200 ml/kg per day), does not contain enough calcium and phosphorus to sustain a high rate of growth for small infants. Gastrointestinal absorption is probably not greater than 65%, and supplementary calcium is needed to sustain optimal calcium balance.

Infants and Children

The data in Table 10 show that body calcium content increases from 27 gm at birth to an average of 830 gm in adult women and 1,110 gm in adult men. Also mentioned earlier was the fact that the bodies of tall adults contain considerably more calcium than those of short adults. The total postnatal growth increment will depend on achieved adult stature and on the age of attainment of full skeletal size. Garn and Wagner[13] estimate this to be age 40 years and Christiansen and co-workers[14] suggest 30 years. The following calculations of growth requirements are offered as examples; the values for adult body calcium are obtained from the data by Cohn and co-workers:[1,2]

tall man (1,290 gm Ca):

$(1,290\text{-}27) \div (20 \text{ yr} \times 365) = 173$ mg per day

$(1,290\text{-}27) \div (30 \text{ yr} \times 365) = 115$ mg per day

short woman (770 gm Ca):

$(770\text{-}27) \div (20 \text{ yr} \times 365) = 102$ mg per day

$(770\text{-}27) \div (30 \text{ yr} \times 365) = 68$ mg per day

Increments in body phosphorus are about half those for calcium (Table 10). Increments in magnesium amount to only 2 to 4 mg per day. Most foods contain generous amounts of both phosphorus and magnesium, so dietary deficiencies of these two elements do not occur in normal individuals, except preterm infants.

The values given here are daily increments averaged over many years; these values are higher during infancy and adolescence than in midchildhood. At the peak of their growth spurt, boys accumulate 290 to 400 mg calcium per day and girls

accumulate 210 to 240 mg per day. The average daily increment from age 10 years to 20 years is 180 to 210 mg and 90 to
110 mg, respectively.[13,14]

Table 11 lists published recommendations for calcium, phosphorus, and magnesium. The differences in the recommendations reflect differences in criteria used to evaluate
need. Breast-fed infants appear to thrive on lower calcium,
phosphorus, and magnesium intakes than those deemed necessary by scientific experts.

Lactation drains the mother's body calcium and phosphorus
(e.g., 34 mg calcium and 14 mg phosphorus for each 100 ml
milk produced). The magnesium drain is only 4 mg per 100 ml
of milk. The last few weeks of pregnancy also require at least
150 mg phosphorus and 250 mg calcium each day for the fetus.
Intestinal calcium absorption is higher in pregnancy, perhaps
high enough to accommodate the mother's increased needs; but
similar data on lactating women are lacking.

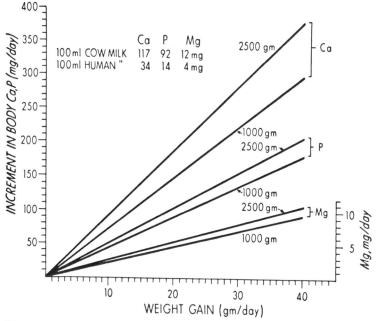

*Figure 7. Increments in body calcium, phosphorus, and magnesium
content as functions of body weight and weight gain, as derived from
analyses of human fetuses. An additional (unknown) quantity is
needed for maintenance. The mineral content of milk is also shown.*[12]

Table 11
Recommended Intakes

Subject	Calcium (mg/day)			Phosphorus (mg/day)		Magnesium (mg/day)	
	FAO/WHO[15,16]	NAS[17]	Canada[18]	NAS[17]	Fomon[19]	NAS[17]	Canada[18]
Infants	500-600*	360-540*	350-500	240-400	120-160	50-70	30-50
Children	400-500	800	500-700	800	—	150-250	60-110
Adolescents							
boys	600-700	1,200	900-1,100	1,200	—	400	220-240
girls	600-700	1,200	700-1,000	1,200	—	300	190-220
Pregnancy	1,000-1,200	+400	+500	+400	—	+150	+15-25
Lactating women	1,000-1,200	+400	+500	+400	—	+150	+80

*Not breast-fed.

Dietary Sources of Calcium

Milk supplies most of the calcium consumed by young infants and an appreciable amount of that consumed by children and adults in the United States, where per capita consumption average is 500 ml daily. However, some individuals are variably intolerant of milk because of allergy or intestinal lactase deficiency. The latter individuals include blacks, Orientals, and American Indians. However, lactose-intolerant individuals can tolerate yogurt much better than milk.[20]

A list of foods reasonably high in calcium is given in Appendix M. Phosphorus and magnesium are both widely distributed in foods.

References

1. Cohn, S.H., Vaswani, A., Zanzi, I., Aloia, J.A., Roginsky, M.S., and Ellis, K.J.: Changes in body chemical composition with age measured by total-body neutron activation. Metabolism, 25:85, 1976.
2. Cohn, S.H.: Personal communication.
3. Widdowson, E.M., and Spray, C.M.: Chemical development in utero. Arch. Dis. Child., 26:205, 1951.
4. Widdowson, E.M., McCance, R.A., and Spray, C.M.: The chemical composition of the human body. Clin. Sci., 10:113, 1951.
5. Mitchell, H.H., Hamilton, T.S., Steggerda, F.R., and Bean, H.W.: The chemical composition of the adult human body and its bearing on the biochemistry of growth. J. Biol. Chem., 158:625, 1945.
6. Forbes, R.M., Cooper, A.R., and Mitchell, H.H.: The composition of the adult human body as determined by chemical analysis. J. Biol. Chem., 203:359, 1953.
7. Forbes, R.M., Mitchell, H.H., and Cooper, A.R.: Further studies on the gross composition and mineral elements of the adult human body. J. Biol. Chem., 223:969, 1956.
8. Neuman, W.F., and Neuman, M.W.: The Chemical Dynamics of Bone Mineral. Chicago: University of Chicago Press, 1958.
9. Newman, J.H., Neff, T.A., and Ziporin, P.: Acute respiratory failure associated with hypophosphatemia. New Engl. J. Med., 296:1101, 1977.
10. O'Connor, L.R., Wheeler, W.S., and Bethune, J.E.: Effect of hypophosphatemia on myocardial performance in man. New Engl. J. Med., 297:901, 1977.
11. Irwin, M.I., and Kienholz, E.W.: A conspectus of research on calcium requirements of man. J. Nutr., 103:1019, 1973.

12. Forbes, G.B.: Nutritional adequacy of human breast milk for premature infants. *In* Lebenthal, E., ed.: Textbook of Gastroenterology and Nutrition in Infancy. Vol. 1. Gastrointestinal Development and Perinatal Nutrition. New York: Raven Press, pp. 321-329, 1981.
13. Garn, S.M., and Wagner, B.: The adolescent growth of the skeletal mass and its implications to mineral requirements. *In* Heald, F.P., ed.: Adolescent Nutrition and Growth. New York: Appleton-Century-Crofts, pp. 139-161, 1969.
14. Christiansen, C., Rödbro, P., and Nielsen, C.T.: Bone mineral content and estimated total body calcium in normal children and adolescents. Scand. J. Clin. Lab. Invest., 35:507, 1975.
15. Calcium Requirements: Report of an FAO/WHO Expert Group. Geneva: World Health Organization, 1962.
16. Passmore, R., Nicol, B.M., Rao, M.N., Beaton, G.H., and Demayer, E.M.: Handbook on Human Nutritional Requirements. WHO Monograph Series No. 61. Geneva: World Health Organization, 1974.
17. Committee on Dietary Allowances and Food and Nutrition Board: Recommended Dietary Allowances, ed. 9, revised. Washington, D.C.: National Academy of Sciences, 1980.
18. Committee for the Revision of the Dietary Standard for Canada: Recommended Nutrient Intakes for Canadians. Ottawa: Canadian Government Publishing Centre, 1983.
19. Fomon, S.J.: Infant Nutrition, ed. 2. Philadelphia: W.B. Saunders Company, 1974.
20. Kolars, J.C., Levitt, M.D., Aouji, M., and Savaiano, D.A.: Yogurt—an autodigesting source of lactose. New Engl. J. Med., 310:1, 1984.

Chapter 13

TRACE ELEMENTS

An element is considered to be a trace element when it constitutes less than 0.01% of total body weight. Trace elements are essential to metabolic processes because they are components of many of the enzyme systems and act either as integral components of metalloenzymes or cofactors for enzymes activated by metal ions. Trace-element deficiencies have been reported in humans and have been shown to be deleterious to health, growth, and development. Because effects of deficiency states frequently are most severe during periods of rapid growth, trace-element deficiencies are of special concern to pediatricians. Currently, 13 trace elements are thought to be nutritionally important for higher animals.[1] These trace elements, in order of importance to children, are: iron, zinc, copper, fluoride, iodine, manganese, selenium, chromium, cobalt, molybdenum, nickel, silicon, and vanadium. All these trace elements will be considered in this chapter, except for iron and fluoride, which are discussed in Chapters 23 and 17.

The Committee on Dietary Allowances of the Food and Nutrition Board, National Research Council, has established Recommended Dietary Allowances for humans for zinc (see Appendix H). This committee also has set ranges of estimated safe and adequate daily dietary intakes for chromium, copper, fluoride, manganese, molybdenum, and selenium. These safe ranges of intake are considered at the lower end of the range to meet nutrient needs or prevent deficiencies, and at the upper end to be below known toxic doses. These ranges take into account nutrient interactions influencing dietary requirements and incomplete knowledge of the requirements. The recommended dietary allowances and the safe and adequate dietary ranges of the major trace minerals discussed in this chapter are shown in Table 12. Also summarized in Table 12 are biochemical actions, effects of deficiency, effects of excess, and good food sources for the trace elements.

Zinc

Zinc functions in many enzyme systems, including carbonic anhydrase, alkaline phosphatase, carboxypeptidase, and alcohol, lactic, and glutamic dehydrogenases. Zinc plays a central role in nucleic acid metabolism; it is needed for the synthesis of both deoxyribonucleic acid and ribonucleic acid. Zinc also is important for taste perception and the hepatic synthesis of retinol-binding protein.[2]

The bioavailability of zinc from human milk is thought to be greater than that from cow's milk and commercial infant formulas.[3,4] However, the absolute amount of zinc absorbed from cow's milk and commercial infant formula is greater than or equal to that from human milk because the zinc content of human milk (1.6 mg/l) is low compared to cow's milk (3.9 mg/l) and commercial infant formulas for term infants (3.7 to 6.0 mg/l).[3] A controversy concerning the nature of substances promoting the absorption of zinc from human milk is still unresolved. A recent study showed that zinc in human milk was bound to both low molecular weight compounds and to proteins in a complex fashion.[5]

All commercial infant formulas for term infants currently contain between 3.7 and 6.0 mg of zinc per liter. Improved growth and higher plasma zinc levels have been reported in male infants but not in female infants fed a cow's milk formula containing 5.8 mg of zinc per liter compared to infants fed a lower zinc formula (1.8 mg/l).[6]

Zinc bioavailability from soy-based formulas may be less than that from cow's milk formulas or human milk.[3,4] The specific factor responsible for this effect has not been determined, but it may be the presence of phytate, a chelator of zinc, in soy formulas.

Studies in animals and humans[7] have demonstrated a competitive interaction between iron and zinc. Zinc absorption in humans is significantly reduced with dietary iron-to-zinc ratios of 2:1 and 3:1 when the iron is inorganic.[7] Heme iron did not affect the absorption of zinc. This competition may be nutritionally significant in commercial infant formulas supplemented with iron.[7]

Zinc deficiency is characterized by growth retardation, hypogeusia, hypogonadism, dermatitis, impaired wound healing, and decreased cell-mediated immunity. Factors important in the development of zinc deficiency include: increased zinc requirements, inadequate dietary intake, alcohol intake, dietary factors or disease states inhibiting zinc absorption, and excessive losses of zinc.[2] In addition, requirements for zinc are increased during periods of rapid growth, in wound healing, and in pregnancy and lactation. The zinc requirement of preterm infants is higher than that of term infants because preterm infants grow more rapidly and their zinc stores are lower at birth than those of term infants.[8] Balance studies have found that preterm infants who are fed pasteurized human milk are in a negative zinc balance until they are 45 days of age.[9]

Individuals not consuming foods high in zinc (such as meat, fish, and whole grains) may not receive an adequate zinc intake (see Appendix N). Infants and children from low-income families are at an increased risk for suboptimal zinc nutrition because of inadequate dietary zinc.[10] Pediatric patients receiving total parenteral nutrition also are at an increased risk for developing zinc deficiency unless an adequate zinc supplement is provided. Children with intestinal malabsorption syndromes are at greater risk for zinc insufficiency because of suboptimal zinc absorption. Excessive loss of zinc in the urine and chronic blood loss also can lead to zinc depletion.

Acrodermatitis enteropathica is a rare, autosomal, recessively inherited genetic defect of zinc absorption that results in acute zinc deficiency.[11] The disease is characterized by skin lesions, diarrhea, and alopecia. Symptoms commence in infancy but are delayed until after weaning if the infant is breast fed. Daily oral zinc supplements (1 to 2 mg of zinc per kilogram of body weight) lead to rapid clinical improvement.

Diagnosis of zinc deficiency is sometimes difficult because plasma or serum zinc values do not always reflect nutritional status. Plasma or serum zinc levels do not reflect total body zinc nutriture in patients with hypoproteinemia or those with active infectious or inflammatory conditions.[12]

Erythrocyte zinc and hair zinc may reflect chronic zinc depletion better than plasma or serum zinc levels. However, to date, the metabolism of zinc in red blood cells and its reflection of total body zinc status has not been adequately assessed.[12] Although hair is a readily accessible tissue, it is more susceptible to environmental contamination than erythrocytes. Hair zinc also depends on the delivery of zinc to the root and the rate of hair growth. Because zinc deficiency can impair hair growth, caution is recommended in using hair zinc to assess zinc status.[12] Low urinary zinc may suggest zinc deficiency.[2] However, both hypozincuria and hyperzincuria have been reported in zinc deficiency.[12] If zinc deficiency is suspected, a trial of zinc supplements (1 mg/kg of body weight per day) may provide a response, but they should not be continued if a response does not occur. The supplement can be administered as a solution of zinc acetate (30 mg zinc acetate in 5 ml of water). Nutritional advice can be valuable in the prevention of zinc deficiency.

Table 12
Trace Elements

Name	Biochemical Action	Effects of Deficiency	Effects of Excess	Daily Requirement	Food Sources
Zinc (Zn)	Component of many enzymes	Anorexia, hypogeusia, retarded growth, delayed sexual maturation, impaired wound healing, skin lesions	Relatively nontoxic; may aggravate marginal copper deficiency	Infants, 3-5 mg; children, adolescents, 10-15 mg	Seafood, liver, meat
Copper (Cu)	Constituent of ceruloplasmin; component of key metalloenzymes; role in connective tissue biosynthesis	Sideroblastic anemia, retarded growth, osteoporosis, neutropenia, decreased pigmentation	Relatively nontoxic; Wilson's disease, liver dysfunction	Safe and adequate range: infants, 0.5-1.0 mg; children, adolescents, 1.0-3.0 mg	Shellfish, meat, legumes
Manganese (Mn)	Activator of metalenzyme complexes important for synthesis of polysaccharides and glycoproteins; constituent of pyruvate car-	Humans, not documented; animals, growth retardation, ataxia of newborn, bone abnormalities, reduced fertility	Relatively nontoxic; neurologic manifestations from industrial contamination has occurred	Safe and adequate range: infants, 0.5-1.0 mg; children, adolescents, 1.0-5.0 mg	Nuts, whole grains, tea

Element	Function	Deficiency	Toxicity	Recommended range	Sources
Selenium (Se)	boxylase and certain superoxide dismutases Component of enzyme glutathione peroxidase	Humans, cardiomyopathy; animals, liver necrosis, muscular dystrophy, exudative diathesis, pancreatic fibrosis	Irritation of mucous membranes (nose, eyes, upper respiratory tract), pallor, irritability, indigestion	Safe and adequate range: infants, 0.01-0.06 mg; children, adolescents, 0.02-0.2 mg	Seafood, meat, whole grains
Chromium (Cr)	Required for maintenance of normal glucose metabolism potentiates the action of insulin	Humans, impairment of glucose utilization; animals, impaired growth, disturbances of carbohydrate, protein, and lipid metabolism	Relatively nontoxic; humans, not well documented; animals, growth retardation, liver and kidney damage	Safe and adequate range: infants, 0.01-0.04 mg; children, adolescents, 0.02-0.2 mg	Meat, cheese, whole grains, brewer's yeast
Cobalt (Co)	Component of vitamin B_{12}	Humans, unknown; animals, anemia, growth retardation	Relatively nontoxic; polycythemia, myocardial degeneration	Not established	Green leafy vegetables
Molybdenum (Mo)	Component of enzymes involved in production of uric acid (xanthine oxidase) and in oxidation of aldehydes and sulfides	Humans, unknown; animals, growth retardation, anorexia	Humans, gout-like syndrome, antagonist of copper	Safe and adequate range: infants, 0.03-0.08 mg; children, adolescents, 0.05-0.30 mg	Meats, grains, legumes

Copper

Copper is an essential component of many proteins, including several metalloenzymes that are important in oxidative metabolism. For example, cytochrome oxidase, which contains one atom of copper, is the terminal enzyme in the electron transport chain. A copper metalloenzyme, lysyl oxidase, is involved in the cross-linking of elastin. More than 90% of the copper in plasma is bound to ceruloplasmin, a glycoprotein containing eight atoms of copper per molecule. Ceruloplasmin has ferroxidase activity and functions in the formation of the Fe (III)-transferrin complex; therefore, it is important in iron transport and availability.

Unmodified cow's milk is a poor source of copper; it contains approximately 0.13 mg per liter. Human milk and commercial infant formulas for term infants are better sources of copper; human milk contains about 0.25 mg of copper per liter,[13] and commercial infant formula contains between 0.4 and 0.6 mg per liter.

Factors predisposing an infant to developing copper deficiency include the following: (1) generalized malnutrition;[2] (2) prolonged diarrhea, especially when the infant is rehabilitated solely on cow's milk;[14] (3) intestinal malabsorption syndromes; (4) premature birth (low hepatic copper stores); (5) prolonged parenteral nutrition without copper supplementation; and (6) Menkes' steely hair syndrome as a result of a genetic defect in copper absorption.[15] Excessive zinc intake impairs copper absorption.

The earliest symptoms of copper deficiency are neutropenia, sideroblastic anemia, and osteoporosis with blurring and cupping of the metaphyses.[16] Other characteristics of copper deficiency include depigmentation of skin and hair and hypotonia with psychomotor retardation. Ataxia occurs in animals, and major vessels rupture because of inadequate cross-linking of the elastin.

Copper deficiency should be suspected in patients with any predisposing factors and if anemia unresponsive to iron therapy, leukopenia, neutropenia, or osteoporosis is present. Low plasma copper or ceruloplasmin levels will confirm the diagnosis. After the infant is 1 to 2 months old, plasma copper levels less than 40 to 50 mg/dl or ceruloplasmin levels less than 15 μg/100 ml should be considered abnormally low.[2] Standards for preterm infants have not yet been established.

Nutritional copper deficiency in infants can be treated effectively with the daily administration of 2 to 3 mg of copper sulfate (400 to 600 μg copper) as a 1% solution. For patients receiving total parenteral nutrition, 20 to 30 μg of copper per kilogram per day should be provided in the infusate. Although the hypocupremia of Menkes' steely hair syndrome can be corrected with parenteral copper administration, copper therapy usually does not reverse the progressive neurologic deterioration. This lack of reversal may be the result of irreversible neurologic damage prior to diagnosis and copper therapy.

Manganese

Manganese is an essential element for many animals and is assumed to be essential for humans. Manganese serves as an activator of many enzyme systems, including hydrolases, kinases, decarboxylases, and transferases.

Although manganese deficiency has not been observed in humans, it has been induced in many animals, including poultry, rats, mice, rabbits, pigs, sheep, and cattle.[17] Manifestations of manganese deficiency in animals are growth retardation, decreased fertility, ataxia of the newborn, and various bone abnormalities.

The toxicity of ingested manganese to animals is low, and concentrations of 1,000 μg/gm of diet must be fed to produce symptoms of toxicity.[17] In humans, toxicity has been reported only in industrial workers exposed to high levels of manganese dust in the air; it has not been observed as a consequence of high dietary intake.

Selenium

The first known physiologic role of selenium was described in 1973; selenium was found to be an integral component of glutathione peroxidase, an enzyme known to metabolize lipid peroxides. Glutathione peroxidase prevents hydroxyl radical formation, which attacks unsaturated membrane lipids.[18] Vitamin E and selenium function cooperatively in protecting biologic membranes because vitamin E acts as a membrane-bound antioxidant.

In humans, a serious cardiomyopathy (Keshan's disease) attributable to selenium deficiency has been described in China.[19,20] A possible case of true selenium deficiency was reported in a woman in New Zealand who had painful neuromuscular symptoms after long-term, total parenteral nutrition.[21] Symptoms improved within 1 week of intravenous selenium administration. Evidence of selenium deficiency was found in an adult patient who developed cardiomyopathy and died while receiving total parenteral nutrition.[22] Selenium deficiency has been demonstrated in experimental animals and livestock raised on selenium-deficient diets.[18] Selenium deficiency showing variable response to vitamin E supplementation includes liver necrosis, muscular dystrophy, pancreatic fibrosis, and exudative diathesis.

Rapidly growing infants, especially preterm infants, may be at risk of selenium insufficiency. However, assessing selenium status in infants is difficult because there are no good indicators of selenium status. Plasma levels of selenium may reflect intake more than stores; selenium intake is correlated with plasma selenium concentrations in infants.[23] Plasma selenium levels of breast-fed infants are higher than those of formula-fed infants. Human milk contains approximately two to three times more selenium than commercial infant formulas (16 μg per liter for human milk versus 5 to 8 μg per liter for formula).[23] Plasma levels of selenium decline in preterm infants fed parenterally with less than 3.2 μg/kg of selenium.[24]

Glutathione peroxidase activity may be the most sensitive indicator of selenium status. Erythrocyte glutathione peroxidase activity appears to decline from birth in preterm infants fed commercial infant formulas; however, the same trends have not been consistently reported in plasma and erythrocyte selenium levels.[25]

Selenium toxicity in humans has been reported in industrial workers exposed to selenium compounds in the form of dust or vapors.[18] However, toxicity resulting from the excessive dietary intake of selenium was not observed in humans until recently.[26] The manifestations of toxicity are pallor, indigestion, and irritability. Both chronic and acute selenium poisoning have been reported in livestock consuming plants with high selenium concentrations. The symptoms of acute toxicity in livestock include respiratory failure, hepatic necrosis, edema, nephritis, and ulceration of numerous tissues. Symptoms of chronic toxicity in livestock are blind staggers and alkali disease.

Other Trace Elements

Chromium functions as a cofactor for insulin. Chromium deficiency is characterized by impaired growth and longevity and by impaired glucose, lipid, and protein metabolism in experimental animals. Chromium deficiency in infants is usually associated with protein-calorie malnutrition.[27] Depletion of chromium also may occur during prolonged parenteral alimentation. Currently, the only reliable indicator of chromium deficiency is the demonstration of a beneficial effect of chromium supplementation.[2]

Cobalt is considered essential for humans only because it is a component of the vitamin B_{12} molecule. Cobalt deficiency has never been demonstrated in humans or laboratory animals, and the requirement of cobalt is considered minute.[17]

The biochemical functions of molybdenum are in the synthesis and function of xanthine oxidase, aldehyde oxidase, and sulfite oxidase. Molybdenum deficiency has not been reported under any natural conditions in humans. However, molybdenum toxicity is a substantial problem in some animals because of the antagonism of molybdenum to copper and because of species differences in tolerance that are not clearly understood.[17] Moderate levels of molybdenum in the diet of humans have been associated with significant urinary losses of copper.[28]

Arsenic, nickel, silicon, and vanadium are other trace elements considered nutritionally important. Human deficiency states have not been demonstrated, and dietary requirements have not been set because of insufficient experience.

Aluminum, although poorly absorbed, can accumulate in patients with renal insufficiency, and this accumulation has been associated with osteomalacia and encephalopathy. Care should be taken when administering aluminum-containing antacids to children with renal insufficiency.

References

1. Mertz, W.: The essential trace elements. Science, **213**:1332, 1981.
2. Hambidge, K.M.: Trace elements in pediatric nutrition. Adv. Pediat., **24**:191, 1977.
3. Johnson, P.E., and Evans, G.W.: Relative zinc availability in human breast milk, infant formulas and cow's milk. Amer. J. Clin. Nutr., **31**:416, 1978.

4. Casey, C.E., Walravens, P.A., and Hambidge, K.M.: Availability of zinc: Loading tests with human milk, cow's milk and infant formulas. PEDIATRICS, 68:394, 1981.
5. Lönnerdal, B., Hoffman, B., and Hurley, L.S.: Zinc and copper binding proteins in human milk. Amer. J. Clin. Nutr., 36:1170, 1982.
6. Walravens, P.A., and Hambidge, K.M.: Growth of infants fed a zinc supplemented formula. Amer. J. Clin. Nutr., 29:1114, 1976.
7. Solomons, N.W., and Jacob, R.A.: Studies on the bioavailability of zinc in humans: Effects of heme and nonheme iron on the absorption of zinc. Amer. J. Clin. Nutr., 34:475, 1981.
8. Shaw, J.C.L.: The absorption of magnesium, copper, zinc and iron by preterm infants in relation to body composition of the foetus. In Visser, H.K.A., ed.: Nutrition and Metabolism of the Fetus and Infant. The Hague: Martinus Nijhoff Publishers, pp. 179-194, 1979.
9. Dauncey, M.J., Shaw, J.C.L., and Urman, J.: The absorption and retention of magnesium, zinc, and copper by low-birth-weight infants fed pasteurized human breast milk. Pediat. Res., 11:1033, 1977.
10. Hambidge, K.M., Walravens, P.A., Brown, R.M., Webster, J., White, S., Anthony, M., and Roth, M.L.: Zinc nutrition of preschool children in the Denver Head Start program. Amer. J. Clin. Nutr., 29:734, 1976.
11. Walravens, P.A., Hambidge, K.M., Neldner, K.H., Silverman, A., van Doorninck, W.J., and Mierau, G.: Zinc metabolism in acrodermatitis enteropathica. J. Pediat., 93:71, 1978.
12. Solomons, N.W.: On the assessment of zinc and copper nutriture in man. Amer. J. Clin. Nutr., 32:856, 1979.
13. Picciano, M.F., and Guthrie, H.A.: Copper, iron, and zinc contents of mature human milk. Amer. J. Clin. Nutr., 29:242, 1976.
14. Graham, G.G., and Cordano, A.: Copper depletion and deficiency in the malnourished infant. Johns Hopkins Med. J., 124:139, 1969.
15. Danks, D.M., Campbell, P.E., Stevens, B.J., Mayne, V., and Cartwright, E.: Menkes's kinky hair syndrome: An inherited defect in copper absorption with widespread effects. PEDIATRICS, 50:188, 1972.
16. Ashkenazi, A., Levin, S., Djaldetti, M., Fishel, E., and Benvenisti, D.: The syndrome of neonatal copper deficiency. PEDIATRICS, 52:525, 1973.
17. Underwood, E.J., ed.: Trace Elements in Human and Animal Nutrition, ed 4. New York: Academic Press, 1977.
18. Shamberger, R.J.: Metabolism of selenium. In Shamberger, R.J., ed.: Biochemistry of Selenium. New York: Plenum Press, pp. 59-75, 1983.
19. Keshan Disease Research Group of the Chinese Academy of Medical Sciences, Beijing: Observations on effect of sodium selenite in prevention of Keshan disease. China Med. J., 92:471, 1979.

20. Keshan Disease Research Group of the Chinese Academy of Medical Sciences, Beijing: Epidemiologic studies on the etiologic relationship of selenium and Keshan disease. China Med. J., **92**:477, 1979.
21. van Rij, A.M., Thomson, C.D., McKenzie, J.M., and Robinson, M.F.: Selenium deficiency in total parenteral nutrition. Amer. J. Clin. Nutr., **32**:2076, 1979.
22. Johnson, R.A., Baker, S.S., Fallon, J.T., Maynard, E.P., III, Ruskin, J.N., Wen, J., Ge, K., and Cohen, H.J.: An Occidental case of cardiomyopathy and selenium deficiency. New Engl. J. Med., **304**:1210, 1981.
23. Smith, A.M., Picciano, M.F., and Milner, J.A.: Selenium intakes and status of human milk and formula fed infants. Amer. J. Clin. Nutr., **35**:521, 1982.
24. Huston, R.K., Benda, G.I., Carlson, C.V., Shearer, T.R., Reynolds, J.W., and Neerhout, R.C.: Selenium and vitamin E sufficiency in premature infants requiring total parenteral nutrition. J. Parent. Enter. Nutr., **6**:507, 1982.
25. Rudolph, N., Preis, O., Bitzos, E.I., Reale, M.M., and Wong, S.L.: Hematologic and selenium status of low-birth-weight infants fed formulas with and without iron. J. Pediat., **99**:57, 1981.
26. Yang, G., Wang, S., Zhou, R., and Sun, S.: Endemic selenium intoxication of humans in China. Amer. J. Clin. Nutr., **37**:872, 1983.
27. Hopkins, L.L., Jr., Ransome-Kuti, O., and Majaj, A.S.: Improvement of impaired carbohydrate metabolism by chromium (III) in malnourished infants. Amer. J. Clin. Nutr., **21**:203, 1968.
28. Deosthale, Y.G., and Gopalan, C.: The effect of molybdenum levels in sorghum (*Sorghum vulgare* Pers.) on uric acid and copper excretion in man. Brit. J. Nutr., **31**:351, 1974.

Chapter 14

VITAMINS

Vitamins are essential cofactors in a wide range of metabolic reactions. These functions are summarized in Table 13. Supplemental vitamins probably are unnecessary for the healthy child more than 1 year old who consumes a varied diet.

Milk from a well nourished mother contains sufficient vitamins for the young, healthy, term infant, except for vitamin D and for vitamin K during the first few days of life.

Most commercial infant formulas contain vitamins in quantities sufficient to meet the recommended daily allowances if the infant consumes 750 ml of formula. Evaporated milk and pasteurized whole cow's milk contain added vitamin D and sufficient vitamin A and most water-soluble vitamins for normal growth. However, infants fed these milks should receive a daily supplement of vitamin C, unless this vitamin was added by the processor.

Recommended daily allowances of vitamins are given in Appendix H, although some will be mentioned here. Infants and children who are ill or receive certain medications may require supplements of specific vitamins. Extra allowances are suggested for pregnant and lactating women.

Vitamin A

The recommended daily allowance of vitamin A, which is stored in the liver, approximates 200 IU per 100 calories (Table 13, Appendix H). Human milk, cow's milk, and commercial infant formulas are excellent sources of vitamin A. Vitamin A toxicity has been reported with as little as 20,000 IU daily for about 1 month.

Vitamin D

Most formulas contain 1.5 μg (62 IU of vitamin D per 100 calories, or 400 IU per liter, as do whole cow's milk (homogenized) and evaporated milks. This is double the estimated requirement of full-term infants. The mandated addition of vitamin D to milk served to reduce greatly, indeed almost eliminate, deficiency rickets in children in the United States. Lactating women must be reminded that human milk does not contain enough vitamin D to prevent rickets. Vitamin D is synthesized in the skin by the action of ultraviolet light (the most effective wave lengths are in the range of 230 to 313 mμ); therefore, the requirement for dietary vitamin D will depend on the amount of exposure to sunlight.

Vitamin D toxicity can occur in infants with intakes of only 2,000 to 4,000 IU daily if continued for several months.

Vitamin E

Full-term infants require approximately 0.5 mg tocopherol equivalent (0.7 IU) per 100 kcal. The requirement for preterm infants is not known, although iron-containing formulas and formulas with higher linoleic acid content require additional vitamin E. Vitamin E may possibly have an effect on the development of retrolental fibroplasia, and deficiency has been associated with hemolytic anemia in preterm infants.

Vitamin K

Most infants born to well nourished mothers will have adequate vitamin stores at birth, except for vitamin K. The newborn infant should be given vitamin K soon after birth (see Chapter 4). Vitamin K is present in most cow's milk formulas, and the bottle-fed infant ordinarily does not need added vitamin K. Breast-fed infants who develop diarrhea of longer than several days' duration should be given an additional intramuscular injection of vitamin K (1.0 mg).

Water-soluble Vitamins

Deficiencies of the water-soluble vitamins are rare in formula-fed infants. In general, the Committee on Nutrition

Table 13
Vitamins*

Name	Characteristics	Biochemical Action	Effects of Deficiency	Effects of Excess	Daily Requirement	Food Sources
Vitamin A (retinol) 1 IU = 0.3 μg retinol	Fat soluble, heat stable; bile necessary for absorption, specific binding protein in plasma; stored in liver	Component of visual purple; integrity of epithelial tissues, bone cell function	Night blindness xerophthalmia, keratomalacia, poor growth, impaired resistance to infection	Hyperostosis, hepatomegaly, alopecia, increased cerebrospinal fluid pressure (also from 13-cis-retinoic acid)	Infants—300 μg; adolescents—750 μg; lactation—1,200 μg	Milk fat, egg, liver
Provitamin A: β-carotene 1/6 activity of retinol	Converted to retinol in liver, intestinal mucosa			Carotenemia		Dark green vegetables, yellow fruits and vegetables, tomato
Biotin	Water soluble; synthesized by intestinal bacteria; deficiency only	Coenzyme: acetyl CoA carboxylase	Dermatitis, anorexia, muscle pain, pallor, alopecia	Unknown	Unknown	Liver, egg yolk, peanuts

	with large intake of egg white, TPN					
Cobalamin (vitamin B₁₂)	Slightly soluble in water, heat stable only at neutral pH, light sensitive; absorption (ileum) dependent on gastric intrinsic factor; Co a part the molecule	Coenzyme component; red blood cell maturation, central nervous system metabolism; methyl-malonyl CoA mutase	Pernicious anemia; neurologic deterioration, methyl-malonic acidemia	Unknown	1-2 μg, all ages	Animal foods, only: meat, milk, egg
Folacin group of compounds containing pteridine ring, p-amino-benzoic and glutamic acids	Slightly soluble in water, light sensitive, heat stable; some production by intestinal bacteria; ascorbic acid involved in interconversions; interference from oral contraceptives, anticonvulsants	Tetrahydrofolic acid the active form; synthesis of purines, pyrimidines, methylation reactions, one carbon acceptor	Megaloblastic anemia, impaired cellular immunity	Only in patients with pernicious anemia not receiving cobalamin	Infants—50 μg; adolescents—400 μg; pregnancy—800 μg	Liver, green vegetables, cereals, oranges

Name	Characteristics	Biochemical Action	Effects of Deficiency	Effects of Excess	Daily Requirement	Food Sources
Niacin (nicotinic acid, amide)	Water soluble, heat and light stable; availability from corn enhanced by alkali; synthesized in the body from tryptophan (60:1), some by intestinal bacteria	Component of coenzymes I and II (NAD, NADP), many enzymatic reactions	Pellagra: dermatitis, diarrhea dementia	Nicotinic acid (not the amide): flushing, pruritus	6.6 mg/1,000 kcal	Meat, fish, whole grains, green vegetables
Pantothenic acid	Water soluble, heat stable	Component of CoA; many enzymatic reactions	Observed only with use of antagonists; depression, hypotension, muscle weakness, abdominal pain	Unknown	Unknown; estimated at 5-10 mg	Most foods

Vitamin	Properties	Function	Deficiency	Toxicity	Requirement	Sources
Pyridoxine (vitamin B$_6$) also pyridoxal, pyridoxamine	Water soluble, heat and light labile, interference from isoniazid; pyridoxal is the active form	Cofactor for many enzymes, e.g., transaminases, decarboxylases	Dermatitis, glossitis, cheilosis, peripheral neuritis. Infants—irritability, convulsions, anemia	Unknown	Infants—0.2-0.3 mg; adults—2 mg	Liver, meat, whole grains, corn, soybeans
Riboflavin	Water soluble, light labile, heat stable; ? synthesis by intestinal bacteria	Cofactor for many enzymes, synthesis FMN and FAD	Photophobia, cheilosis, glossitis, corneal vascularization, poor growth	Unknown	0.6 mg/1,000 kcal	Meat, milk, egg, green vegetables, whole grains
Thiamine (vitamin B$_1$)	Heat labile; absorption impaired by alcohol, requirements a function of carbohydrate intake; synthesis by intestinal bacteria	Coenzyme for decarboxylation, other reactions as thiamine pyrophosphate	Beriberi: neuritis, edema, cardiac failure, hoarseness, anorexia, restlessness, aphonia	Unknown	0.5 mg/1,000 kcal	Liver, meat, milk, whole grains, legumes

Name	Characteristics	Biochemical Action	Effects of Deficiency	Effects of Excess	Daily Requirement	Food Sources
Ascorbic acid (vitamin C)	Easily oxidized, especially in presence of copper, iron, high pH; absorption by simple diffusion	Exact mechanism unknown: functions in folacin metabolism, collagen biosynthesis, iron absorption and transport, tyrosine metabolism	Scurvy	Massive doses may lead to temporary increase in requirement, predispose to kidney stones	Infants—35 mg; adolescents—45 mg	Citrus fruits, tomatoes, cabbage, potatoes, human milk
Vitamin D (D_2-activated calciferol; D_3-activated dehydro-cholesterol) 1 IU = 0.025 μg	D_2 from diet, D_3 from action of ultraviolet on skin; hydroxylated sequentially in liver and kidney to form 1,25-di-hydroxychole-calciferol, the	Formation of calcium transport protein in duodenal mucosa, facilitates bone re-sorption, phosphorus	Rickets, os-teomalacia	Hypercal-cemia, azotemia, poor growth, vomiting, nephrocal-cinosis	All ages, 10 μg (400 IU)	Fortified milk, fish, liver, salmon, sardines, mackerel, egg yolk, sunlight

Vitamin	Metabolism	Function	Deficiency		RDA	Sources
	active compound; regulated by dietary calcium, PTH; now called a hormone; anticonvulsant drugs interfere with metabolism	absorption; synthesis of Ca-binding protein in epithelial cells				
Vitamin E (1 IU = 1 mg α-tocopherol acetate)	Stored in adipose tissue, transported with β-lipoproteins; absorption dependent on pancreatic juice and bile (iron may interfere); requirement increased by large amounts of polyunsaturated fats	Antioxidant, role in red blood cell fragility; stabilizes biological membranes, prevents peroxidation of unsaturated fatty acids	Hemolytic anemia in premature infants; otherwise, no clear-cut deficiency syndrome in man	Unknown	Infants—4 mg; adolescents—15 mg	Cereal seed oils, peanuts, soybeans, milk fat, turnip greens

Name	Characteristics	Biochemical Action	Effects of Deficiency	Effects of Excess	Daily Requirement	Food Sources
Vitamin K (napthoquinones)	Fat soluble, bile necessary for absorption, synthesis by intestinal bacteria	Blood coagulation: Factors II, VII, IX, X	Hemorrhagic manifestations	Water-soluble analogs only: hyperbilirubinemia	Newborn—single dose of 1 mg; thereafter, 5 μg/day; older infants, children—unknown	Cow's milk, green leafy vegetables, pork, liver

*Adapted from Barness, L.A.: Vitamins in nutrition. *In* Practice of Pediatrics, Vol. 1, rev. ed., Hagerstown, Maryland: Harper and Row, Chapter 28, 1974; and Forbes, G.B.: *In* Hoekelman, R.A., Blatman, S., Brunell, P.A., Friedman, S.B., and Seidel, H.M., ed.: Principles of Pediatrics: Health Care of the Young, New York: McGraw-Hill, pp. 138-139, 1978.

agrees with the recommended daily allowances of the National Research Council of the National Academy of Sciences.

Vitamin dependency states are inborn errors of metabolism in which pharmacologic doses of vitamins may ameliorate signs of the disease. These states have been described for thiamine, pyridoxine, folic acid, vitamin B_{12}, biotin, niacin, riboflavin, ascorbate, and vitamin D.

Vitamin requirements for preterm infants are not well specified. At present, recommendations are the same as those for full-term infants (see Chapter 4). Megavitamin therapy is discussed in Chapter 33.

The infant, child, and adolescent eating a diet consisting of fruits, vegetables, animal protein source, cereals or bread, and dairy products (fortified with vitamin D) consumes sufficient vitamins to meet daily allowances, particularly after the rapid growth periods.

Children eating only vegetables and no dairy products, meat, or eggs require a supplemental source of vitamin B_{12}. Folic acid may be in a form difficult to absorb in some diets, so children receiving special diets or those with diseases which increase folic acid requirement (e.g., hemolytic anemia, malabsorption) should be periodically examined for folic acid deficiency or given a 0.1 to 0.5 mg daily supplement of folic acid.

Some evidence exists for an increased need of thiamine, riboflavin, pyridoxine, ascorbate, folic acid, vitamin E, and vitamin B_{12} in those taking oral contraceptives. Further data are needed before a general recommendation is possible. This may have relevance for the teen-age girl, particularly during pregnancy. Excessive alcohol intake increases the need for thiamine.

Toxic effects from large intakes of water-soluble vitamins are mentioned in Chapter 33. Recommended allowances are given in Table 13 and in Appendix H.

Chapter 15

INFANT NUTRITION AND THE DEVELOPMENT OF GASTROINTESTINAL FUNCTION

The enormously complex yet efficient gastrointestinal mechanisms required for the absorption of nutrients and the maintenance of health are well developed at birth. However, in specific areas normal developmental changes in gastrointestinal function are important for the nutrition of the small preterm infant and the infant compromised by surgery or disease. This chapter will discuss the functional aspects of gastrointestinal development and focus on the continuum of development which begins *in utero* and extends until 1 year of age.[1,2]

Swallowing, Sucking, and Gastrointestinal Motility

The gastrointestinal tract *in utero* plays a major role in the regulation of amniotic fluid volume. Fetal swallowing of the amniotic fluid may be demonstrated as early as 16 to 17 weeks of gestation; by term, it equals nearly 45 ml per day, or nearly one-half the total amniotic fluid volume. At this time, the amniotic fluid contains enough protein (nearly 600 mg/dl) to supply as much as 0.6 gm/kg per day of protein as a nutrient source.

In contrast to the early development of the ability to swallow, sucking matures between 30 and 34 weeks of gestation. Immaturity in the coordination of breathing, sucking, swallowing, and gastric emptying in the preterm infant may severely limit enteral nutritional intake. Control of the lower esophageal sphincter may be incomplete in preterm and newborn term infants, and significant gastroesophageal reflux frequently is demonstrated. Delayed gastric emptying also is an important clinical problem in preterm infants. Instillation of formula by tube directly into the stomach or proximal small intestine is usually an effective technique in infants with enteral feeding limited by small gastric volumes, delayed gastric emptying, or reflux. Nonnutritive sucking (on a pacifier) during tube feedings has been shown to accelerate the development of an effective suck, speed gastric emptying, and shorten the transition to nipple feeding; and it may have a significant effect on the utilization of nutrients.[3]

Although a normal distribution of ganglion cells throughout the intestine has been shown to be present as early as 24 weeks of gestation, large intestine motility may not be fully coordinated in the preterm infant, which can result in stool retention and/or functional obstruction and further complicate enteral nutrition. Additional studies delineating the role of gastrointestinal hormones and environmental and nutritional factors on gastrointestinal motility are needed to determine the most efficacious methods to maximize the enteral delivery of nutrients.

The Development of Absorptive Mechanisms

Carbohydrates

Carbohydrate digestion occurs principally at the surface of the mucosal cell. Therefore, both enzyme activity and the surface area of the intestine must be sufficient to accommodate the dietary load of carbohydrate in the diet before carbohydrate absorption and digestion can proceed efficiently. Between 6 weeks of gestation and birth, the surface area of the intestinal mucosa increases nearly 100,000-fold, with the small intestine achieving a length nearly two and a half times the length of the infant at birth. The development of lactase activity is delayed in comparison to sucrase and does not reach maximal levels until 34 to 38 weeks of gestation. Few preterm infants demonstrate a clinical intolerance to lactose, even though lactose malabsorption may be documented by hydrogen excretion in breath. In addition to hydrogen, bacterial metabolism of carbohydrate in the colon produces short-chain fatty acids, which are absorbed and utilized; this reduces fecal water loss and conserves the energy content of the carbohydrate. Clinically evident carbohydrate intolerance frequently is a harbinger of disease or injury to the gastrointestinal tract rather than the result of immaturity.

Starch digestion is initiated within the lumen of the intestine by alpha-amylases. In infants 6 months old and younger, pancreatic amylase is absent or present in negligible amounts. Thus, other alpha-amylases (e.g., salivary, human milk) have become recognized as important determinants of the infant's ability to digest starch. Salivary amylase is at low levels at birth and rises rapidly to one third of adult levels by 3 months of age. Human milk also contains a high concentration of alpha-amylase. Both salivary and human milk amylases are acid resistant and are stable in the newborn infant's gastric environment; this suggests these enzymes may be important amylolytics in the neonate.[4] Glucoamylase, an intestinal brush-border amylase, is also present at birth, and these enzymes may together compensate for the lack of pancreatic amylase in newborn infants.

A variety of carbohydrate sources are well tolerated by preterm and full-term infants. Lactose is the logical choice for most healthy, full-term infants. Lactose-free formulas most commonly provide carbohydrate in the form of sucrose, corn syrup solids, or glucose polymers. Most full-term and preterm infants are readily able to digest sucrose. Corn syrup solids, glucose polymers, and maltodextrins, which are partially digested or hydrolyzed starches, are well tolerated even by stressed infants. However, the adequacy of starches as the sole carbohydrate source in the neonate is not established.

Lipids

Lipid absorption in the neonate is an inefficient process. Preterm infants 32 to 34 weeks of gestation absorb as little as 65 to 75% of the intake. However, full-term infants may absorb up to 90% of the intake. Adult levels of lipid absorption (>95%) are not routinely achieved until 4 to 6 months of age (Fig. 8). Lipids are the nutrient of highest caloric density; therefore, it is important to understand the mechanisms of fat absorption and to explain the variations in the efficiency of absorption of various lipids (i.e., human milk versus other fats).

The initial step of fat digestion in the newborn infant involves hydrolysis of triglyceride by the lipolytic triad of lingual lipase, human milk lipase, and pancreatic lipase.[9] Secreted by the serous lingual glands, lingual lipase has been found to be active as early as 25 weeks of gestation, has a pH optimum of 4.0 to 5.5, and is partially specific for the fatty acid on the number three position of the triglyceride molecule. It acts intragastrically to hydrolyze dietary triglyceride predominately to free fatty acids and partial glycerides. Human milk lipase is present in significant amounts throughout lactation in both preterm and term milks. It is inactivated by pasteurization (>60°C), but it is stable at stomach pH (>3.5) and active in the duodenum (pH optimum, 8.0 to 9.5), where it hydrolyzes tri-, di-, or monoglycerides to free-fatty acids and glycerol in a nonstereospecific manner. A low concentration of bile salt is required for activity, and it enhances the resistance of the lipase to proteolysis and heat. Milk lipase facilitates the hydrolysis of milk fat by pancreatic lipase because it degrades monoglycerides, a product of pancreatic lipase action. At a pH optimum of 6.5, pancreatic lipase exerts its activity with colipase and hydrolyzes triglyceride to 2-monoglycerides and free-

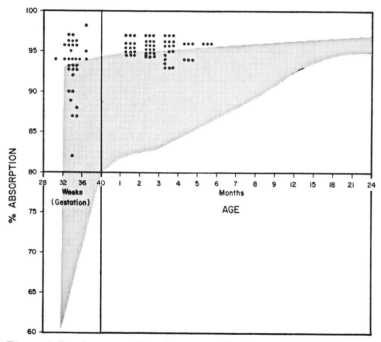

Figure 8. Development of fat absorption. Shaded area equals the range for the percentage of fat absorption for normal preterm and full-term infants fed commercial infant formulas or a normal diet for age. • *represents infants fed human milk. (Adapted from Weijers et al.,[5] Watkins et al.,[6] Järvenpää,[7] and Alemi et al.[8])*

fatty acids. Pancreatic lipase is present by 16 weeks of gestation, reaches a low plateau (about 5% of adult) at 23 weeks, and remains unchanged until term; its activity increases fivefold in the first weeks of life and increases 20-fold at some time between 1 and 9 months of age. Pancreatic enzyme secretion increases in response to exogenous cholecystokinin administration in newborn infants. For optimal activity, the products of lipase action must be incorporated into mixed micelles with bile salts, facilitating transport to the mucosa and absorption. Micelle formation requires that bile salts be present at or above a critical concentration, termed the critical micellar concentration (CMC, approximately 2 to 3 mM).

Maintenance of intraluminal bile salt concentrations sufficient for micellar formation requires a critical mass of bile acids and an efficient recirculation of the bile salt pool (Fig. 9). In the preterm (32 to 36 weeks of gestation) infant, the bile salt pool is approximately one-half to one-third that of full-term infants, and the intraluminal bile salt concentration is at or below the CMC.[10] Both pool size and intraluminal concentration increase dramatically during the first month of life, with a corresponding improvement in the efficiency of fat absorption. In the preterm infant, intestinal losses of bile salt have been proposed as contributing to the decreased pool size. However, maturation of the hepatic and intestinal components of the enterohepatic circulation are equally important in producing the increases in bile salt pool size and intraluminal concentrations observed with postnatal age. Human milk feeding also has been shown to enlarge the bile salt pool, suggesting that dietary factors independent of postnatal maturity also may contribute significantly to the enlargement of the bile salt pool.[6]

Lipid uptake, triglyceride synthesis, and chylomicron formation within the intestinal mucosal cell are poorly studied at present; however, chylomicrons have been demonstrated in the serum of newborn infants after 2 to 3 days of age. Studies in immature animals indicate that fatty acid acylation within the enterocyte and the distribution of the intestinal fatty acid-binding protein are increased by large fat loads to the distal intestine; this aspect of lipid absorption may yet prove limiting for the small infant.

These observations have stimulated the design of commercial infant formulas from which the fat is absorbed as efficiently as with human milk fat. Various mechanisms have been postulated to explain this increased efficiency. Human milk triglyceride structure and the degree of fatty acid saturation may be particularly important. Because saturated fatty acids are poorly solubilized within the intestine and poorly absorbed from the intestine, they require bile acid micelles for efficient absorption. For this reason, triglycerides composed principally of long-chain, saturated lipids frequently are poorly tolerated by infants. Vegetable oils, which contain triglycerides composed of highly unsaturated fatty acids, are more easily solubilized and absorbed; therefore, they now are used in most infant formulas. In addition, saturated lipids frequently form insoluble calcium soaps within the intestinal lumen. A high calcium intake may increase steatorrhea in newborn infants; conversely, formulas which contain a high content of saturated lipids diminish calcium absorption.

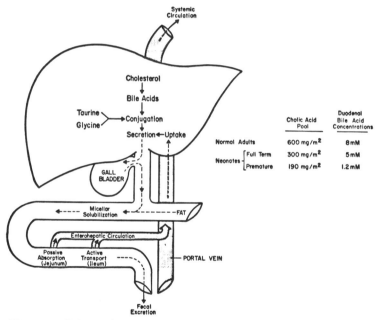

Figure 9. Bile acid metabolism and function. The two primary bile acids (cholic acid and chenodeoxycholic acid) are synthesized by the liver from cholesterol and conjugated with taurine or glycine. Bile acids then are concentrated in the gallbladder and secreted into the intestine. Intraluminal concentrations are frequently less than the critical micellar concentration in the preterm infant, which significantly reduces the solubilization and absorption of fat. Immaturity of both hepatic and intestinal components of the enterohepatic circulation contribute to this reduction. (Adapted from Watkins et al.[10])

Medium-chain triglycerides readily form emulsions that are rapidly hydrolyzed by both lingual and pancreatic lipases and undergo a different metabolism within the intestinal mucosa cell; they are bound directly to albumin in the portal circulation and transported directly to the liver. Most commercial formulations for preterm infants now contain medium-chain triglycerides, and an improvement in lipid absorption has been observed.

Other nutritionally significant nonpolar lipids in the diet include the vitamins A, D, E, and K and cholesterol. Detailed studies of these nutrients' capacity for absorption in the immature infant are lacking; however, most experimental data demonstrate that they require solubilization within bile salt micelles for efficient absorption. Thus, these vitamins may be poorly absorbed by cholestatic or small preterm infants. This is demonstrated by the high requirements for vitamin E in the rapidly growing preterm infant. Vitamin E requirements also depend on the iron content of the milk and the type and degree of saturation of dietary fats. Current recommendations are to provide 0.5 mg tocopherol equivalents of vitamin E in an aqueous form per gram of linoleic acid, and to maintain a vitamin E:polyunsaturated fatty acid ratio which is at least 0.5 mg per gram.

Protein

Protein digestion is initiated in the stomach by pepsin. Pepsin secretion parallels acid secretion, both of which are present by 20 weeks of gestation. Pepsin secretion is highest during the first days of life, then falls to reach its lowest level between 10 and 30 days of age, after which there is a slow increase paralleling weight gain. Even in the first days of life, the mean gastric pH achieved during feeding exceeds the pH optimum for pepsin activity (1.8 to 3.5). Lowering of the proteolytic activity may serve to facilitate the absorption of intact antibody protein from colostrum but does not appear to impair nitrogen absorption. The intraluminal phase of protein digestion involves the hydrolysis of dietary protein by pancreatic trypsin and chymotrypsin, both of which are present in adequate amounts as early as 26 to 28 weeks of gestation. Trypsin secretion in response to exogenous pancreozymin and secretin administration is blunted in the preterm infant when compared to older children. Trypsin activation occurs in the presence of bile salts by interaction with enterokinase, a brush-border enzyme. The developmental curve for enterokinase activity is similar to that observed for lactase. Enterokinase deficiency has been reported but is rare; and sufficient trypsin is present for the initial hydrolysis of protein in most newborn infants. Peptides of varying lengths and solubility remain after intraluminal proteolytic digestion. These peptides then are either further hydrolyzed by brush-border peptidases or absorbed directly. Peptidase activity is present early in gestation, and the levels appear to be unaffected by gestational age. Accordingly, the use of peptides as a nutritional source is being explored. The use of amino acids, which are absorbed at the brush border by specific carrier-mediated, transport mechanisms believed to function effectively at term, also is being evaluated.

The quality and quantity of protein supplied to a newborn infant also has important effects on nutrition and, perhaps, on development of the gastrointestinal tract. Studies have demonstrated that whey-predominant formulas are more digestible, and they are better suited to meeting the amino-acid requirements and physiologic limitations of the preterm infant than casein-predominant formulas.[11]

Immunoglobulins/Macromolecules

The absorption of intact immunoglobulins from the intestine is quantitatively significant in the rodent and other animal species which do not acquire gamma globulin transplacentally. Specific mucosal receptors have been identified which facilitate immune gamma-globulin absorption and are present for the first 2 to 3 weeks after delivery. After this period, circulating immunoglobulin levels are adequate, immunoglobulin synthesis is intact, and intestinal protein absorption is less prominent. Gastrointestinal absorption of immunoglobulins in the human infant does not contribute significantly to the circulating immunoglobulin pool. However, the mucosal barrier is immature in the newborn period, particularly in preterm and small-for-dates infants, and is vulnerable to penetration by potentially harmful intraluminal substances. Intact foreign protein, specifically bovine serum albumin, is absorbed by the human infant. Human milk contains antibodies and viable leukocytes as well as substances which can interfere with bacterial colonization and prevent antigen penetration. Despite some evidence for the absorption of the intact protein, no consistent data suggest that either human milk or colostrum is required to initiate local protective mechanisms in the intestine or to maximize the nutrition of small preterm infants.

Vitamin B_{12}

Vitamin B_{12} absorption in the neonate is more efficient than in the adult and may be intrinsic-factor independent. Although this possibility has not been verified in the human, intrinsic-factor independent B_{12} absorption occurs in the newborn rat by pinocytosis of carrier protein. Intrinsic factor-dependent B_{12} absorption gradually develops during the first several months of life. Infants need a sustained intake of B_{12} because of their rapid growth; therefore, infants whose intake is inadequate or in whom B_{12} malabsorption occurs secondary to ileal resection may become B_{12} deficient as early as 6 to 8 months of age.

Minerals

Absorption of minerals depends largely on specific, carrier-mediated transport and localized absorptive capacities within the gastrointestinal tract. Because the majority of mineral accretion occurs during the last trimester, the preterm infant is at high risk for mineral deficiencies because of low stores. Several minerals (most notably iron, calcium, and zinc) appear to be absorbed passively early in postnatal life in experimental animals, with the gradual development of active, carrier-mediated transport mechanisms.[12] The passive transport of calcium is sensitive to the presence and abundance of other nutrients such as lactose and fatty acids.[13,14] There appear to be mineral transport factors unique to human milk which facilitate absorption of iron and zinc. Young animals absorb iron, lead, calcium, and strontium much better than adults,[12,15] and the fact that human infants readily absorb lead[16] means they are at greater risk than adults.

References

1. Grand, R.J., Watkins, J.B., and Torti, F.M.: Development of the human gastrointestinal tract: A review. Gastroenterology, **70**:790, 1976.
2. Lebenthal, E., and Lee, P.C.: Review article. Interactions of de-

terminants in the ontogeny of the gastrointestinal tract: A unified concept. Pediat. Res., **17**:19, 1983.
3. Bernbaum, J.C., Pereira, G.R., Watkins, J.B., and Peckham, G.J.: Nonnutritive sucking during gavage feeding enhances growth and maturation in premature infants. PEDIATRICS, **71**:41, 1983.
4. Heitlinger, L.A., Lee, P.C., Dillon, W.P.., and Lebenthal, E.: Mammary amylase: A possible alternate pathway of carbohydrate digestion in infancy. Pediat. Res., **17**:15, 1983.
5. Weijers, H.A., Drion, E.F., and Van De Kamer, J.H.: Analysis and interpretation of the fat-absorption coefficient. Acta Paediat. Scand., **49**:615, 1960.
6. Watkins, J.B., Järvenpää, A.-L., Szczepanik-Van Leeuwen, P., Klein, P.D., Rassin, D.K., Gaull, G., and Räihä, N.C.R.: Feeding the low-birth weight infant: V. Effects of taurine, cholesterol and human milk on bile acid kinetics. Gastroenterology, **85**:793, 1983.
7. Järvenpää, A.-L.: Feeding the low-birth-weight infant: IV. Fat absorption as a function of diet and duodenal bile acids. PEDIATRICS, **72**:684, 1983.
8. Alemi, B., Hamosh, M., Scanlon, J.W., Salzman-Mann, C., and Hamosh, P.: Fat digestion in very low-birth-weight infants: Effect of addition of human milk to low-birth-weight formula. PEDIATRICS, **68**:484, 1981.
9. Jensen, R.G., Clark, R.M., deJong, F.A., Hamosh, M., Liao, T.H., and Mehta, N.R.: The lipolytic triad: Human lingual, breast milk and pancreatic lipases: Physiological implications of their characteristics in digestion of dietary fats. J. Pediat. Gastro. Nutr., **1**:243, 1982.
10. Watkins, J.B., Szczepanik, P., Gould, J.B., Klein, P., and Lester, R.: Bile salt metabolism in the human premature infant. Preliminary observations of pool size and synthesis rate following prenatal administration of dexamethasone and phenobarbital. Gastroenterology, **69**:706, 1975.
11. Räihä, N.C.R., Heinonen, K., Rassin, D.K., and Gaull, G.E.: Milk protein quantity and quality in low-birthweight infants: I. Metabolic responses and effects on growth. PEDIATRICS, **57**:659, 1976.
12. Ghishan, F.K., Jenkins, J.R., and Younoszai, M.K.: Maturation of calcium transport in the rat small and large intestine. J. Nutr., **110**:1622, 1980.
13. Ghishan, F.K., Stroop, S., and Meneely, R.: The effect of lactose on the intestinal absorption of calcium and zinc in the rat during maturation. Pediat. Res., **16**:566, 1982.
14. Barnes [sic], L.A., Morrow, G., III, Silverio, J., Finnegan, L.P., and Heitman, S.E.: Calcium and fat absorption from infant formulas with different fat blends. PEDIATRICS, **54**:217, 1974.
15. Forbes, G.B., and Reina, J.C.: Effect of age on gastrointestinal absorption (Fe, Sr, Pb) in the rat. J. Nutr., **102**:647, 1972.
16. Ziegler, E.E., Edwards, B.B., Jensen, R.L., Mahaffey, K.R., and Fomon, S.J.: Absorption and retention of lead by infants. Pediat. Res., **12**:29, 1978.

Chapter 16

PARENTERAL NUTRITION*

Clinical experience has demonstrated the value of optimal nutritional status in resisting the effects of trauma and disease as well as in improving response to medical and surgical therapy. The metabolic demands of rapid growth and the low nutritional reserves in infancy make the potential benefit of good nutrition to critically ill pediatric patients even greater.

This statement is not meant to be a comprehensive review of parenteral nutrition nor a guideline for specific techniques. It is intended to provide an update on the "state of the art" of parenteral alimentation. Details concerning the physiology, techniques for approach, and efficacy of parenteral nutrition are given elsewhere.[1,2]

In spite of the many formulas and feeding techniques available, several gastrointestinal and medical problems arise in infants that preclude or severely limit the use of the intestine for nutritional support. Since the first successful use of total parenteral nutrition in a malnourished infant in 1944, the use of total or supplemental parenteral nutrition has become a common practice. Premature infants with severe respiratory disease, congenital anomalies of the gastrointestinal tract, or inflammatory disease of the intestinal mucosa (necrotizing enterocolitis) are frequently candidates for this form of nutritional support. Older infants with intractable diarrhea, short bowel syndrome, severe malnutrition, or inflammatory bowel disease also have been successfully rehabilitated with parenteral feedings. Extensive body surface burns, malignancies, cardiac failure, and renal failure are examples of disorders outside the gastrointestinal tract in which parenteral nutrition support has been useful. Specific formulations and procedures are available for these latter situations and have been reviewed elsewhere.[3]

In certain settings, particularly larger hospitals with increased numbers of more complicated patients receiving parenteral nutrition, a nutritional support team may be beneficial in providing optimal care. An interdisciplinary team consisting of medical, nursing, dietary, pharmacy, and surgical staff

---

*Adapted from Committee on Nutrition: Commentary on parenteral nutrition, PEDIATRICS, **71**:547, 1983.

with expertise in parenteral nutrition provides invaluable con-
sultative services in the management of these patients.

Catheters

Parenteral nutrition can be carried out via peripheral veins
using standard peripheral intravenous catheters and solutions
with an osmolality of 300 to 900 mosmol/l. When solutions of
higher osmolality are used, larger veins with a high blood flow
volume must be used to avoid sclerosis and inflammation of the
wall of the vein.

Strict asepsis is always mandatory during catheter placement. The catheters are made of a flexible material such as
silicone elastomer, polyurethane, or stiffer polyethylene. They
are generally placed, under anesthesia, in the subclavian or
internal jugular vein and advanced toward the right atrium.
Certain of these catheters can be introduced percutaneously
into the subclavian vein. The more flexible catheters must be
introduced through a hollow needle, or they can be placed by
incising the skin and subcutaneous tissue to expose the vein or
by creating a subcutaneous tunnel into a superficial neck vein
and advancing the catheter toward the right atrium. The
placement of flexible catheters in the preterm infant has a
lower incidence of vein perforation and thrombosis. On occasion when jugular or subclavian sites have been unavailable,
veins that run toward the inferior vena cava, such as the inferior epigastric veins, are alternate choices. Regardless of the
site, roentgenographic confirmation of the intravascular
placement of the catheter is mandatory before parenteral nutrition solutions are infused.

A number of complications directly related to the catheter
may occur. Malposition of a central venous catheter outside the
vein, with infusion of hypertonic solutions into the pleural or
pericardial space, may be life threatening. A rapid decrease in
serum glucose or the acute onset of circulatory or respiratory
compromise should signal this complication. Hemorrhage, associated with erosion of central veins or of the wall of the right
atrium, also has been reported. Pneumothorax and brachial
plexus injuries are relatively common complications of per-
cutaneous subclavian line insertion. Air embolus may occur.
Air-eliminating filters and properly secured tubing junctions

may help prevent this. Catheter emboli have occurred from rupture of silicone elastomer catheters perfused under extremely high pressures or from the tips of polyethylene catheters sheared off when the catheter was pulled back through the hub of the needle used to insert it. Thrombophlebitis may be observed in peripheral veins receiving hypertonic solutions. Skin slough is a rare but serious complication of extravasation of the parenteral solution into the interstitial space.

A major complication is catheter-related sepsis. Fever alone is not an indication for removal of a parenteral nutrition catheter. Other sources of infection should be searched for; if none are found, removal of the catheter then should be considered. Signs of sepsis in the neonate include lethargy, hyperbilirubinemia, temperature instability, and intolerance to previously tolerated glucose and lipid loads. Careful placement of the central catheter and strict adherence to established guidelines for catheter care and maintenance considerably decrease the incidence of catheter-related complications.

Metabolic complications caused by the composition and administration of the infusate will be considered as the various caloric sources are discussed. A suggested schedule for monitoring parenteral nutrition is shown in Table 14.

Composition of Solutions for Infants and Children

Protein

Current solutions supply nitrogen requirements as crystalline amino acids. Infants have demonstrated adequate growth with this source of protein. Commercial preparations are available as concentrated 3.5 to 10% mixtures of crystalline amino acids which can be diluted to meet nutritional requirements of infants at different ages. None of the solutions available in the United States has a composition qualitatively identical with that of the amino acid composition of human milk, which has been used as the standard for the formulation of enteral mixtures promoting optimal growth in healthy infants. Also, the commercial solutions do not contain cysteine, although separate preparations of cysteine which can be added to the solutions are available. Cysteine may be an essential amino acid in preterm infants with low activity of hepatic cystathionase, which converts methionine to cysteine. Taurine, which is formed from cysteine and is present in human milk, also may be important for these preterm infants and is absent from commercial solutions. None of the available solutions contains carnitine, which is required for the optimal oxidation of fatty acids.

In spite of the recently recognized potential deficiencies, infants have tolerated the available solutions and have grown well while using them. Most metabolic complications related to amino acids in the solutions, including azotemia and acidosis, have occurred when the infants received more than 4 gm of

Table 14
Suggested Monitoring Schedule During
Total Parenteral Nutrition

Variable Monitored	Suggested Frequency	
	Initial Period*	Later Period†
Serum electrolytes	3-4 times/wk	2-3 times/wk
Serum urea nitrogen	3 times/wk	2 times/wk
Serum calcium, magnesium, phosphorus	3 times/wk	2 times/wk
Serum glucose	‡	‡
Serum acid-base status	3-4 times/wk	2-3 times/wk
Serum ammonia	2 times/wk	weekly
Serum protein (electrophoresis or albumin/globulin)	weekly	weekly
Liver function studies	weekly	weekly
Hemoglobin	2 times/wk	2 times/wk
Urine glucose	daily	daily
Clinical observations (activity, temperature, etc.)	daily	daily
WBC count and differential count	as indicated	as indicated
Cultures	as indicated	as indicated
Serum triglyceride	as indicated	as indicated

*Initial period is period before full glucose intake is achieved, or any period of metabolic instability.
†Later period is period during which patient is in a metabolic steady state.
‡Blood glucose should be monitored closely during the period of glucosuria (to determine the degree of hyperglycemia) and for 2 to 3 days after cessation of parenteral nutrition (to detect hypoglycemia). In the latter instance, frequent Dextrostix determination constitutes adequate screening.

protein equivalent per kilogram per day. Complications are rarely encountered with the recommended intake of 2 to 3 gm of protein equivalent per kilogram per day. Hyperammonemia, seen with earlier solutions, now rarely occurs with the increased amounts of arginine and decreased quantities of glycine in the formulations. Hyperchloremic metabolic acidosis, another problem noted with earlier crystalline amino acid solutions, has been ameliorated by the substitution of acetate for chloride in the salts of lysine and the use of basic salts of histidine.

Carbohydrate

Glucose (dextrose), fructose, galactose, sorbitol, glycerol, and ethanol all have been used as a source of carbohydrate calories in infants. Presently, nearly all centers use glucose as the principal carbohydrate. A small amount of glycerol present in lipid solutions contributes to carbohydrate calories. The other carbohydrate sources have fallen out of favor because they have no advantage over glucose and can produce serious complications in preterm infants.

The quantity of glucose in the infusate that preterm infants will tolerate is variable. Infusing glucose at 5 mg/kg per minute and advancing to 15 mg/kg per minute over a 2-day period may reduce the intolerance seen when large amounts of glucose are infused initially. This is accomplished by increasing the concentration of glucose in the solution while keeping the volume of infusate constant at between 100 to 150 ml/kg per day, depending on the infant's fluid requirements. A suggested protocol to gradually increase the amount of glucose given the infant is shown in Table 15. Acute consequences of glucose intolerance are serum hyperosmolality and osmotic diuresis. Both of these situations can be avoided by careful serum monitoring. Hypoglycemia is generally related to the sudden cessation of the total parenteral nutrition solution. In adult postsurgical patients, there appears to be no correlation between glucose clearance and the rate of oxidation of glucose.[4] An increase in the glucose infusion rate from 4 to 7 mg/kg per minute is associated with an increased rate of glucose oxidation; but, at higher infusion rates, fat is synthesized from the glucose without a further increase in glucose oxidation or energy derived therefrom. Although similar studies have not been completed in infants, this suggests that higher glucose loads delivered by solutions containing more than 20% glucose at 150 ml/kg per day may not be beneficial to infants and may

Table 15
Suggested Protocol for a 3 kg Infant on Central Parenteral Nutrition Solutions Containing Amino Acids*·†

Formulation	Volume (ml/kg/da)	kcal/ 24 hr	kcal/ kg/da	Amino Acids (kg/da)
Pediatric 10% dextrose solution	100	126 (122)‡	42 (40.6)	1.4
Pediatric 10% dextrose solution	150	189 (153)	63 (51)	3.0
Pediatric solution 15% dextrose (central)	150	266 (230)	89 (77)	3.0
Pediatric solution 20% dextrose (central)	150	342 (306)	114 (102)	3.0
Pediatric solution 25% dextrose (central)	150	419 (383)	140 (128)	3.0

*From *Pediatric Parenteral Nutrition Manual*.[10] If glucose intolerance develops: (1) the rate of infusion can be lowered, then increased slowly over several hours; (2) intravenous fat emulsion can be started. Ten percent fat emulsion supplies 1.1 kcal/ml (0.122 gm/ml) and will allow use of lower glucose loads while maintaining adequate fluid volumes. Fat emulsion contains 87% wt/vol water, and this should be counted in the total daily fluid intake. Twenty percent fat emulsion provides 0.222 gm fat per milliliter, 2 kcal/ml, and is 77% wt/vol of water (20% fat emulsions should be used with care). *Note*: Begin intravenous fat emulsion at 0.5 gm/kg per day, given over 20 to 24 hours, and increase the volume over 96 hours to a maximum of 4 gm/kg per day or 45% of total calories, whichever is reached first. Essential fatty acid requirements can be met by 0.5 gm/kg per day once to twice a week. All caloric calculations use 3.4 calories per gram of intravenous dextrose, due to water of hydration. Weight gain of more than 50 gm per day more likely represents edema than cell growth and suggests the need for a more concentrated solution to provide adequate calories while limiting fluid intake.

†Catheter is placed in central vein and dextrose 5% in water is infused following roentgenographic confirmation that catheter is in proper position.

‡Values in parentheses are nonprotein calories.

contribute to the fatty infiltration of the liver seen with prolonged parenteral nutrition. The use of added insulin is difficult because of unpredictable responses to this hormone.

Lipids

The composition, use, and complications of intravenously infused fat emulsions have been discussed.[5] Briefly, in addition
to being a concentrated source of energy and providing essential fatty acids, parenteral lipid solutions are iso-osmolar.

When lipid and amino acid-glucose solutions are infused
simultaneously into the same vein, the patient receives a
higher calorie, lower osmolar solution than with a glucose-
amino acid solution alone. The use of "Y" connector tubing
proximal to the Micropore filter to infuse lipids simultaneously
with, but separately from, the glucose-amino acid solution
(containing vitamins, minerals, electrolytes, and trace elements) has greatly improved the effectiveness of peripheral
intravenous nutrition and increased its use substantially in
nutritional support.

The requirement for linoleic acid (essential fatty acid requirement) can be achieved by supplying 0.5 to 1 gm/kg per
day of intravenous lipid. Preterm infants have adequate lipoprotein lipase to metabolize serum triglyceride concentrations
of 100 mg/dl. When triglyceride levels exceed 100 mg/dl, deposition of lipid may occur in reticuloendothelial cells or along
vascular endothelial surfaces. The easier ways of determining
lipid tolerance, visual inspection and nephelometry, correlate
well with serum chylomicron concentration; but they do not
correlate well with the glyceride or free fatty acid concentrations. Unfortunately, the latter chemical determinations are
costly, require relatively large volumes of blood, or may not be
readily available. The slow (20 to 24 hours) infusion of up to 4
gm/kg per day of intravenous lipid should minimize the chance
of lipid intolerance. Under some circumstances (i.e., sepsis,
hyperbilirubinemia, pulmonary hypertension), the lowest dose
that meets essential fatty acid requirements should be used.

Vitamins, Minerals, and Trace Elements

Vitamins, minerals, and trace elements must be supplied in
parenteral solutions. Metabolic complications have been de-

scribed for deficiencies and excesses of some of these nutrients. Intravenous dose requirements are not fully known. Current recommendations are derived from oral requirements and knowledge of enteric absorption. Guidelines for multivitamin and essential trace element preparations for parenteral use have been established.[6,7] No currently available formulation meets all recommendations. Therefore, a combination that most closely approaches these needs should be used. Certain nutrients are not available and/or approved for continuous intravenous administration in the United States (iron, B_{12}, vitamin K). Therefore, intramuscular or bolus infusions are necessary to meet needs until suitable, low-risk preparations are available.

Gastrointestinal Effects of Parenteral Nutrition

The single most problematic gastrointestinal complication of total parenteral nutrition is the development of liver disease, presenting clinically as hepatomegaly and jaundice and histologically as cholestasis, hepatocellular necrosis, and, in far advanced cases, as cirrhosis or hepatic failure.[8] Since 1971, liver disease has been recognized in approximately one third of preterm infants receiving total parenteral nutrition. The etiology remains obscure.[9] Toxic effects of the amino acid and lipid solutions have been proposed, although not corroborated on further study. The appearance of liver disease with elevations in levels of transaminases, bilirubin, and alkaline phosphatase usually occurs after 2 weeks of total parenteral nutrition; it frequently is progressive and leads to fibrosis and, in a few infants, hepatic failure. These infants frequently are compromised by a number of intercurrent illnesses, including sepsis and severe respiratory distress. It has been difficult to separate these factors from the effects of parenteral nutrition on the development of hepatic dysfunction. The longer the infusions are administered, the greater the risk of cholestasis.

Much less is known about the long-term effects of total parenteral nutrition on gastric, pancreatic, and small bowel structure and function. Studies in animals have documented pancreatic hyposecretion and intestinal mucosal atrophy, which are reversible on resumption of enteric feeding. The few studies from human subjects suggest that exocrine pancreatic secretion and gastric parietal cell mass are decreased, and the mucosa of the small intestine atrophies during total parenteral nutrition. However, amino acids infused intravenously stimulate gastric acid secretion, but much less than if amino acids are infused into the stomach. These effects disappear over a variable period of time after a return to enteral nutrition. Although similar studies have not been done in preterm infants, clinical experience suggests that enteric functions in preterm infants also return to normal with time.

Enteral Feedings

Initiation of enteral feedings should begin as soon as the gastrointestinal tract is functional. Initially, enteral feedings may be a supplement to parenteral nutritional support, which should not be discontinued until the patient is tolerating enteral feedings well enough to meet nutritional requirements.

Summary

Nutritional requirements of young infants, both preterm and full term, can be met better by recognizing the absorptive and digestive limitations present. When gastrointestinal disease is superimposed on an immature digestive system, special support frequently is needed to maintain adequate growth. This support can be offered as parenteral nutrition or with specialized enteral feeding techniques and formulations.

Because parenteral solutions are formulated to provide complete nutritional support, they may be used for short as well as extended periods of time. Recommendations for use include:

1. Careful catheter placement and confirmation of position by roentgenogram; strict adherence to aseptic techniques and established guidelines of catheter care; and laboratory and clinical monitoring of patients for intolerance.

2. Protein, in the form of crystalline amino acids, should be provided at a rate of 2 to 3 gm/kg per day. The concentration of carbohydrate, as glucose (dextrose), should be advanced in a methodical manner to ensure tolerance. Essential fatty acid requirements can be met by infusing 0.5 to 1 gm/kg per day of intravenous lipid. The slow infusion of up to 4 gm/kg per day of intravenous lipid should maximize tolerance. Vitamins, min-

erals, and trace elements are essential nutrients and should be contained in parenteral nutrition solutions.

3. The transition to enteral nutrition should begin as soon as possible, with continuation of parenteral nutrition until full nutritional support is achieved via the gastrointestinal tract.

4. Continuous monitoring of nutritional status is mandatory to assure the adequacy of nutritional support. In some settings, a nutritional support team with expertise in parenteral nutrition can help provide optimal care.

References

1. Goodgame, J.T.: A critical assessment of the indications for total parenteral nutrition. Surg. Gynecol. Obstet., 151:433, 1980.
2. Wretlind, A.: Parenteral nutrition. Nutr. Rev., 39:257, 1981.
3. Fischer, J.E., ed.: Total Parenteral Nutrition. Boston: Little, Brown and Company, 1976.
4. Wolfe, R.R., Allsop, J.R., and Burke, J.F.: Glucose metabolism in man: Responses to intravenous glucose infusion. Metabolism, 28:210, 1979.
5. Committee on Nutrition: Use of intravenous fat emulsions in pediatric patients. PEDIATRICS, 68:738, 1981.
6. American Medical Association, Department of Food and Nutrition, 1975: Multivitamin preparations for parenteral use: A statement by the Nutrition Advisory Group. J. Parent. Enter. Nutr., 3:258, 1979.
7. American Medical Association: Guidelines for essential trace element preparations for parenteral use: A statement by the Nutrition Advisory Group. J. Parent. Enter. Nutr., 3:263, 1979.
8. Cohen, M.I.: Changes in hepatic function. *In* Winters, R.W., and Hasselmeyer, E.G., ed.: Intravenous Nutrition in the High Risk Infant. New York: John Wiley and Sons, pp. 293-305, 1975.
9. Sondheimer, J.M., Bryan, H., Andrews, W., and Forstner, G.G.: Cholestatic tendencies in premature infants on and off parenteral nutrition. PEDIATRICS, 62:984, 1978.
10. Pediatric Parenteral Nutrition Manual. Boston: Children's Service, Massachusetts General Hospital, 1983.

Chapter 17

NUTRITION AND ORAL HEALTH

Although the oral cavity presents no special nutritional needs over and above those required for general health, the mouth can reflect many nutritional disorders which have more general implications. The teeth, which are the most highly calcified structures in the body, serve as permanent records of nutritional and metabolic disturbances occurring during their formation. Also, a child's dietary habits may predispose to one of the most widespread diseases beyond infancy, dental caries. This chapter will discuss the role of nutrition in odontogenesis, oral soft tissue health, and dental caries. The final section deals with fluoride supplementation, including the Academy's fluoride dosage schedule.

Odontogenesis

Tooth formation begins as early as 6 weeks *in utero* with the formation of the dental lamina. Hard tissue formation is initiated at 14 weeks *in utero* and continues into the third decade with the final root development of third molars. At birth, much of the enamel of the primary (deciduous) incisor crowns is formed (Table 16). Severe maternal and neonatal nutritional deficiencies may disturb this process, although these deficiencies are rarely seen in individuals from developed countries. Vitamin A, C, and D deficiencies and protein deprivation have been associated with hypoplastic defects of enamel in humans and rats.[1,2] These defects not only are esthetic problems, but they also may predispose the teeth to caries. Iron deficiency has been implicated as a caries-contributory factor in rats, but a similar relation between iron deficiency and caries in humans has not been established.

Any ill effects from maternal malnutrition on the oral health of fully breast-fed infants also are rare in developed countries. Supplementation of an adequately balanced maternal diet during pregnancy or lactation is not necessary for proper dental development.

Prenatal Fluoride

In 1966, the Food and Drug Administration banned the advertising and marketing of fluoride products which claimed to

Table 16
Calcification of Primary Teeth*

Primary Tooth	Hard Tissue Formation Begins (weeks *in utero*)	Amount of Enamel Formed at Birth	Enamel Completed Months After Birth	Eruption Age (mo)
Maxillary				
Central incisor	14	$5/6$	1½	10
Lateral incisor	16	$2/3$	2½	11
Canine	17	$1/3$	9	19
First molar	15½	cusps united; ½ to ¾ crown height	6	16
Second molar	19	cusps united; $1/5$ to ¼ crown height	11	29
Mandibular				
Central incisor	14	$3/5$	2½	8
Lateral incisor	16	$3/5$	3	13
Canine	17	$1/3$	9	20
First molar	15½	cusps united	5½	16
Second molar	18	cusps united	10	27

*Adapted from, Lunt, R.C., and Law, D.B.: A review of the chronology of calcification of deciduous teeth. J. Amer. Dent. Assn., **89**:599, 1974.

provide caries protection to offspring if taken during pregnancy. At this time, the practice of prenatal fluoride administration, although not harmful to the mother or fetus, cannot be supported on the basis of controlled scientific evidence. Sufficient dietary fluoride passes through the placenta to aid in the mineralization of enamel and bone.

Craniofacial Development

Animal studies have shown that caloric restriction and ascorbate deficiency can result in dental malocclusion.[3,4] Recently, Corruccini and Beecher[5] demonstrated a relation between malocclusion and soft diets in monkeys. According to these authors, when a society's diet shifts to soft, processed foods, the transition from predominately good to bad human occlusion can occur in as short a time span as one generation. Certainly, more research is needed to uncover the underlying factors in the relation between nutrition, diet, and craniofacial development.

Diet and Dental Caries

Three major factors are necessary for the initiation of dental caries: a susceptible tooth, cariogenic bacteria, and sugar. Sucrose has been found to be the most cariogenic sugar, followed by glucose, maltose, lactose, fructose, sorbitol, and xylitol. Cariogenic streptococci break down sucrose into glucose and fructose, which are further polymerized to dextrans and levans, respectively. These sticky polymers aid in the retention of the bacterial plaque on the tooth surface. One by-product of the fructose-levan process is lactic acid, which dissolves the enamel and leads to cavity formation.

In addition to the presence of sugar in the diet, other factors have a relation to dental caries, such as the frequency of eating. Plaque which comes into contact with sugar can produce acid for at least 20 minutes. Therefore, limiting the number of times sugar is ingested will reduce the acid challenge to the teeth. Plaque between the teeth, which is less accessible to the buffering effects of saliva, may produce acid for up to 2 hours, however. The physical nature of the food also has a bearing on its cariogenicity. Some forms of sugar, such as cakes and toffee, are highly retentive and remain on the teeth longer than sugars in solution. These retentive forms have a higher cariogenic potential.[6] Even bread is retentive enough that salivary amylase can degrade the starch into sugar. Sugar in solution can promote an acid challenge to the teeth, but it is rapidly cleared from the mouth.

Coarse brown sugar and coarse refined sugar may be less cariogenic than powdered refined sugar; but honey, which has been recommended as a sucrose substitute, is about equal to sucrose in cariogenicity. Furthermore, honey's sticky consistency may prolong oral clearance times and increase its acid-forming potential.

Certain foods have been studied for protective factors. Fats, for example, offer caries protection by coating the teeth, changing the surface activity, and reducing the retention of sugar and even plaque. Fats also may decrease sugar solubility and have toxic effects on oral bacteria. Protein elevates salivary urea levels and increases the buffering capacity of the saliva. Foods rich in protein and fat (e.g., cheese or nuts) may help elevate plaque pH after a carbohydrate challenge. Phosphates have been thought to have cariostatic properties. Inorganic phosphates have provided caries protection in rats. However, studies on humans have not been as promising.

For years, fibrous foods such as apples and celery have been called "nature's toothbrush." But these foods do not have a "detergent" or toothbrush action. They may help in removing gross food debris from teeth, but they are ineffective as plaque removers. But they are beneficial in stimulating salivary flow which can buffer up to 90% of the acids produced by plaque.

Recommendations

Dietary control of caries is only one part of a complete preventive program. A preventive regime also includes effective daily cleaning of the teeth and rendering the teeth less susceptible to decay through exposure to fluoride. Elimination of all sugar from the diet is neither desirable nor feasible. Rather, supervision of between-meal snacks and substitution of less cariogenic snack foods should be promoted. If possible, sugar intake should be restricted to mealtimes, when salivary flow is high; and toothbrushing should follow.

Professional dental care should begin by the time a child is 3 years old. Many dentists, particularly pedodontists, prefer to see children at an even earlier age. By seeing the child at age 2 or younger, much can be done to institute preventive home care and reduce the chance that early restorative treatment will be necessary.

Pediatricians are well aware of the devastating effects of nursing bottle caries. This distinctive pattern of decay is a result of giving a child a bottle of milk, formula, or juice at naps or bedtime. The teeth most severely affected are the upper incisors, frequently to the extent that extraction of these teeth is required in children as young as 18 months old. Obviously, parents should be warned of the possible dangers inherent in this practice.

Oral Soft Tissue Health

The gingiva, tongue, and oral mucosa are sensitive indicators of several vitamin deficiencies, although some are rare occurrences. The first indication of a vitamin deficiency may be changes in the oral cavity.

Vitamin A deficiencies may lead to decreased salivary flow and decreased taste acuity; keratotic lesions may appear. Vitamin K deficiency may lead to oozing of blood from the gingival sulcus. Bleeding, of course, is not diagnostic of vitamin K deficiency, and the diagnosis of this deficiency must be supported by other clinical signs and laboratory tests.

Oral changes are usually the first to occur in vitamin B-complex deficiencies. Nicotinic acid deficiencies cause hypertrophy and atrophy of the filiform papillae of the tongue; give it a bald, red appearance; and leave it susceptible to injury and infection. The patient may experience a burning sensation in the mouth, with soreness of the lips and tongue. Riboflavin deficiency is one cause of angular cheilosis. Inflammation of the lateral margins of the tongue also may be present.

The relation between thiamin deficiencies and oral signs and symptoms is less clear. Oral hypersensitivity, burning sensations, and decreased taste acuity have been reported. Folic acid deficiencies can produce a smooth, red tongue and ulcerations on the buccal mucosa, pharynx, esophagus, and lateral borders of the tongue. Gingival inflammation and a superimposed necrotizing ulcerative gingivitis may accompany the other findings. Cobalamin deficiencies produce the characteristic burning and painful tongue with ulcerations. No oral findings have been associated with pyriodoxine deficiencies.

Vitamin C deficiencies are rare. Associated oral findings include swollen, bluish-red gingiva; acute, necrotizing, ulcerative gingivitis; and mobile teeth.

No oral soft tissue findings have been associated with deficiencies of vitamins D and E.

Recommendations

Adequate, balanced diets need no special supplementation for the maintenance of oral soft tissue health.

Fluoride Supplementation

One of the greatest discoveries in the field of public health was the relation between naturally occurring fluoride in drinking water supplies and reduced susceptibility to dental caries in the corresponding population. It was quickly recognized that an adjustment of the fluoride level of fluoride-deficient water supplies could provide excellent caries protection while minimizing the risk of fluoride mottling (enamel fluorosis). This practice has been the subject of some of the best controlled epidemiologic studies in medicine. Caries reductions of 50 to 60% are well documented.[7,8]

Fluoride supplementation for children residing in nonfluoridated areas is potentially as beneficial as consuming optimally fluoridated water; but the caries reduction figures usually are somewhat less than the 50 to 60% reported. The aim of fluoride supplementation is to approximate the daily fluoride intake that would be derived from drinking optimally fluoridated water (about 1.0 mg/l). Supplementation provides exposure to the ion only once per day and probably is less effective than the multiple daily exposures from fluoridated drinking water. The effectiveness is further limited by the difficulty in motivating parents to supervise the supplementation daily from shortly after birth to age 16 years when the permanent second molars are erupted. Even with these compromises, fluoride supplementation is a relatively inexpensive and beneficial means of reducing the caries experience of patients who live in communities with nonfluoridated water supplies.

Two major factors must be considered in establishing the proper dose of supplemental fluoride: the patient's weight and the exposure to fluoride from dietary and other sources. These factors are more easily translated into age and fluoride concentration of the patient's water supply.

Dietary Fluoride

The major source of fluoride for infants is formula diluted with fluoridated water. In 1979, formula manufacturers in the United States began to reduce the fluoride level of the water used in the manufacturing process, so ready-to-feed and liquid concentrates are uniformly low in fluoride (about 0.1 mg F per kilogram in the final product). Human milk and cow's milk contain only traces of fluoride.

Recent studies[9,10] indicate that prepared infant foods and beverages contain fluoride in previously unsuspected amounts. The levels vary considerably, even for different samples of a given product from the same manufacturer. Nevertheless, these products are a potentially significant source of fluoride for infants who live in areas with nonfluoridated water supplies. Another source of fluoride for young children is fluoridated toothpaste, much of which is swallowed during toothbrushing. These previously unrecognized sources led to the reduction in recommended supplementation dosages by the Committee on Nutrition[11] in 1979.

Because these sources of fluoride are so variable, they cannot be reliably estimated for any patient. Neither can water consumption, which also can vary tremendously from one child to another. However, the fluoride concentration of a patient's water supply is accepted as the best indicator of dietary exposure to fluoride.

Age

The optimal intake of fluoride from all sources is estimated to be 0.05 mg fluoride per kilogram body weight per day. Obviously, a supplementation regime based on body weight would be the most desirable, although it also is the most complicated. Therefore, the dosage regime is geared to the patient's age for simplicity.

Dose

The dose regime (Table 17) is the same as given in 1979. The dose schedule was lowered in 1979 because of findings of enamel fluorosis in children from communities with nonfluoridated water supplies who were given supplements at the previously recommended levels. The fluorosis seen was primarily not of esthetic concern, but it did indicate that fluoride intake from other sources was increasing. The 1979 schedule balances a reduced risk of fluorosis with maximal protection against caries.

Two aspects of fluoride supplementation that have engendered considerable discussion are the requirements of breast-fed infants and the use of fluoride during the first 6 months of life. Because breast-fed infants frequently consume little or no water, it has been suggested that they should receive fluoride supplements whether or not they live in optimally fluoridated communities. Human milk, as is true with cow's milk, contains little fluoride, even in areas with fluoridated water supplies.[9] However, the frequency of caries was identical in a study comparing infants who were breast-fed to those who were fed powdered cow's milk formula diluted with naturally fluoridated

Table 17
Supplemental Fluoride Dosage Schedule
(mg/da*)

Age	Concentration of Fluoride in Drinking Water (ppm)		
	<0.3	0.3-0.7	>0.7
2 wk-2 yr	0.25	0	0†
2-3 yr	0.50	0.25	0
3-16 yr	1.00	0.50	0

*2.2 mg sodium fluoride contains 1 mg fluoride.
†0.25 mg fluoride should be given to infants at age 6 months who are still being breast-fed exclusively.

water. Other studies in naturally fluoridated communities also suggest that, after weaning, the fluoride obtained from an optimally fluoridated water supply is sufficient to decrease the prevalence of caries in permanent teeth.[8] These studies do not completely answer the contention that the prevalence of caries might be reduced further by providing fluoride to breast-fed infants during a period when their fluoride intake might otherwise be particularly low and when mineralization of unerupted teeth is taking place. This issue is not of paramount importance when breast feeding is only maintained for a few months; however, with more than 6 months of exclusive breast feeding, fluoride administration seems advisable.

For formula-fed infants, some physicians have suggested that fluoride supplementation should not start until the infant is 6 months old because variations in feeding regimens complicate the selection of an appropriate dosage.[12,13] However, some clinicians argued that supplementation should start shortly after birth because the period of mineralization of unerupted deciduous teeth includes early infancy. In weighing these opposing views, the Committee on Nutrition favors initiating fluoride supplementation shortly after birth in breast-fed infants (0.25 mg fluoride per day) and according to the fluoride content of the drinking water in formula-fed infants. This regimen should have a beneficial effect during a period of active mineralization of bone and teeth, and starting a regimen in early infancy might facilitate long-term compliance. In addition, the Committee on Nutrition recognizes the basis for the view that satisfactory reduction in the prevalence of caries can be accomplished by initiating fluoride supplementation as late as 6 months of age.

Fluoride-vitamin Combinations

When an indication exists for vitamin supplementation, fluoride-vitamin preparations are more convenient and economical than separate preparations. The use of these combinations also may enhance compliance. There is no evidence that the fluoride in these combinations is less available or less effective than fluoride given separately. The wider range of dose combinations currently being manufactured makes it relatively easy to provide the appropriate dose of all components.

Prescriptions

Prescriptions for supplemental fluoride should be specific about when and how the supplement is to be delivered. Fluoride given on an empty stomach is 100% bioavailable.[13] Fluoride administered with milk or a calcium-rich meal will be incompletely absorbed. The best time for the parent to administer the supplement is at bedtime, after the teeth have been cleaned and no more food or drink is given. For infants, the supplement should be given between feedings.

The maximum amount of fluoride to be prescribed at any one time is 120 mg (254 mg sodium fluoride). This amount, if ingested by a small child, would not produce acute toxicity. For accidental ingestions of larger amounts, vomiting should be induced and milk given to bind any fluoride remaining in the stomach.

Providing the proper dose is only the first step in effective supplementation. Counseling the parents in the rationale and benefits of fluoride supplementation also is important. Properly motivated, the parents will be able to reduce significantly the potential effects of a prevalent disease.

References

1. Sweeney, E.A., Cabrera, J., Urrutia, J., and Mata, L.: Factors associated with linear hypoplasia of human deciduous incisors. J. Dent. Res., **48**:1275, 1969.
2. Glick, P.L.: Mineralization of the teeth: Prenatal and postnatal nutrient requirements. In Wei, S.H.Y., ed.: Pediatric Dental Care. New York: Medcom, Inc., pp. 13-17, 1978.
3. Tonge, C.H., and McCance, R.A.: Normal development of the jaws and teeth in pigs and the delay and malocclusion produced by calories deficiencies. J. Anat., **115**:1, 1973.
4. Alfano, M.C., Miller, S.A., and Drummond, J.F.: Effect of ascorbic acid deficiency on the permeability and collagen biosynthesis of oral mucosal epithelium. Ann. N.Y. Acad. Sci., **258**:253, 1975.
5. Corruccini, R.S., and Beecher, R.M.: Occlusal variation related to soft diet in a nonhuman primate. Science, **218**:74, 1982.
6. Gustafsson, B.E., Quensel, C.E., Lanke, L.S., Lundqvist, C., Grahnen, H., Bonow, B.E., and Krasse, B.: The Vipeholm dental caries study: The effect of different carbohydrate intake on caries

activity in 436 individuals observed for five years. Acta Odontol. Scand., **11**:232, 1954.

7. Arnold, F.A., Jr., Dean, H.T., Jay, P., and Knutson, J.W.: Effect of fluoridated public water supplies on dental caries prevalence. Tenth year of the Grand Rapids-Muskegon study. Pub. Health Rep., **71**:652 and 1136, 1956.

8. Ast, D.B., Smith, D.J., Wachs, B., and Cantwell, K.T.: Newburgh-Kingston caries-fluorine study, XIV. Combined clinical and roentgenographic dental findings after ten years of fluoride experience. J. Amer. Dent. Assn., **52**:314, 1956.

9. Singer, L., and Ophaug, R.: Total fluoride intake of infants. PEDIATRICS, **63**:460, 1979.

10. Adair, S.M., and Wei, S.H.Y.: Fluoride content of commercially prepared strained fruit juices. Pediat. Dent., **1**:174, 1979.

11. Committee on Nutrition: Fluoride supplementation: Revised dosage schedule. PEDIATRICS, **63**:150, 1979.

12. Ericsson, Y., and Ribelius, U.: Wide variations of fluoride supply to infants and their effect. Caries Res., **5**:78, 1971.

13. Ekstrand, J., Alvan, G., Boreus, L.O., and Norlin, A.: Pharmacokinetics of fluoride in man after single and multiple oral doses. Eur. J. Clin. Pharmacol., **12**:311, 1977.

Chapter 18

COMMUNITY NUTRITION SERVICES FOR CHILDREN

Promoting the nutritional health of children is a common goal of the nutrition services offered by a wide variety of public and private agencies, organizations, and individuals in communities across the nation. These include state health departments; local health agencies such as city and county health departments, community health centers, health maintenance organizations, and outpatient clinics at hospitals; voluntary health agencies such as the diabetes and heart associations; social service agencies; elementary and secondary schools, colleges, and universities; nutritionists and dietitians in private practice; and business and industry.

This chapter summarizes some of the community nutrition services to assist physicians and other health care workers in understanding the scope and benefits of such programs and how to use them effectively.

Nutrition Services Provided Through Federal, State, and Local Health Agencies

Each year Congress appropriates funds for a variety of health programs, many of which are targeted to mothers and children. Such programs, administered at the national level by the Department of Health and Human Services (DHHS), include the Maternal and Child Health Services Block Grant Programs; the Preventive Health Services Block Grant Programs; the Early, Periodic Screening, Diagnostic and Treatment Program under Medicaid; Indian Health Services; and programs such as the community health centers and migrant health projects which serve underserved and disadvantaged populations. In addition to federal support, considerable state and local funds also support child health programs.

Although nutrition services were introduced into public health programs as early as the late 1920's, Title V of the Social Security Act of 1935 initiated the federal/state partnership for maternal and child health that served as the major impetus for the development of nutrition services for mothers and children.[1] Today more than 2,000 public health nutritionists are employed in federal, state, and local public health agencies; they serve as members of health care teams and have the responsibility of assessing community nutrition needs as well as planning and directing the nutrition services.

Nutrition Services—A Component of Health Care

Efforts are made to provide a basic core of nutrition services for children in community health programs. These include:

1. assessment of the child's nutritional status and needs;
2. nutrition counseling to help patients and their families understand and implement nutrition recommendations, including prescribed diets for specific conditions;
3. nutrition education for patients and their families, physicians and nurses, and the community at large;
4. treatment of nutrition-related conditions; and
5. follow-up and referral, as necessary, to provide assistance in obtaining adequate food, prescribed dietary supplements, special feeding equipment, and other services required to maintain or improve nutritional status.

Health Agencies—A Nutrition Resource

Federal, state, and local health agencies—particularly those employing public health nutritionists—can be helpful resources for physicians for such nutrition services as:

1. technical consultation and practical information in nutrition, including information on community resources;
2. direct nutrition care;
3. nutrition education;
4. provision of special dietary products; and
5. continuing education and training in nutrition.

Up-to-date information about the science of nutrition and its practical application in patient care is available from public health nutritionists in health agencies. A basic core of nutrition services is provided for children as a component of health care in maternity clinics, child health care clinics, crippled children's services, primary care, and specialized projects such as adolescent clinics, intensive newborn infant care programs, mental retardation programs, and so forth.

In addition, many state and local health agencies are extending direct nutrition care services, particularly nutrition counseling, on a fee-for-service basis to physicians in the community. Hospital-based dietitians frequently refer patients who require continuing nutrition follow-up to state or local health department nutritionists. Individuals and families with complex nutrition problems related to inborn errors of metabolism, chronic illness, and handicapping conditions, as well as the physicians caring for them, frequently find these nutrition services helpful. Many health agencies offer classes on specific aspects of nutrition. These classes usually are open to clinic patients as well as others referred by physicians in the community. Agencies sponsor radio and television programs on nutrition topics as well as a wide range of publications for the lay public (which may be available in quantity for physicians to use for health education). Many of these publications are available in foreign languages.

To help physicians and nurses keep abreast of scientific advances in nutrition, food technology, and related areas, federal, state, and local health agencies frequently sponsor nutrition seminars and workshops—usually in cooperation with professional organizations and education institutions.

Through state maternal and child health programs, crippled children's services, or the Special Supplemental Food Programs for Women, Infants, and Children (WIC), provision is made for special foods required for the treatment of inborn errors of metabolism. These foods usually are expensive and may need to be continued for a number of years. Physicians should contact the maternal and child health program of their state health department for information about patient eligibility for these foods and procedures for obtaining them.

Other Community Nutrition Resources

In addition to federal, state, and local health agencies, voluntary agencies such as visiting nurse associations, diabetes and heart associations, health maintenance organizations, and hospital outpatient departments frequently employ nutrition personnel. They usually provide technical consultation in nutrition to physicians and nurses and nutrition counseling to patients and other agencies in the community. An increasing number of dietitians also have established independent practices as registered dietitians.

Food Assistance Programs

National policy has long provided for publicly supported food assistance programs to safeguard the health of individuals whose nutrition status is compromised because of poverty or complex physiological, social, or other type of stress, i.e., school children, refugees and migrants, pregnant women, and infants. The National School Lunch Act of 1946 provided for a major federal role in food service for school children. There currently are two major types of food assistance programs operated nationally by the U.S. Department of Agriculture (USDA): the Family Nutrition Program (Food Stamp) and the Special Nutrition Programs which include the Child Nutrition Programs and the Supplemental Food Programs. Table 18 lists the present expenditures of the various programs.

Family Nutrition Program—Food Stamp Program

The Food Stamp Program differs from the Special Nutrition Programs in that it applies to the family unit rather than the individual, and all age groups are included.

Authorized as a permanent program in 1964, the Food Stamp Program is the largest of all food assistance programs. The 1982 Amendments to the Food Stamp Act extended the program through 1985. The program provides monthly benefits to low-income households to help purchase an adequate diet. Nearly 50% of the recipients are children less than 18 years old. Criteria for participation include requirements such as the following: able-bodied applicants must meet certain work requirements; all households may have up to $1,500 worth of countable resources; households of two or more individuals may have up to $3,000 if one member is 60 years old or older; and only households with gross monthly incomes at or

below 130% of the poverty line and net income after deductions
of 100% of the poverty line may qualify for food stamps, unless
the household contains elderly or disabled members. Income
limits vary by household size, are based on federally established poverty lines, and are adjusted each July to reflect
changes in the cost of living. Food stamp allotments as of Oc-
tober 1983 were $139 per month for a family of two and $253
for a family of four. Stamps can be used to buy food at authorized stores. They cannot be used to buy alcohol, tobacco, or
nonfood items such as soap or paper supplies.

Child Nutrition Programs

The child Nutrition Programs include the School Nutrition
Programs, Child Care Food Program, and the Summer Food
Service Program. These programs help support food services
for children in public and nonprofit private schools as well as
group care programs for children such as residential institutions and center- or home-based day care programs.

Table 18
Food Assistance Programs

Program	Average Monthly Participation (est.)	Program Expenditures Fiscal Year 1982 (est.)
Food Stamp Program*	22 million	$10.8 billion
School Lunch Program	23 million	$3 billion
School Breakfast Program	3.4 million	$321 million
Special Milk Program	—	$21 million
Child Care Food Program	833,000	$318 million
Summer Food Assistance Program	1 million	$93 million
Commodity Supplemental Food Program	126,000	$26 million
Special Supplemental Food Program for Women, Infants, and Children (WIC)	2.2 million	$954 million
Total		$15.5 billion

*Does not include Puerto Rico from July 1 to September 30, 1982.

School Nutrition Programs

The National School Lunch, School Breakfast, and Special Milk Programs in most states are administered by the state education agency, which enters into agreements with officials of local schools or school districts to operate nonprofit food services. About 90% of all schools in the United States are participating in the National School Lunch Program. Participating schools receive cash assistance to help purchase food and pay labor costs as well as direct donations of agricultural food commodities. Any public or nonprofit private school of high school grade or under is eligible. Public and licensed nonprofit, private residential child care institutions such as orphanages, homes for retarded children, juvenile detention centers, and temporary shelters for runaway children also are eligible.

To assure that the nutrition goals of the program are met, minimum meal pattern requirements are specified, and these are periodically updated by the USDA. The lunch is designed to provide about one third of the Recommended Dietary Allowances for age. Recent regulatory changes have provided for more flexibility in the quantities and types of foods offered in the meal pattern, e.g., skimmed milk, unflavored low fat milk, flavored whole milk, or buttermilk can be offered as a choice for those who do not wish regular whole milk.

Participating schools must agree to serve meals at a reduced price or free to children who are unable to pay the locally established full price. Children who can pay full price are expected to do so. Local school officials determine the individual eligibility of each child for reduced-price or free meals on the basis of family size and income. Each year the Secretary of Agriculture issues uniform national standards for free and reduced-price eligibility based on national poverty guidelines. Although federal subsidies continue to be provided for meals served to children from all income levels, recent legislation has shifted emphasis to directing more of the program benefits to needy children.

The Special Milk Program reduces the cost of each half-pint of milk served to children by providing for cash reimbursement at an annually adjusted rate. A school district can choose to provide milk free to children who meet the eligibility guidelines. This program is available only to schools that do not participate in the National School Lunch, School Breakfast, or Commodity Programs.

Child Care Food Program

The Child Care Food Program provides cash reimbursement and/or commodities for the provision of meals and snacks to institutions providing nonresidential child care for children. Institutions eligible to participate include child care centers, settlement houses, neighborhood and Head Start centers, and institutions providing day care for the handicapped and their families, or group day care homes. Proprietary day care centers can participate only when at least 25% of their enrolled children are receiving benefits through Title XX, the Social Services Program.

Subsidies are provided for two meals and one snack per day for children less than 12 years old. Meals must meet USDA specified requirements. Family or group day care homes are paid a fixed reimbursement, depending on the type of meals served. Day care centers are reimbursed for meals at rates depending on the type of meal and eligibility of children for free, reduced-price, or paid meals.

Summer Food Assistance Program

The Summer Food Assistance Program provides nutritious meals for preschool and school-aged children in recreation centers or summer camps, during vacations in areas operating under a continuous school calendar, or in areas with poor economic conditions. Meals are served free and must meet minimum standards established by the USDA. Sponsors of the program must be either public or private-nonprofit school food authorities; state, local municipal, or county governments; or public, private-nonprofit residential summer camps.

Supplemental Food Programs

Special Supplemental Food Programs for Women, Infants, and Children

Since its initiation in 1972, the WIC program has grown from $20 million to more than $1 billion yearly in authorized funds.

The WIC program differs from all other federal food assistance programs in its close association with health care services. These services are defined as ongoing, routine pediatric and obstetric care (such as infant and child care and prenatal and postpartum examinations or referral for treatment). Designed to provide specified food and nutrition education to low-income pregnant and postpartum women, lactating mothers, infants, and children up to 5 years old who are determined to be at nutritional risk, the program must be operated as an adjunct to good health care. Health care is usually provided by state and local public and private, nonprofit health or human service agencies as well as the private sector.

The USDA provides annual grants to state health departments or comparable agencies and to Indian groups. Program funds are allocated to state agencies on the basis of a formula which considers food costs and administrative costs. Eighty percent of the funds must be used for food; about 20% is available for administrative costs. The latter costs include start-up and outreach, developing and printing food vouchers, auditing, nutrition education, certification, and monitoring. None of the funds can be used for health care services other than certifying for eligibility for the program. Eligibility for the program is determined by health professionals on the basis of nutrition risk criteria. Also, persons must meet income guidelines established by the state agency, which cannot exceed the income criteria established for reduced-price meals under the National School Lunch Program, namely, 185% of the income poverty guidelines, nor be less than 100% of the poverty guidelines. Approximately 75% of the current participants are children from birth to 5 years old.

Participants are provided monthly food packages, primarily through the use of a food voucher which can be redeemed at certain retail stores for specified items. In some instances, participants receive food through a home delivery or warehouse distribution system. Foods provided include infant formula, cereal, and juice for infants, and milk, cheese, eggs, juice, cereal, and beans or peanut butter for children and pregnant or lactating women. Nonlactating, postpartum women receive a similar package, except that some quantities are reduced and legumes are not provided. The average monthly cost per participant in fiscal year 1982 was approximately $29.00 for the food package and $7.00 for administrative costs, or a total of about $36.00.

Nutrition education is considered a benefit of the program to be provided at no cost to the participants. Efforts are made to adapt the education activities to the individual participant's nutritional needs, cultural preferences, and education levels.

Commodity Supplemental Food Program

The Commodity Supplemental Food Program (CSFP) is being continued, at local option, in several states. Providing commodity supplemental foods and nutrition education to low-income pregnant, lactating, and postpartum women and to infants and children to age 6 years, the CSFP is designed to supplement participants' diets. Although it has many of the characteristics of the WIC program, there are some differences. These include differences in the variety of foods provided (i.e., canned meat or poultry and canned vegetables) plus the types of foods provided in WIC; distribution of actual foods rather than vouchers for redemption at the grocery store; and more flexible ties to health care (i.e., health care is encouraged but not mandated, except if it was in existence prior to 1978). Simultaneous participation in WIC and CSFP is prohibited. The supplemental foods are distributed to state agencies or Indian tribes, groups responsible for administering the program. Each state selects local, private, nonprofit agencies to administer the program at the local level. The local agencies determine eligibility of applicants, distribute the supplemental foods, and provide nutrition education. Federal funds provide for some of the administrative costs such as outreach, warehousing of food, and transportation to obtain food if necessary.

Where To Seek Food Assistance for Patients

Food assistance programs are usually administered at the local level by several agencies:

1. local school authority—School Lunch Program, School Breakfast Program, Summer Food Service Program, Special Milk Program, and the Child Care Food Program;

2. state and local, public or private, nonprofit health agency and Indian tribes or groups recognized by the U.S. Department of the Interior—Supplemental Food Program for Women, Infants, and Children;

3. local social services or welfare department—Food Stamp Program.

Summary

As the key provider of child health care, the physician has a major role in assuring that nutrition services for children include assessment of their nutritional status, provision of a safe food supply adequate in quality and quantity, nutrition counseling, and nutrition education for children and parents. As the primary expert on health in the community and a concerned citizen, the physician can provide significant leadership in the formulation of sound nutrition policy and training of legislators, administrators, and others who influence the community's response to the nutritional needs of its children.

Reference

1. Egan, M.C.: Public health nutrition services: Issues today and tomorrow. J. Amer. Diet. Assn., **77**:423, 1980.

Chapter 19

CURRENT LEGISLATION AND REGULATIONS REGARDING INFANT FORMULAS

The manufacture of commercial infant formulas is regulated by the Food and Drug Administration according to specifications in the Code of Federal Regulations; they also are voluntarily monitored by guidelines developed and adopted by manufacturers.[1] The scope and authority of federal regulation of commercial infant formula manufacture were broadened with passage of the Infant Formula Act of 1980, PL 96-359, which became law on September 26, 1980.[2] When fully implemented, the provisions of this law will strengthen the Food and Drug Administration's regulations concerning composition and quality assurance of commercial infant formulas. Parts of the Infant Formula Act will be described.

Nutrient composition of commercial infant formula is based largely on recommendations of the Committee on Nutrition of the American Academy of Pediatrics. The composition is specified, with provision that the Secretary of the Department of Health and Human Services (DHHS) may (1) revise the list of nutrients, (2) revise the required levels for any nutrients, (3) establish requirements for quality factors for nutrients, and (4) establish quality control procedures to assure that a commercial infant formula provides the specified nutrients and to establish requirements for retaining records. Some formulas designed and labeled for use by preterm infants or those with inborn errors of metabolism or other unusual medical or dietary problems currently are exempt from these requirements.

The Infant Formula Act specifies that each manufacturer verify all currently produced formulas and that new or reformulated products for normal infants meet the prescribed standards for nutrient composition, quality of components, and processing methods. Records authenticating the quality of formulas must be maintained for 1 year longer than their shelf life. A manufacturer must promptly notify the Secretary of DHHS of noncompliance or risk to human health if there is reasonable knowledge that a formula does not provide the required nutrients or is otherwise adulterated or misbranded.[2] The Secretary of DHHS will determine the scope of recalls appropriate for the degree of risk to human health. Regulations to implement recalls will be proposed by the Food and Drug Administration. After review of existing requirements of labeling of infant foods, the Secretary of DHHS may recommend legislative or administrative action regarding labeling of infant formulas.[2]

In addition to the provisions of the Infant Formula Act, manufacturers must continue to comply with current and proposed regulations for quality control procedures, labeling of infant formulas, good manufacturing practice, and, in the case of fluid formulas, regulations governing the production of thermally processed, low-acid foods packaged in hermetically sealed containers. The Code of Federal Regulations specifies requirements for personnel, buildings and facilities, equipment, production and process controls, and record maintenance. Inspection of raw materials and ingredients to ensure suitability for incorporation into human food is also specified in this code.

Guidelines for assurance of the safety of food in the Code of Federal Regulations include specifications on control of microbial contamination. Similarly, the Codex Alimentarius Commission and the United Nations Protein Advisory Group[3] have recommended microbiologic and sanitary standards for the production and use of powdered and liquid commercial infant formulas.

Strict adherence to guidelines for microbiologic safety is standard practice for the infant formula industry. Infant gastrointestinal disorders caused by enteric bacterial or viral pathogens from commercial infant formulas are extremely infrequent. Proper feeding techniques should be stressed to hospital nursery personnel and new mothers by pediatricians and paramedical personnel. The most important measures for control of microbial growth continue to be effective cleansing of bottles and nipples and storage in a cool place.

Open dating of powdered, concentrated, and ready-to-feed infant formula containers is a standard practice of manufacturers belonging to the Infant Formula Council. The dating is prominently displayed or stamped on the container and normally indicates an expiration or "use before" date.

References

1. Infant Formula Council: Memorandum of a meeting with the Food and Drug Administration, December 4, attachment 3. (Docket No.

80N-0025.) Rockville, Maryland: Food and Drug Administration Hearing Clerk, 1979.
2. United States Congress: Infant Formula Act of 1980. Washington, D.C.: United States Capitol Health Documents Room. Public Law 96-359, September 26, 1980.
3. United Nations Protein Advisory Group: Guideline for the sanitary production and use of dry protein foods. (PAG guideline No. 11.) New York: United Nations, 1972.

Nutrition in Disease

Chapter 20

ASSESSMENT OF NUTRITIONAL STATUS

The assessment of nutritional status involves the application of clinical appraisal, anthropometry, and easily available clinical laboratory tests supplemented as indicated with more specific tests for deficiencies of specific nutrients.

The Use of Growth Charts

Growth is a predictable attribute of healthy children. The growth charts used in this handbook were prepared by the National Center for Health Statistics (NCHS). (See Appendix A, which includes growth charts for preterm infants.) Ideally, the data on which growth charts should be based are longitudinal observations on a well defined, healthy population. However, few such data are available for children in the United States, and the data which are available were collected nearly a generation ago.[1]

The NCHS growth charts were derived from longitudinal studies of a selected population less than 3 years old and from cross-sectional data on large numbers of infants and children who participated in national surveys. The data were then smoothed by computer techniques and presented as percentiles. Recumbent length is given on the 0 to 3 years old chart, and standing height is given on the 2 to 18 years old chart. Be aware that a growth chart is only a measuring device which should be used to separate normal from abnormal growth patterns.

The conclusions from data plotted on a growth chart are only as good as the accuracy of the measurements and the precision with which the subject's age is known. Figure 10 shows a suitable board for measuring recumbent length. Note that the back of the patient should be straight, the knees straight, and the gaze directly upward. Experienced personnel should be able to reproduce length measurements to less than a centimeter. Figure 11 shows a simple apparatus for measuring standing height. The right angles between the measuring stick and the head board and between the head board and the wall are critical. The extension rods on most clinical scales are not reliable. A stadiometer which gives direct readings[2] reduces the clerical errors in recording the measurements. Measurement should be made to the nearest 5 mm. Scales which permit accuracy to the nearest 0.1 kg are satisfactory except for very small infants undergoing research studies. The date, height or length, weight, and head circumference should be recorded on the growth chart and the age calculated in years, months, and days for infants (years and months for children) before the points are plotted on the chart. This approach makes it possible to replot the data at a later time if the age, for instance, has been miscalculated. The head circumference measurement should be the largest occipital-frontal circumference. Several measurements should be made to determine which one is largest. A number of satisfactory cloth and plastic tapes are available. The physician who wishes to use the measurements should assume responsibility for the proper training of the staff. Growth rate is a sensitive bioassay for nutritional status and certain hormonal functions; and the more care which is taken in measurement technique, the better will be the assessment of growth velocity.

Because the growth charts are a compilation of data derived from many children, individual variations from the lower percentiles to the higher ones, and vice versa, are obscured. At present there are no clear-cut guidelines in interpreting a shift from one percentile to another. However, the infant whose weight goes from the 50th percentile to the 90th in a few

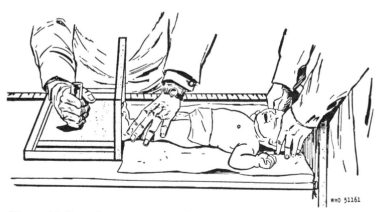

Figure 10. Length measurement of an infant. (Adapted from Jelliffe[10].)

months is in danger of becoming obese. Also, steady progress of a small infant along the 5th percentile may well be normal for that infant.

Serial measurements are always easier to interpret than single measurements. When single measurements fall above the 95th or below the 5th percentile, the statistical chance that the child is abnormal is 1 to 20. Parental height has an influence on linear growth of children, and charts using mid-parent stature have been published[3] (see Appendix B). For practical purposes, however, short parental stature is rarely the cause of length or height below the 5th percentile. Low-birth-weight infants do not fit well onto the NCHS charts during infancy, and the deviations need to be learned by the observer when the perinatal growth charts based on gestational age[4] (see Appendix C) are outgrown. Although weight gain may come in spurts, any change in linear growth should at least raise a suspicion that a growth disturbance might be present. This should lead to follow-up measurements.

The measurement of skinfold thickness* and of arm circumference (mid arm) has been used to obtain quantitative data on body fat and muscle mass.[5] Despite its seeming simplicity, the procedure for taking these measurements requires more training than those for taking height and weight.† Skinfold thickness measurements are most useful in the management of infants and children with under and over nutrition and in the follow-up of disease states associated with changes in body composition.

Workers in underdeveloped areas believe these measurements, especially midarm circumference, have an advantage over weight in that the increment in arm circumference during childhood is in relative terms much less than is the increment in weight; hence, the former is helpful in children whose birth date is not known precisely. The reason lies in the fact that subcutaneous fat thickness declines during late infancy and early childhood as muscle mass increases. Appendix D contains tables of percentile distributions for midarm cir-

*Suitable calipers are: the Harpenden caliper, H.E. Morse Company, Holland, Michigan; the Holtain-Harpenden, Holtain Ltd., Brynberian, Crymmych, Pembrokeshire, Wales; and the Lange caliper, Cambridge Scientific Industries, Inc., Cambridge, Maryland.

†The measurement is made by grasping the subcutaneous tissue between thumb and forefinger, gently shaking to exclude underlying muscle and stretching it just far enough to permit the jaws of the spring-actuated caliper to impinge on the tissue. Because the caliper jaws compress the tissue, the caliper reading diminishes for a few seconds, then the dial is read. The usual sites are the triceps region midway between shoulder and elbow, and at the tip of the scapula.

cumference, arm muscle circumference, arm muscle area (really muscle + bone area), arm fat area, and a nomogram for

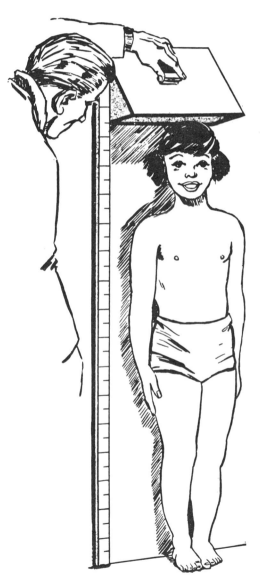

Figure 11. Height measurement of a child more than 2 years old. (Adapted from Jelliffe[10].)

calculating muscle circumference and area from measurements of arm circumference and triceps skinfold.

Although some have suggested that the ratio of arm circumference to head circumference‡ could be of additional help in assessing malnutrition, a recent trial found no advantage over weight for age.[6]

Assessment by History

In addition to the medical history, information about the eating habits and food intake of an infant or child is helpful in determining the nutritional status. Although it may require the skills of a dietitian to elicit information which can be translated into precise calories and specific amounts of nutrients, the physician should learn to evaluate the caloric intake and determine whether or not the child is eating a relatively balanced diet. It is important to ask about what the child drinks as well as what he or she eats; milk is an excellent source of nutrients.

Laboratory Assessment

The initial laboratory assessments of nutritional status are a measure of hematologic status and a measure of protein nutrition. This can be as simple as the determination of the microhematocrit and the total serum protein concentration using a refractometer from the plasma portion of the hematocrit tube. If venous blood is obtained, the hematology profile and an automated battery of biochemical tests give similar information and more detail in both areas. Normal values will be found in Appendix V. The absence of anemia usually will exclude nutritional anemias such as iron deficiency and folate and vitamin B_{12} deficiency. Red cell size is valuable in the differential diagnosis of anemias (see Chapter 23). The total serum protein determination is interpretable only if the globulins can be assumed to be normal. Albumin is a better measure of protein nutrition because it has a shorter biologic half-life than the globulins. Low albumin concentrations will occur when albu-

‡Ratio >0.31 indicates health, 0.31 to 0.25 indicates mild to moderate malnutrition, <0.25 indicates severe malnutrition.

min is lost from the body in large amounts as in nephrosis, exudative enteropathies, and from burned tissue. The so-called "visceral" proteins synthesized in the liver which have even shorter half-lives than albumin (such as retinol binding protein, prealbumin, and transferrin) are gaining acceptance as measurements of protein status in the nutritional assessment of adults.

Increasing evidence that immunologic abnormalities such as loss of delayed hypersensitivity, reduction in T lymphocyte numbers, and changes in lymphocyte response to *in vitro* stimulation by phytohemagglutinins are valid clinical measurements of nutritional status has been presented.[7] Their use in infants and children has not yet been extensive.

Tests for specific deficiencies such as iron deficiency and rickets are becoming more sophisticated using complex and often relatively unavailable tests for such substances as ferritin and vitamin D metabolites. Textbooks on nutrition should be consulted because a detailed discussion is beyond the scope of this handbook.

Clinical Assessment

Careful inspection of the patient remains a valid method of nutritional assessment. A recent test in adult surgical patients showed that a careful history and physical examination "is a reproducible and valid technique for evaluating nutritional status . . . ."[8] Obesity and wasting are obvious, although they need to be confirmed by the growth chart. Observation is a useful screening test for gross changes in body composition. Edema and dehydration, excess or inadequate subcutaneous fat, and increase or decrease of the muscle mass can be detected. The skin changes of zinc or essential fatty acid deficiencies can be recognized. The tongue and lips frequently reflect changes in the rest of the gastrointestinal mucosa. Rickets has reappeared, and craniotabes and beading of the ribs are helpful signs. The clinical signs and symptoms of specific vitamin or mineral deficiencies are not pathognomonic, nor are those of nutrient excess.[9] Exceptions are the changes in growth velocity which are the result of energy excess or deficiency, the skeletal abnormalities of rickets, the xerophthalmia of vitamin A deficiency, and the "bayonet" deformity of the costochondral junctions in scurvy. Appropriate laboratory tests as well as roentgenographic examinations can be helpful in diagnosis.

Unfortunately, many hospital laboratories lack facilities for determining vitamin levels in blood or urine; however, serum alkaline phosphatase and phosphorus (which are readily available) are sensitive indicators of rickets. It should be remembered that almost all nutrient deficiencies result in growth failure.

The value of a therapeutic trial should not be forgotten: the symptoms of scurvy and thiamin, niacin, pyridoxine, and vitamin K deficiencies respond rather quickly to specific therapy, as does the anemia caused by iron, folate, or vitamin B_{12} deficiency.

References

1. Van Wieringen, J.C.: Secular growth changes: 1. *In* Falkner, F., and Tanner, J.M., ed.: Human Growth: 2. Postnatal Growth. New York: Plenum Press, pp. 445-473, 1978.
2. Tanner, J.M., and Whitehouse, R.H.: Clinical longitudinal standards for height, weight, height velocity, weight velocity, and stages of puberty. Arch. Dis. Child., **51**:170, 1976.
3. Garn, S.M., and Rohmann, C.G.: Interaction of nutrition and genetics in the timing of growth and development. Pediat. Clin. N. Amer., **13**:353, 1966.
4. Lubchenko, L.O., Hansman, C., and Boyd, E.: Intrauterine growth in length and head circumference as estimated from live births at gestational ages from 26 to 42 weeks. PEDIATRICS, **37**:403, 1966.
5. Frisancho, A.R.: Triceps skin fold and upper arm muscle size norms for assessment of nutritional status. Amer. J. Clin. Nutr., **27**:1052, 1974.
6. Sen, V., and Sharma, R.: Midarm/head circumference ratio in the assessment of protein-energy malnutrition. Indian J. Pediat., **47**:213, 1980.
7. Chandra, R.K.: Immunocompetence as a functional index of nutritional status. Brit. Med. Bull., **37**:89, 1981.
8. Baker. J.P., Detsky, A.S., Wesson, D.E., Wolman, S.L., Stewart, S., Whitehall, J., Langer, B., and Jeejeebhoy, K.N.: Nutritional assessment: A comparison of clinical judgment and objective measurements. New Engl. J. Med., **306**:969, 1982.
9. Solomons, N.W., and Allen, L.H.: The functional assessment of nutritional status: Principles, practice and potential. Nutr. Rev., **41**:33, 1983.
10. Jelliffe, D.B.: The Assessment of the Nutritional Status of the Community (Monograph Series No. 53). Geneva: World Health Organization, 1966.

Chapter 21

PROTEIN-CALORIE MALNUTRITION

Protein-calorie malnutrition has become a commonly accepted term to describe the changes seen when the food supply is deficient in calories and/or protein, when nutrients are not ingested in adequate amounts, or when diseases involving digestion, absorption, or appetite interfere with the assimilation of food. The spectrum of protein-calorie malnutrition will be discussed here with emphasis on environmental causes such as inadequate food sources, altered behavior patterns, and several disease states which appear to produce the same end result.

Infant Malnutrition

Millions of infants and children throughout the world suffer and die each year for lack of adequate nourishment. The highest incidence of this morbidity and mortality is in the technically underdeveloped countries where social, economic, sanitary, and educational factors are important contributors.[1] The decrease in breast feeding in the absence of a cheap, acceptable, and sanitary substitute is perhaps the most important single factor. Intercurrent infections, particularly of the gastrointestinal tract, are a major contributor to morbidity and mortality.

The clinical syndromes range from moderate growth failure (a common occurrence in underdeveloped countries) to more severe conditions such as marasmus and kwashiorkor. The former results from an inadequate intake of a suitable diet; the latter results from a diet with a low protein:energy ratio, frequently with protein of poor biologic quality. Intermediate forms known as marasmic-kwashiorkor also are seen. Growth retardation, weight loss, psychic changes, muscular atrophy, pellagroid dermatitis, hair changes, edema, hypoproteinemia, fatty liver, gastrointestinal changes, and a host of other more subtle abnormalities are present in various combinations. The duration of the malnutrition and its degree of severity influence the pattern of changes and the association of water-soluble and fat-soluble vitamin and mineral deficiencies in each infant.[2,3] Treatment consists of feeding adequate amounts of both calories and protein in a form accepted and tolerated by the infant and measures to combat intercurrent infection. Although the mortality rate is high, the response of the infants and young children who do recover is gratifyingly rapid. Nitrogen is retained with great efficiency, and "catch-up" growth readily occurs. The ratio of protein to calories in the diet need be no different from that in normal diets; 10 to 15% of calories should come from protein. Prevention of infant malnutrition is one of the largest challenges faced by child health workers in the world. Diarrhea, which frequently accompanies severe malnutrition, is discussed in Chapter 22, and the interaction between nutrition and infection is discussed in Chapter 30.

Failure To Thrive

Failure to thrive secondary to so-called environmental deprivation is a broad term used to describe a distortion of physical, social, emotional, or other aspects of somatic and psychic growth in poorly mothered children. The term implies more than simply failure to grow.[4] Infants and children with this condition have values for height and weight below the 5th percentile on the NCHS Growth Charts (see Appendix A). Their families are characterized by marital strife and financial instability. Public welfare assistance is common, as is overcrowded and substandard housing. These social factors, emotional instability, and inadequate mothering result in a harsh, nonnurturing environment. The children frequently are temperamental and difficult to care for. They are either intensely irritable or immobile and unresponsive. Their behavior affects that of their caretakers.

Two current hypotheses have been proposed to explain the changes in weight and length. Some clinicians[5] have presented evidence that undereating is the main etiologic factor; this theory is supported by the prompt gain in weight which frequently follows the removal of the child from the home. However, a neuroendocrine derangement secondary to emotional deprivation has been another hypothesis. No study has attempted to establish the relative roles played by the two factors. The developmental and multidisciplinary nature of the problem makes it a difficult research endeavor.

The child suspected of failure to thrive should be hospitalized for observation in a controlled environment. Usually no organic disease is present. However, this cannot be taken for granted, and appropriate studies should be performed. In some instances[4] the syndrome is superimposed on another disease process. Because of the secondary malnutrition, studies of intestinal absorption should be delayed until after 10 to 14 days of feeding, when many of the gastrointestinal symptoms will have disappeared. There is a fine line between failure to thrive and child abuse.

Treatment of the infant or child with failure to thrive usually is a slow process. Adequate nourishment and a loving and supportive environment are necessary.

Inflammatory Bowel Disease

Because diet therapy has only a minor role in the treatment of inflammatory bowel disease, patients should not be crippled further with stringent diets unless some condition such as lactase deficiency is present, as it is in about 20% of the population from which these patients come. Nevertheless, growth failure occurs in about 25% of patients.[6] Studies on energy balance in growth failure show that the energy needs for recovery are equal to the energy needs for maintenance, plus those for growth, plus the deficit which has accumulated. The sum of these factors may be about 40% above the usual intake of the patients. There are a limited number of means by which these energy deficits occur. The most common one is a poor appetite with an inadequate intake. There are excessive losses of blood cells, proteins, calcium, zinc, and magnesium. Malabsorption occurs in about one third of the patients, leading to steatorrhea and malabsorption of folic acid and iron. It has been more difficult to document increased requirements, except in the presence of fever.

Cessation of linear growth, lack of weight gain, retarded bone maturation, and delayed sexual maturation are common. No clear endocrine mechanism has been found to explain the growth failure. In a recent study,[6] the most common finding was a lack of adequate caloric intake with only occasional evidence of severe malabsorption or excessive losses. The response to adequate caloric intake by the parenteral route, when administered over a month's time, gave a growth response in some of the patients. To be effective in linear growth, parenteral nutrition must be instituted before puberty. However, bowel rest in combination with adequate nutrition, whether enteral or parenteral, is not a panacea for severe bleeding, intestinal obstruction, and other surgical complications except as a preparation for surgery, in which case postoperative healing is improved. The problems of understanding the growth retardation seen in inflammatory bowel disease were reviewed in a recent publication.[7]

Cystic Fibrosis

Another disease in which growth failure is common is cystic fibrosis. The growth failure has been more closely related to the degree of pulmonary disease than to the malabsorption,[8] and the malabsorption cannot be totally corrected by pancreatic replacement therapy. The fact that calories are the most important nutrient is emphasized in two recent publications in which increased caloric intake was associated with at least a temporary improvement in nutritional and pulmonary status.[9,10] The provision of an adequate, balanced diet is as important in the management of this disease as the use of pancreatic enzymes and antibiotics.

Anorexia Nervosa

Anorexia nervosa, a widely studied and all too frequently occurring psychosomatic disorder, comes to the attention of the physician when the degree of emaciation appears to threaten the life of the patient. The body tolerates malnutrition in different ways, depending on (1) the patient's weight and state of health at the onset of the illness, (2) the speed of the weight loss, (3) the use of cathartics, and (4) the amount of vomiting. The changes in a patient with anorexia nervosa have much in common with the experimental findings in human starvation. Keys and co-workers in 1950[11] found the following changes when the weight loss exceeded 25%: (1) social isolation, (2) decreased verbalization of feelings, (3) a depressed effect, (4) food preoccupation, (5) increased compliance, (6) apathy, and

(7) unusual eating behavior when refed. These changes can be attributed to the state of starvation and occur in individuals without manifest psychologic disorders.

Evaluation of patients with anorexia nervosa from a purely medical viewpoint begins with an estimate of the rate of weight loss because chronic starvation is better tolerated than acute starvation. Physical examination shows many changes which can be attributed to starvation. Most common are skin changes resembling poor hygiene, which is rarely a problem. There may be much lanugo. Hypothermia frequently is present, and a temperature of 38°C may represent a high fever. Bradycardia, bradypnea, and hypotension reflect the low metabolic rate. Murmurs and electrocardiographic changes are common, despite the absence of structural heart disease. The occurrence of edema is difficult to explain because the serum albumin and renal and liver function are usually normal.[12] Physical signs of vitamin deficiency rarely are seen.

Laboratory changes frequently noted are a low vitamin A concentration and a high serum carotene. Lutenizing hormone is usually depressed. The glucose tolerance curve may show a flat response or a diabetic-like curve. There is reduced xylose excretion after an oral dose, perhaps reflecting an atrophied intestinal mucosa. The blood urea nitrogen frequently is increased. Bone marrow hypoplasia frequently is present, with low white blood cell and platelet counts; but anemia is rare. By contrast, the serum proteins are usually normal, including the immunoglobulins. The electrolyte changes are limited to hypochloremic alkalosis in the presence of vomiting; this condition is well tolerated and disappears when the vomiting ceases. Resistance to infection is reduced.

The mortality rate has been estimated as between 5 and 10%. The most important decision to be made by the physician responsible for the patient's medical management is to determine the point at which further weight loss becomes dangerous to survival and nutritional intervention becomes necessary. Intervention can take the form of feeding nutritionally complete mixtures by either enteral or parenteral routes. A weight gain of 3 to 4 kg may be followed by a decrease in social isolation and unusual food habits; however, the long-term prognosis remains guarded for many patients.

The all important role of psychiatric management of this disease is beyond the scope of this chapter. Although some patients can be managed satisfactorily by the pediatrician, many will require the collaboration of a psychiatrist.

References

1. Gómez, F., Ramos-Galván, R., Cravioto, J., and Frenk, S.: Prevention and treatment of chronic severe infantile malnutrition (kwashiorkor). Ann. N.Y. Acad. Sci., 69:969, 1958.
2. Béhar, M., Viteri, F., Bressani, R., Arroyave, G., Squibb, R.L., and Scrimshaw, N.S.: Principles of treatment and prevention of severe protein malnutrition in children (kwashiorkor). Ann. N.Y. Acad. Sci., 69:954, 1958.
3. Olson, R.E., ed.: Protein-Calorie Malnutrition. New York: Academic Press, 1975.
4. Barbero, G.J., and Shaheen, E.: Environmental failure to thrive: A clinical view. J. Pediat., 71:639, 1967.
5. Whitten, C.F., Pettit, M.G., and Fischhoff, J.: Evidence that growth failure from maternal deprivation is secondary to undereating. J.A.M.A., 209:1675, 1969.
6. Grand, R.J.: Model for the treatment of growth failure in children with inflammatory bowel disease. In Suskind, R.M., ed.: Textbook of Pediatric Nutrition. New York: Raven Press, pp. 483-492, 1981.
7. Davidson, M., ed.: Growth retardation among children and adolescents with inflamatory bowel disease. New York: National Foundation for Ileitis and Colitis (295 Madison Ave.), 1983.
8. Lapey, A., Kattwinkel, J., di Sant' Agnese, P.A., and Laster, L.: Steatorrhea and azotorrhea and their relation to growth and nutrition in adolescents and young adults with cystic fibrosis. J. Pediat., 84:328, 1975.
9. Shepherd, R., Cooksley, W.G.E., and Cooke, W.D.D.: Improved growth and clinical, nutritional, and respiratory changes in response to nutritional therapy in cystic fibrosis. J. Pediat., 97:351, 1980.
10. Parsons, H.G., Beaudry, P., Dumas, A., and Pencharz, P.B.: Energy needs and growth in children with cystic fibrosis. J. Pediat. Gastroenterol. Nutr., 2:44, 1983.
11. Keys, A., Brožek, J., Henschel, A., Mickelsen, O., and Taylor, H.L.: The biology of human starvation, Vol. 1 and 2. Minneapolis: University of Minnesota Press, 1950.
12. Silverman, J.A.: Medical consequences of starvation: The malnutrition of anorexia nervosa; caveat medicus. Neurobiology and Neurology Vol. 3. Anorexia nervosa: Recent developments in research. New York: Alan R. Liss, pp. 293-299, 1983.

Chapter 22

CHRONIC DIARRHEA AND MALABSORPTION

Chronic diarrhea is one of the most common complaints in pediatrics. It is defined as "excessive" fecal output for more than 2 weeks. The term "excessive" is usually left open to interpretation because accurate stool volume measurements are not done on outpatients; however, stool volumes greater than 20 to 50 ml/kg per day are considered excessive.

Most infants with chronic diarrhea are less than 3 years old and do not show significant malabsorption. Many of them have the irritable bowel syndrome.[1] The term "nonspecific diarrhea" has been proposed for these patients,[2] with the term "intractable diarrhea" reserved for those with malabsorption, growth retardation, or dehydration. Thus, extensive diagnostic study is not needed if the presence or absence of malabsorption can be diagnosed with a few office screening tests. After the age of 5 years, children with chronic diarrhea are more likely to have malabsorption and require more extensive evaluation.

Evaluation of the Infant and Child with Chronic Diarrhea

History

The chronologic order of signs and symptoms during the development of diarrhea may have significance, e.g., introduction of cow's milk (milk allergy), cereals and bread (celiac disease), or table sugar (sucrase deficiency; fructose intolerance); persistence after acute onset (acquired transient disaccharidase deficiency); and affected siblings (nonspecific diarrhea). It is important to find out whether the diarrhea is diet induced (e.g., afternoon and evening stools are more liquid than morning stools).

Reports suggest that two components of the dietary history frequently are not emphasized: the ratio of fat to carbohydrate calories and the volume of ingested liquids. Cohen and co-workers[3] noted that some infants had been inadvertently placed on a low-fat diet, and that the diarrhea was controlled on a diet containing 40% of the calories as fat. Greene and Ghishan[4] have reported that diarrhea can be promoted by excessive fluid intake. Fifteen of 85 children less than 2 years old without malabsorption consumed more than 60 oz of liquid each day. The most common liquids were Gatorade and Kool-Aid, but excessive amounts of fresh and canned juices also were consumed. The diarrhea resolved after restricting the volume of intake.

Physical Examination

Physical examination early in the course of diarrhea may not show abnormalities. However, with continued malabsorption the rate of weight gain is soon affected. Thus, the single most helpful test is the growth chart. A recent decline in the rate of weight gain is an important clue.

Excessive bowel gas, which may be the result of bacterial action on unabsorbed nutrients, frequently causes some abdominal distention in toddlers. Frequently, patients who have celiac disease, cystic fibrosis, or bacterial overgrowth in the small intestine pass foul-smelling flatus during a long examination.

Macroscopic Examination of the Stools

A macroscopic examination of the stool may be misleading and, except for grossly oily stools, general impressions should be confirmed by microscopic examination of the stool or by chemical tests.

Microscopic Examination of the Stools

Microscopic examination of the stool is a most useful test which can be quickly and easily performed in the physician's office. This procedure alone usually can identify patients who have significant malabsorption or invasive disease of the colon and provides a cheap and logical approach to management. Examination for fat is best done with one or two drops of water well mixed with a small amount of stool. A coverslip is applied to give a thin as well as a thick area for examination. With significant steatorrhea, large and small droplets of lipid are present throughout the thick area of stool and are obvious to a lesser degree in the thinner area. Sudan stains have been recommended; but, because of the time necessary for proper staining and the need for heat to cause absorption of the stain, this stain is not suggested for office use. For experience in identifying the appearance of abnormal amounts of fecal fat, examinations of stool from newborn infants or patients with cystic fibrosis are helpful.

A drop of methylene blue mixed thoroughly with the stool and examined through a coverslip will provide enough nuclear staining to identify the presence of polymorphonuclear leukocytes. With invasive bacterial disease or chronic inflammatory disease, there are literally "sheets of polys" to be seen throughout the smear; only a few neutrophils are seen in stools from patients with viral enteritis.

Giardia lamblia cysts can be identified with a simple wet preparation. However, more experience is generally required for accurate identification of giardia than is necessary to identify fat and neutrophils. Newer methods of concentrating the cysts make it more likely these cysts will be identified by hospital laboratories than by a simple office examination.

Examination for Carbohydrate

An examination for carbohydrate is particularly helpful in diagnosing carbohydrate malabsorption in a young infant. Most commercial infant formulas contain 30 to 50% of the calories as lactose, sucrose, or corn syrup solids. Unless bacterial action in the large bowel has converted the malabsorbed carbohydrate to organic acids and produced an acid pH of stool, these sugars can be detected easily by Clinitest (reducing sugars) or test-tape analysis (glucose only). Sucrose does not give a positive Clinitest unless it is first hydrolyzed by 0.1 N HCl and heat.[1] Malabsorbed sugars or the organic metabolites produced by bacteria are osmotically active and produce watery stools, whereas fat malabsorption alone may be associated with excessive but normally formed stools.

Bacterial Cultures

Bacterial cultures should be performed. In addition to shigella, salmonella, and enterotoxic strains of *Escherichia coli,* campylobacter and yersinia organisms can cause diarrhea from direct invasion of bowel epithelium or by production of endotoxins. Staphylococci and clostridia may be found in enterocolitis.

Sweat Chloride

Analysis of sweat for chloride and/or sodium content should be done in any child with excessive stool fat or failure to gain weight normally.

Fecal Fat

A 72-hour stool sample is necessary to quantitate the degree of fat malabsorption. The fecal fat content should not exceed 5% of the ingested fat.

Immunoelectrophoresis

Serum immunoelectrophoresis may identify the rare patient with an immunodeficiency.

Tolerance Tests

Carbohydrate tolerance tests are difficult to perform in infants and children and frequently are more difficult to interpret. Analysis of breath for hydrogen is a noninvasive way to detect excessive carbohydrate reaching the lower small bowel and colon. Both carbohydrate malabsorption and contamination of the small bowel by bacteria give high values.

Although it has several limitations, the 1-hour xylose tolerance test is helpful in the evaluation of infants less than 3 years old who may have mucosal damage. After a 6-hour fast, 5 gm of D-xylose is given by mouth and a blood sample is obtained exactly 60 minutes later. A rise of less than 20 mg/dl is abnormal and warrants an intestinal biopsy.

Roentgenograms

A roentgenographic examination is indicated if there is clinical or laboratory evidence to suspect inflammatory bowel disease or undiagnosed malabsorption.

Common Causes of Persistent Diarrhea

Postgastroenteritis Syndrome with Persistent Diarrhea and Malabsorption

Secondary changes in intestinal mucosal morphology with abnormal digestive and absorptive function occur with many gastrointestinal disorders. In most, the etiology is believed to be infectious in origin (e.g., viral, bacterial, or parasitic). These infections frequently occur in infants and children, and diarrhea with malabsorption caused by a secondary decrease in disaccharidase activities is more common than diarrhea caused by a genetic deficiency of the enzymes. The intestinal villi may be blunted, and there may be inflammatory cell infiltration of the lamina propria. The resulting decrease in disaccharidase activities causes lactose and, occasionally, sucrose intolerance. The loss of absorptive surface area plus the decrease in disaccharidase activities frequently are sufficient to cause substantial carbohydrate malabsorption and diarrhea. In addition, the mucosal transport of nutrients also may be diminished. Most secondary mucosal abnormalities are reversible, and a normal diet eventually can be reinstituted.

Management should be dietary. Anticholinergic agents should be avoided because they may produce intestinal stasis and secondary entercolitis. Lactose-free feedings usually are adequate, but restriction of sucrose also may be required. The severity of water losses is proportional to the osmotic load, which is a reflection of the amount of sugar ingested at any one time. Thus, dilution of the formula and frequent feedings of a small volume may be of additional help during the recovery period. The possible contribution of ingested amino acids to this osmotic load should be considered in choosing the diet.

Most patients can be gradually weaned to more normal feedings in 1 to 3 weeks.

Chronic, Nonspecific Infantile Diarrhea Without Protein-calorie Malabsorption

Also termed the irritable colon syndrome, toddler diarrhea, or the "sloppy stool" syndrome, chronic, nonspecific infantile diarrhea without protein-calorie malabsorption accounts for the majority of young children referred to gastroenterologists for persistent or intermittent loose stools. There is a growing number of children in the United States who have this syndrome. Recent findings suggest this increased incidence is caused, at least in part, by variations in diet. For this reason, it might be appropriate to separate the patients with chronic, nonspecific diarrhea into two categories: (1) patients who improve with dietary manipulation, and (2) patients who continue to have diarrhea in spite of dietary manipulation. In either category, the diarrhea usually begins when the patient is between 6 months and 1 year old; it is associated with no other symptoms, the intestinal morphology is normal, and there is normal growth, unless the patient has been placed on a calorie-restricted diet.

Patients who improve with dietary manipulation frequently have a history of acute enteritis, probably of infectious origin, but continue to have persistent watery stools well beyond the expected period of recovery. Characteristically, a good dietary history will reveal the following: (1) stools are intermittently normal, (2) weight percentile exceeds height percentile, (3) watery stools are more frequent in the afternoon and evening, (4) caloric intake is substantially greater than calculated needs, and/or (5) fluid intake is excessive or consists of large amounts of juices or hypertonic drinks. Patients with a low intake of dietary fat occasionally may be seen. By adjusting the diet to a more balanced intake and giving specific instructions to limit the volume of fluids (Gatorade, Pedialyte, and so forth) to the amounts needed, these patients show remarkable improvement.

The typical patient who does not improve with dietary manipulation is one who was colicky as an infant and has three to six mucus-containing stools per day with equal numbers in the morning as compared to evening. A family history of unusual bowel habits such as irritable colon syndrome in parents is common, and there is a similarly affected sibling in up to 50% of the patients. Investigations should be done to exclude malabsorption and infection. The parents and patients can profit from a patient and understandable explanation of the condition.

Gradual but complete recovery by 3 to 4 years is to be expected, although follow-up examinations should be planned to ensure adequate growth.

Milk Intolerance

Diarrhea and/or vomiting after milk feedings in the neonate may represent the first symptoms of lactose intolerance, monosaccharide intolerance, galactosemia, or certain inborn errors of protein metabolism. Although these disorders should be considered, they are extremely unusual. The more common of the milk-related illnesses is sensitivity to milk protein. In the United States, the incidence of this sensitivity is reportedly between 0.3 and 7%, and it reportedly is higher in children with eczema, asthma, or chronic rhinorrhea.

The clinical features appear when the infant is between 2 days and 4 months old and tend to disappear spontaneously when the patient is between 2 and 3 years old. Explosive diarrhea with volume depletion has been noted in some instances, but more commonly the diarrhea is chronic and associated with vomiting or colic. Chronic malabsorption may lead to weight loss, hypoproteinemia, and edema. Mucus in the stool is frequent, and gross or occult blood is present in up to 80% of patients.

No laboratory test is diagnostic, and the diagnosis of milk protein sensitivity depends on the fulfillment of three clinical criteria: (1) symptoms subside within 48 hours after removal of milk from the diet, (2) symptoms consistently reappear within 48 hours after reintroduction of milk to the diet, and (3) a similar response occurs after three consecutive challenges. These criteria do not differentiate the more unusual causes of milk intolerance (e.g., galactosemia). Skin testing and the presence of circulating milk antibodies have shown poor correlation with gastrointestinal milk allergy.

Milk-induced colitis appears to be a separate entity, which

primarily involves colonic epithelium. It usually occurs in young infants; is associated with chronic diarrhea; and is characterized by passage of blood, mucus, and, at times, sheets of colonic epithelial cells and leukocytes. Sigmoidoscopy reveals hemorrhagic, friable mucosa similar to ulcerative colitis. However, milk-induced colitis can be differentiated from ulcerative colitis because it resolves within 48 to 72 hours after milk elimination.

Treatment is the elimination of milk and milk products from the diet. Occasionally, improvement may not be dramatic because of secondary intestinal damage or a coexisting intolerance to other proteins (e.g., egg or soy bean). Because of the increased prevalence of sensitivity to soy protein in infants with milk protein sensitivity, a protein hydrolysate formula should be given if soy protein formula is not tolerated.

Pancreatic Exocrine Insufficiency

Pancreatic exocrine insufficiency occurs with the following diseases, of which cystic fibrosis is the most common:

1. cystic fibrosis of the pancreas,

2. Shwachman-Diamond syndrome (pancreatic insufficiency with bone marrow hypoplasia),

3. severe malnutrition,

4. congenital lipase deficiency.

These conditions produce steatorrhea and fat malabsorption by deficiency of the pancreatic lipase. Other pancreatic enzymes also may be deficient. Therefore, treatment involves replacement of pancreatic enzymes by exogenous lipase and other pancreatic enzymes. Dietary fat need not be restricted, although a moderate limitation to 30 to 40 gm of fat daily will allow for relatively normal stools. Fat absorption cannot be restored to normal in patients with cystic fibrosis, even with excessive doses of preparations such as Pancrease, Viokase, and Cotazyme. Therefore, the aim of therapy should be to provide seminormal stools without the manifestations of under- or overdosage. These include, (1) in older children, the meconium ileus equivalent with abdominal pain, palpable abdominal masses, and, rarely, signs of intestinal obstruction with underdosage; and (2) perianal skin breakdown in the infant with overdosage. The dose of pancreatic enzyme replacement must be adjusted to stool frequency and consistency. Viokase, ¼ to 1 teaspoon in an infant and one to four tablets in an older child, may be required with each feeding or meal. Some pancreatic supplement should be given with between-meal snacks as well as with meals. Rigid dietary restriction should be avoided. Up to 200 kcal and 4 to 5 gm protein per kilogram daily may be required for catch-up growth. Multivitamin supplementation is desirable. Infants should be given vitamin K, 5 mg three times weekly, until the dietary treatment is established. A water-soluble, vitamin E preparation should be administered. In addition, steatorrhea is commonly associated with malabsorption of trace minerals; for this reason, supplemental zinc is recommended.

Medium-chain triglycerides (8-10 carbons) are better absorbed than the usual long-chain, dietary fats (18-22 carbons). The medium-chain triglyceride diet may be used for patients with cystic fibrosis who fail to gain adequately or who have abdominal pain, liver disease, or rectal prolapse.

Celiac Disease—Gluten-sensitive Enteropathy

Celiac disease produces nutrient malabsorption because of a loss of mucosal cell microvillus surface area and impaired activity of mucosal cell enzymes secondary to mucosal damage induced by wheat or rye gluten.[1] Although it is not known whether the damage is the result of toxic metabolites or represents an immune complex disease, the histologic abnormality of the small intestine is characteristic. Definitive diagnosis is based on recovery of the intestinal mucosa on a gluten-free diet and recurrence of symptoms following ingestion of gluten. The mucosal atrophy resembles that seen in malnutrition and severe allergic reactions. In some instances, tolerance is acquired or the body's reaction to gluten disappears. Lifelong treatment is the usual expectation.

The gluten-free diet is simple to prescribe but difficult to follow. All foods containing flour or cereal derived from wheat or rye should be excluded from the diet. Rice, corn, and potato flour are well tolerated. The use of oats and barley is controversial, but they probably should be excluded from the diet. Many prepared foods, even some flavorings, contain gluten; so the parents should read the labels carefully. The services of a dietitian can be helpful.

Dietary Management of Malabsorption

Many preparations on the market for formula feeding of adults are nutritionally complete. However, some of these preparations contain too much protein and sodium for infants and children less than 4 years old (see Appendix J). When formulas free of milk, lactose, soy protein, or sucrose are needed for infants and children less than 4 years old, nutritionally complete infant formulas are more appropriate than products designed for use by adults. Appropriate diets which will meet the needs of infants and children with malabsorption problems can be devised with the help of a pediatric dietitian.

References

1. Davidson, M., and Wasserman, R.: The irritable colon of childhood (chronic nonspecific diarrhea syndrome). J. Pediat., **69**:1027, 1966.
2. Lo, C. W., and Walker, W.A.: Chronic protracted diarrhea of infancy: A nutritional disease. PEDIATRICS, **72**:786, 1983.
3. Cohen, S.A., Hendricks, K.M., Eastham, E.J., Mathis, R.K., and Walker, W.A.: Chronic nonspecific diarrhea: A complication of dietary fat restriction. Amer. J. Dis. Child., **133**:490, 1979.
4. Greene, H.L., and Ghishan, F.K.: Excessive fluid intake as a cause of chronic diarrhea in young children. J. Pediat., **102**:836, 1983.

Chapter 23

IRON DEFICIENCY

Iron-deficiency anemia is most common in young children who are between 6 months and 3 years old; it increases in prevalence again in the teens. Routine screening for anemia is usually done on infants between 9 and 15 months old. It may be indicated again at the time of a preschool checkup when children are 5 to 6 years old and again when they are 12 to 14 years old, particularly among disadvantaged populations. Anemia is defined as a lower-than-normal concentration of hemoglobin or hematocrit. By convention, the lower limit of normal is set 2 S.D. below the mean for a normal population of the same age, or at the 2.5th percentile. The limits of normal at various ages for hemoglobin, hematocrit, and mean corpuscular volume (which is also useful in the diagnosis of iron-deficiency anemia) are shown in Appendix V.

Iron deficiency is by far the most common cause of anemia. Thus, the prevalence of anemia will generally provide an estimate of the prevalence of iron deficiency. In the individual patient, this impression always must be confirmed by additional laboratory tests or by documenting improvement in the anemia in response to a therapeutic trial of iron (see the section in this chapter entitled Diagnosis). Other common causes of anemia are thalassemia minor, infection, and chronic disease. Nutritional deficiencies of folic acid, vitamin B_{12}, vitamin E, and copper also may cause anemia. However, these deficiencies are rare; and they usually are detected by other means.

Iron Metabolism

Iron is a constituent of hemoglobin, myoglobin, the cytochromes, and a number of other proteins which function in the transport, storage, and utilization of oxygen. When the supply of dietary iron is inadequate, storage iron is depleted before hemoglobin and other metabolically functioning iron compounds become decreased.

The adult male absorbs about 1 mg of iron per day, an amount equivalent to iron losses through desquamation of intestinal and skin cells. About the same amount of iron must be absorbed during infancy and childhood, despite a lower caloric intake, to allow for a normal increase in total body iron during rapid growth.

The accumulation of body iron is regulated by the mucosal cell of the intestine. This cell, by virtue of its 2- to 3-day life span, constitutes a temporary holding zone for iron between the intestinal lumen and the blood. When iron stores are abundant, iron is taken up and largely retained by the mucosal cell, to be returned later to the luminal contents by desquamation. In contrast, as iron stores become depleted, more iron crosses the mucosa into the circulation and little is retained by the mucosal cell.

The dietary source of iron strongly influences absorption. The range of iron absorption from a variety of foods averages from less than 1% to more than 20%. Food of vegetable origin is at the lower end of the range, dairy products are in the middle, and meat is at the upper end. About 4% of the iron in fortified formulas and about 10% of the minute amount of iron in unfortified formulas is absorbed. The absorption of reduced iron of small particle size when used to fortify infant cereals is estimated to be about 4%. Infants absorb about half of the iron in human milk. Normally the diet contains 5 to 20 times the amount of iron absorbed.

There are two types of iron in food. Most of the iron in infant diets is in the form of nonheme iron, and a much smaller proportion is present as heme iron (primarily in meat). Heme iron is relatively well absorbed, regardless of the nature of the meal in which it is consumed. Nonheme iron is less well absorbed, and absorption is strongly influenced by the other foods ingested at the same meal. Ascorbic acid and an unknown component of meat are among the most potent enhancers of nonheme iron absorption from the meal as a whole. Tea and milk tend to inhibit nonheme iron absorption from the meal with which they are consumed.

The common etiologic factors in the development of iron deficiency are an insufficient dietary intake of iron, dilution of body iron by rapid growth, and blood loss. Intestinal blood loss can be a contributing factor in the development of anemia in infants, but it rarely is associated with the gross anatomic lesions (e.g., ulcer or carcinoma) which are more common in adults.

Developmental Factors in the Susceptibility to Iron Deficiency

In the full-term infant, iron-deficiency anemia is uncommon before the infant is about 4 to 6 months old because of the abundance of the iron stores at birth and the normal, postnatal decrease in the production of hemoglobin. After the iron stores are consumed, there is a dependence on dietary iron to provide for a rapid rise in total body hemoglobin. Preterm infants and twins have low iron stores at birth that are in proportion to their smaller size. Because their rate of growth is more rapid than that of full-term infants, their iron stores may be depleted by the time they are 2 to 3 months old.

Iron deficiency is most common when children are between 6 months and 3 years old because the rate of growth is rapid and milk is a major source of calories. Milk contains only about 1.5 mg of iron per 1,000 kcal, in contrast to the 6 mg per 1,000 kcal in the average mixed diet. The consumption of large amounts of fresh or pasteurized cow's milk occasionally is associated with occult intestinal blood loss, which contributes significantly to the development of iron deficiency. This type of blood loss usually ceases when sterilized cow's milk formula or soy-based formula is substituted for fresh cow's milk, whether or not iron is administered. This suggests an intestinal sensitivity to a protein component of milk, such as lactalbumin, which can be denatured or modified by heat processing. The iron content of human milk is similar to that of cow's milk; however, because more of the iron from human milk is absorbed, the maintenance of breast feeding confers substantial protection against the development of iron deficiency in full-term infants.

In the preschool-aged and preadolescent child, iron nutrition generally becomes improved because there is greater opportunity to obtain iron from a mixed diet. In adolescence, the prevalence of mild iron-deficiency anemia increases because of acceleration in the rate of growth and the onset of menstruation. Among susceptible age groups, iron deficiency is most prevalent among disadvantaged populations. In parts of the world in which hookworm infestation is a problem, severe iron-deficiency anemia remains common throughout childhood.

Blood loss from anatomic lesions should be suspected when anemia persists or recurs after iron therapy has been administered, when intestinal blood loss persists despite substitution

of processed formula for fresh cow's milk, or when anemia is
severe.

Recommendation for Infants

Iron supplementation from one or more sources should start
when full-term infants are between 4 and 6 months old and in
preterm infants no later than 2 months of age. Convenient
sources of iron are iron-fortified, commercial infant formula
and/or two servings a day of iron-fortified infant cereal. Iron-
fortified infant cereal is the preferred iron source for breast-fed
infants. Either source provides an adequate supply of iron
(about 1 mg/kg per day) for full-term infants. In preterm infants who are formula-fed, iron-fortified formula usually provides adequate iron. Breast-fed preterm infants should receive
iron in the form of ferrous sulfate drops at a dose of 2 to 3
mg/kg per day (of elemental iron) to a maximum of 15 mg per
day. If iron-containing drops are used, no more than 1 month's
supply should be kept in the home to reduce the risk of accidental poisoning. The maintenance of breast feeding for 6 months
or more protects against the development of iron deficiency in
full-term infants; however, preterm infants fed human milk
require iron-containing drops after 2 months of age and iron-
fortified cereal when solid foods are started.

Commercial infant formula and other sterilized milk products are preferable to fresh milk as substitutes for human-milk
feeding during the first 9 to 12 months of life because excessive
ingestion of unprocessed cow's milk may contribute to iron deficiency by increasing gastrointestinal blood loss. The volume
of milk or formula should not exceed 1 liter per day to encourage the introduction of iron-rich solid foods and set the pattern
for a more varied diet.

Children and Adults

Iron absorption is strongly influenced by the combination of
foods in each meal. Meals from which iron is well absorbed are
those rich in meat and/or ascorbic acid. A major source of iron
is iron-fortified cereal and flour products. Tea and milk, which

tend to decrease the absorption of iron from foods, will have less influence on iron availability if they are ingested between meals.

Prevention of iron deficiency is a particularly complex and urgent problem in developing countries where hookworm infestation and the predominance of unfortified cereals in the diet are responsible for a high prevalence of iron deficiency.

Diagnosis

The symptoms of iron deficiency are nonspecific and become apparent only with severe anemia. They include pallor, fatigue, and decreased exercise tolerance. Iron deficiency also may impair intellectual performance and resistance to infection, but these effects are not likely to be apparent in individual patients. Mild iron deficiency is usually diagnosed on the basis of routine laboratory screening or as part of the evaluation of a child seen for an intercurrent infection. The goal should be to diagnose iron deficiency and start treatment at the same visit, thereby reducing cost and inconvenience and increasing the likelihood of compliance with the treatment regimen. Be aware that iron deficiency frequently indicates shortcomings in the diet requiring correction.

Screening Tests

The laboratory tests commonly used in the diagnosis of iron deficiency can be grouped conveniently into screening and confirmatory tests. The primary screening tests are the hemoglobin and hematocrit. The hemoglobin is the preferred of the two methods because it seems to be more sensitive in diagnosing iron-deficiency anemia. When the blood count is done by electronic counter, the mean corpuscular volume serves as an ancillary screening method. Hemoglobin, hematocrit, and mean corpuscular volume all change substantially during development. Therefore, age-specific reference standards such as the tables and percentile curves in Appendix V should be used. Low or low-normal values may warrant either further laboratory tests or a therapeutic trial of iron. It is important to take into consideration the relatively poor reproducibility of hemoglobin and hematocrit obtained from skin puncture blood. When the results are borderline, it frequently is preferable to repeat the study on venous blood rather than to proceed to additional laboratory tests.

Therapeutic Trial or Confirmatory Tests

In most clinical settings that involve infants and children, nutritional iron deficiency is the predominant cause of mild anemia. In mild iron-deficiency anemia, additional laboratory tests may yield a confusing combination of positive and negative results. A therapeutic trial of iron may be the most practical course if the child is otherwise well. A therapeutic trial can consist of 3 mg iron per kilogram per day as ferrous sulfate for about 1 month. In a 10 kg infant, this is equivalent to 30 mg iron, an amount well tolerated as a single, before-breakfast dose. In children, the iron is better administered in two doses given between meals. If there are gastrointestinal side effects, a lower dose and/or a three-dose per day regimen can be tried. The therapeutic trial must be monitored by repeat laboratory studies after about 1 month, ideally on venous blood. By this time, the hemoglobin response should be about two-thirds complete. If there has been a more than 1 gm/dl hemoglobin increase, the presumption is that iron-deficiency anemia was present, and treatment should be continued for about 4 months to allow for complete repair of anemia and restoration of iron stores. In mild anemia (hemoglobin more than 10 gm/dl), the reticulocyte response is usually of such small proportion that it is not practical to monitor this as early evidence of a therapeutic response. In the rare instances in which anemia is still present after 1 month of iron therapy, poor compliance may be an explanation; a more extensive diagnostic evaluation is indicated.

Other laboratory tests for iron deficiency include serum ferritin, iron/iron-binding capacity, and erythrocyte protoporphyrin. The concentration of serum ferritin in infants more than 6 months old is normally equal to or greater than 10 μg per liter. The concentration of serum ferritin corresponds roughly to the magnitude of iron stores. Consequently, the assay is useful for estimating iron reserves in normal individuals as well as those with a deficiency or an overload. Because iron stores are normally marginal in childhood, particularly during infancy and adolescence, an isolated finding of a low serum ferritin level falls into the ambiguous area between iron deficiency and the normal developmental depletion of iron reserves. Iron depletion manifested only by a low serum ferritin may correct itself without treatment, particularly in late infancy when the rate of growth slows and if the contribution of milk to the diet is decreased.

Virtually all iron in the serum is normally bound to transferrin. The decrease in serum iron and increase in total iron-binding capacity (TIBC) in iron deficiency result in a decreased transferrin saturation (serum iron/iron-binding capacity), a value that is of greater diagnostic use than the serum iron level alone. Serum iron concentrations show day-to-day as well as diurnal variation, with higher values in the morning. Thus, blood for this determination is best obtained early in the day. Because of these and other biologic variations, there is substantial overlap between deficient and normal values. Infants more than a few months old and young children normally have lower transferrin saturations than adults. A value less than 10% suggests iron deficiency.

Protoporphyrin is a compound that combines with iron to produce heme. When iron deficiency restricts hemoglobin production, abnormally high values are found. Values above 3 μg per gram hemoglobin (30 μg/dl blood or 75 μ/dl erythrocytes) are abnormal. The assay is a technically simple and rapidly performed fluorometric procedure.

The diagnosis of moderate or severe iron-deficiency anemia can be made easily using the criteria for hemoglobin, mean corpuscular volume, and one of the confirmatory tests. A reticulocyte response 1 to 2 weeks after therapy has been initiated is helpful in confirming the diagnosis. In severe iron-deficiency anemia (hemoglobin less than 10 gm/dl), evidence of occult intestinal blood loss should be sought, particularly in infants.

Differential Diagnosis

Iron-deficiency anemia can be difficult to distinguish from the anemia of chronic disease or infection, especially because the two often coexist. Both can be characterized by mild anemia, an elevated erythrocyte protoporphyrin, and a low serum iron concentration. In simple iron deficiency, TIBC is normal or elevated; in chronic disease, TIBC is normal or depressed. A depressed serum ferritin (less than 10 μg/l) is diagnostic of iron deficiency, whereas infection and chronic disease are associated with normal or elevated values. Because laboratory tests frequently fail to distinguish iron deficiency in the presence of infection and chronic disease, a therapeutic trial with iron may be indicated.

The other common cause of microcytic anemia is thalassemia minor. Thalassemia minor is not characterized by a decrease in serum ferritin or transferrin saturation. The erythrocyte protoporphyrin level is normal in thalassemia minor, somewhat elevated in iron deficiency, and often considerably elevated in lead poisoning. The use of any of these diagnostic methods or a therapeutic trial permits the detection of most instances of iron deficiency; the quantitation of hemoglobins A_2 and F is reserved for patients suspected of having beta thalassemia trait. A hemoglobin value of less than 10 gm/dl with a low mean corpuscular volume is almost always associated with iron deficiency rather than thalassemia trait.

Bibliography

Dallman, P.R., Siimes, M.A., and Stekel, A.: Iron deficiency in infancy and childhood. Amer. J. Clin. Nutr., 33:86, 1983.

Chapter 24

INBORN ERRORS OF METABOLISM

Recent decades have witnessed the discovery of a large number of conditions involving errors in protein, carbohydrate, or fat metabolism. These conditions usually share the following features: (1) an extremely low incidence, ranging from 1/12,000 to 1/200,000 births in the United States; (2) a genetic basis, usually autosomal recessive; (3) an abnormality in intermediary metabolism, gastrointestinal absorption, or membrane transport. Specific enzyme defects have been identified for some conditions, and a few have been localized to particular chromosomes (example: the gene for galactosemia is on the long arm of chromosome 9). This chapter will discuss the metabolic errors which have nutritional significance.

The primary defect is an alteration in DNA structure. This alteration manifests itself in one of several ways; the common denominator is disrupted cell and organ function. For example, the absence of phenylalanine hydroxylase results in an overproduction of by-products of phenylalanine metabolism, and these by-products are toxic to the central nervous system. Familial hypercholesterolemia is caused by a disorder in the cellular feedback regulation of cholesterol metabolism. Disordered membrane transport is manifested at the renal level in cystinuria and at the gastrointestinal level in disaccharidase deficiencies. An example of cell membrane dysfunction is familial hypophosphatemic rickets.

A few inborn errors, such as essential fructosuria and essential pentosuria, are asymptomatic, but many result in symptoms and signs of organ dysfunction, including the central nervous system. However, these symptoms and signs may not be present in the immediate neonatal period, a fact which has led to the development of screening tests for neonates. All states now require that a sample of blood be taken from each neonate to be tested for phenylketonuria, and many states require tests for hypothyroidism, maple syrup urine disease, histidinemia, homocystinuria, galactosemia, and adenosine deaminase deficiency.

Any tests that are positive should be repeated. When a screening test is positive, arrangements should be made to refer the patient to a physician who is able to perform a definitive test for the disorder in question. In the meantime, the diet should be low in protein (1.0 gm/kg per day, or less) if aminoaciduria is suspected and devoid of lactose if galactosemia is suspected.

Special diets are available for the management of phenylketonuria, maple syrup urine disease, homocystinuria, tyrosinosis, and histidinemia. Galactosemia requires that all sources of lactose be removed from the diet (soy formulas and protein hydrolysate formula are lactose free). Other conditions (e.g., pyridoxine dependency) may be helped by additional vitamins or alterations in dietary protein, fat, or carbohydrate. Careful monitoring of the diet and biochemical and clinical status is essential, as are the services and advice of a facility which specializes in the management of inborn errors of metabolism. Long-term benefits and essentially normal health can now be achieved by those with some types of inborn errors who receive proper treatment soon enough.

Genetic counseling is an obvious requirement because parents should be made aware of the risk associated with subsequent pregnancies. Procedures for prenatal diagnosis of galactosemia, some aminoacidurias, and at least one type of familial hypercholesterolemia are now feasible (a list of these disorders, some of which involve nutritional management, has been compiled by Stanbury et al.[1] Efforts also are being made in the detection of heterozygotes. Examples are the reduced tolerance to an administered load of phenylalanine in those with the gene for phenylketonuria and leukocyte enzyme assays in those who are carriers of acid lipase deficiency (Wolman's disease).

One problem is the welfare of the fetus carried by a woman with an inborn error of metabolism. For example, pregnant women who have phenylketonuria must maintain a serum phenylalanine level well below 15 mg/dl while ensuring adequate nutrition.

Additional inborn errors of metabolism may be discovered in the future, and some of these may involve nutritional considerations. Future problems include challenges for biochemists in elucidating the underlying defect, for geneticists in working out the inheritance pattern, for nutritionists in devising appropriate therapy, and for clinicians in diagnosing and managing these patients.

Specialized formulas for inborn errors of metabolism are available from multiple sources. The Committee on Nutrition has a task force which is updating previous information.

Reference

1. Stanbury, J.B., Wyngaarden, J.B., Fredrickson, D.S., Goldstein, J.L., and Brown, M.S., ed.: The Metabolic Basis of Inherited Disease, ed. 5. New York: McGraw-Hill, 1983.

Bibliography

Committee on Nutrition: Special diets for infants with inborn errors of amino acid metabolism. PEDIATRICS, 57:783, 1976.
Levy, H.L., and Waisbren, S.E.: Effects of untreated maternal phenylketonuria and hyperphenylalaninemia on the fetus. New Engl. J. Med., 309:1269, 1983.
Rudolph, A.M., and Hoffman, J.I.E., ed.: Pediatrics, ed. 17. Norwalk, Connecticut: Appleton-Century-Crofts, 1982.

Chapter 25

DIABETES MELLITUS

In the last few years, those who care for children and adolescents with Type I or insulin-dependent diabetes mellitus have developed a clearer and more rational understanding of what is meant by good control, of how it is assessed, and of the principle factors which influence it.[1,2] Dietary regulation is one factor. The intake of energy, its expenditure in physical exercise, and the amount of insulin given are the most important variables in the management of diabetes. The role of dietary management can be understood only in relation to all the other factors.

The child who develops diabetes and the child whose disease is poorly controlled need an intensive, detailed learning experience, frequently in a hospital, to acquire an understanding of the disease and its day-to-day management. Parents must be involved in this learning process. The dietitian or nutritionist who is part of the diabetes care team plays an important role in this process.

There is an increasing appreciation of the beneficial effects of stricter control on long-term outcomes of children with diabetes. The essentials of good control can be summarized as follows:

1. control of symptoms, e.g., polyuria, polydipsia, and polyphagia;

2. control of hyperglycemia and acidosis;

3. normal physical and emotional growth, sexual maturation, and a normal lifestyle;

4. maintenance of blood sugar levels in the range of 80 to 180 mg/dl;

5. maintenance of a serum cholesterol level less than 210 mg/dl and an overnight fasting serum triglyceride level of less than 130 mg/dl;

6. maintenance of a stable glycohemoglobin (HgbA$_{1c}$) level of less than 3% above the normal value;

7. in children who refuse finger pricks, the achievement of a urine glucose concentration 1% or less and a 24-hour urine glucose excretion of less than 20 gm/M^2 per 24 hours, or 7% of the dietary intake of carbohydrate (finger prick samples should be obtained to document hypoglycemic reactions).

The assessment of the degree of control has been changed in

the last few years by the availability of assays of blood glycohemoglobin levels and by instruments for blood-glucose monitoring at home. The type of monitoring has been hastened by two disparate factors: (1) third party acceptance of the cost of glucose monitoring devices, and (2) the understanding that, particularly in teen-agers and especially in girls, the renal threshold for glucose may be variable enough so urine tests are an unreliable reflection of blood glucose.[3]

The use of highly purified pork insulins or of synthetic human insulins plays a relatively small role in improving control, except in a few selected patients. The same may be said for insulin pumps, which have enjoyed a recent vogue but which may lead to hyperinsulinemia with the adverse metabolic effect this entails. Much more important are the roles of correct insulin dose, of lack of stress,[4] and of regular exercise in promoting serum glucose homeostasis.[5]

Within the framework of the foregoing considerations, the role of diet in achieving good control can be summarized as follows. From a practical standpoint, the existing family eating patterns, including cultural and economic factors, must be understood. It may be necessary to try to modify the eating pattern so it is based on three meals plus a midmorning snack, an afternoon snack, and a bedtime snack to spread the load of ingested carbohydrate. The total calories should be age and sex appropriate. The distribution of calories should not be rigid but should conform reasonably to a diet that derives about 50 to 60% of energy from carbohydrate, 30 to 38% from fat, and 12 to 20% from protein. It seldom is necessary to weigh meals, but consistency is extremely important. There is a need to have meals and snacks at about the same time each day and to eat about the same amount and the same kind of foods. A suitable scheme appears to be one of giving approximately 20% of total calories at breakfast, 5% at midmorning, 30% at lunch, 10% at midafternoon, 25% at dinner, 10% in the evening, and an additional snack of protein and carbohydrate in anticipation of extra physical activity. Children and their parents also must develop a reasonable understanding of the food "exchange" system[6] (Appendix T). They should be taught to use judgment in the purchase of foods and to read labels, especially the wording having to do with added sugar.

Some other considerations need to be incorporated into eating patterns. One is an understanding of the hypoglycemic effect of exercise; snack times may have to be adjusted to cover exercise, and the insulin dose may have to be reduced or the food intake increased. A second consideration is the use of protein and fat in the bedtime snack, which helps to prevent low blood sugar levels during the night.

Young people with diabetes are vulnerable to hypertriglyceridemia and hypercholesterolemia. The long-term significance of these abnormalities is still debated; but, until their significance is resolved, measurements should be taken annually and dietary changes instituted (see Chapter 27) to maintain homeostasis of blood lipids. The use of polyunsaturated vegetable oil margarines instead of butter, of 2% milk, and of polyunsaturated cooking oils is recommended. Special dietetic foods, with the possible exception of artificial sweeteners, should not be encouraged for young diabetics. They are expensive and unnecessary. Most important, they differentiate the affected child from the rest of the family.

The popularity of fad diets (see Chapter 33) has extended to the treatment of diabetes, with a varying degree of scientific basis. Brewer's yeast as a source of the glucose tolerance factor and guar gum to delay the absorption of glucose have been used, but they have not been demonstrably effective in young diabetic patients. The use of alternative sweeteners such as aspartame in drinks and other products has been beneficial for children who have diabetes. Sorbitol and fructose can be metabolized without forming glucose if sufficient insulin is present and the child is in good diabetic control. A high-fiber, moderate-fat diet in which carbohydrate is given as complex carbohydrates appears to be beneficial. Perhaps as the different functions and properties of different fibers and carbohydrates become known, more progress will be made in this area. Recent studies suggest there is a spectrum of biologic responses to different complex and simple carbohydrates with so much overlap they cannot be distinguished as separate groups. Responses to single carbohydrates are attenuated when they are given as part of a meal.[7]

Obesity in the child with diabetes deserves the same attention and presents the same problems as it would in a person without diabetes. At the same time, it brings the added burden of relative insulin resistance. There is a small subset of diabetic adolescents who have Type II, or maturity onset diabetes. These patients are usually overweight, and girls are more frequently involved than boys. This type of diabetes usually can be benefited by weight reduction and carbohydrate restriction.

Alcohol and drug intakes can cause considerable difficulty in teen-agers with diabetes. Initially, alcoholic beverages usually result in increased blood sugar levels. Later, hypoglycemia will be more likely because of sleeping late the next day, missed snacks, and a reduction in gluconeogenesis.

Many people believe there is a strong relationship between diet and diabetes so parents, relatives, and friends frequently see an exaggerated role for diet in control of diabetes. The food intake of the young patient with diabetes should be adapted to the individual. Consistency in time, amount, and distribution of calories is necessary. Carbohydrate intake needs to be spread throughout the day, which also will even out hypoglycemic periods. There also is a need for a modest adaptation of fat intake to lessen the risks of developing hyperlipidemia. The benefit of precise control is emphasized by a recent study of Type I diabetes; the width of muscle capillary basement membranes was shown to decrease along with levels of glycosylated hemoglobin, in contrast to patients managed by conventional means.[8]

References

1. Drash, A.: The control of diabetes mellitus: Is it achievable? Is it desirable? J. Pediat., 88:1074, 1976.
2. Brouhard, B.H.: Control and monitoring for the child with insulin-dependent diabetes mellitus. Amer. J. Dis. Child., 137:787, 1983.
3. Moffitt, P.S.: Interpretation of glycosuria in the teenage diabetic patient. Diabetes Care, 3:112, 1980.
4. Chase, H.P., and Jackson, G.G.: Stress and sugar control in children with insulin-dependent diabetes mellitus. J. Pediat., 98:1011, 1981.
5. Skyler, J.S.: Diabetes and exercise: Clinical implications. Diabetes Care, 2:307, 1979.
6. Exchange Lists for Meal Planning. New York: American Diabetes Association, and Chicago: American Dietetic Association, 1976.
7. Crapo, P.A., and Olefsky, J.M.: Food fallacies and blood sugar. New Engl. J. Med., 309:44, 1983.
8. Raskin, P., Pietri, A.O., Unger, R., and Shannon, W.A., Jr.: The effect of diabetic control on the width of skeletal-muscle capillary basement membrane in patients with Type I diabetes mellitus. New Engl. J. Med., 309:1546, 1983.

Chapter 26

HYPOGLYCEMIA

An impaired ability to sustain normal blood glucose levels, a common metabolic problem in infancy and childhood, can result from many causes (Table 19). Determination of the cause of hypoglycemia is extremely important. Appropriate treatment for a child with one type of hypoglycemia may be harmful to a child with another type. Also, the physician should be familiar with tests for the laboratory diagnosis of hypoglycemia. Vague or bizarre symptoms, a psychiatric disturbance, or a learning disorder might alert a physician to the possibility of hypoglycemia. But hypoglycemia should not be diagnosed without the demonstration of blood glucose levels well below the normal range for age.

The neonate, who is abruptly cut off from its exogenous and plentiful source of glucose at the moment of birth, must rely on endogenous sources of glucose until oral feedings are established. The problem is more acute for preterm infants (especially those who are small for gestational age) inasmuch as liver glycogen stores are meager until about 35 weeks of fetal life. Rates of glucose flux in infants (production and utilization) are about threefold those for adults per unit of body weight. Glucose flux is linearly related to estimated brain weight and not to body weight, an observation in keeping with Cornblath and Schwartz's hypothesis[1] that the greater relative brain size of infants places them at risk for hypoglycemia.

Neonatal Hypoglycemia

Hypoglycemia is a significant cause of morbidity and mortality in newborn infants. It may be caused by many pathologic conditions; but, in a significant number of infants, no etiologic factors are apparent. Hypoglycemia is self-limiting in many infants; the blood glucose level stabilizes within a few hours or days of birth, and there are no recurrences (transient neonatal hypoglycemia). In a few infants, hypoglycemia may be secondary to severe central nervous system abnormalities, e.g., congenital brain defects or cerebral trauma. An occasional infant will have recurrent or persistent hypoglycemia lasting more than 7 days. These infants need a thorough investigation to determine the cause, e.g., hormone deficiency or excess (especially hyperinsulinism) or hereditary defects of carbohydrate or amino acid metabolism.

Definition

Blood glucose levels in newborn infants are usually lower than in older children and adults. Hypoglycemia is defined as two plasma or serum glucose levels <25 mg/dl in a preterm or low-birth-weight term infant (<2.5 kg), <35 mg/dl in a normal weight or full-term infant up to 72 hours of age, and <46 mg/dl thereafter. Other authorities consider 40 mg/dl as the lower limit. Because glycolysis is rapid in blood from neonates, samples must be processed quickly unless a glycolytic inhibitor is used. Serum glucose values are about 15% higher than those for whole blood (example, whole blood, 50 mg/dl; serum, 58 mg/dl). Methods for rapid assessment of blood glucose ranges which can be performed at the bedside are now available.

Clinical Features

Most infants with hypoglycemia appear normal at birth; but, within 6 to 72 hours, they develop muscular tremors, anorexia, irritability, cyanotic or apneic spells, and convulsions. Most infants become asymptomatic after the administration of intravenous glucose; in the few who do not, the symptoms probably are not caused by hypoglycemia.

Hypoglycemia generally occurs within 1 to 2 hours after birth in infants of mothers with diabetes.

Some infants with transient hypoglycemia, especially infants of mothers with diabetes, may have no symptoms associated with hypoglycemia; others may have only minor symptoms (e.g., "jitteriness" and tenseness) which disappear after intravenous glucose is given.

Pathogenesis

Factors which may contribute to the pathogenesis of neonatal hypoglycemia include lack of oxidizable substrate because of deficient carbohydrate stores at birth potentiated by postnatal starvation; relative organ hypercellularity, oxygen lack, and chilling, all of which contribute to a degree of hyper-metabolism; and defective gluconeogenesis caused by late maturation of one or more enzyme systems. Infants of mothers who have gestational diabetes have hyperinsulinism, and there is evidence that hyperinsulinism also may operate in infants of mothers who have diabetes.

Diagnosis

No symptoms are pathognomonic of hypoglycemia in the neonatal period. Convulsions, cyanosis, and apneic episodes also may be seen in infants with cerebral birth injury, sepsis, cardiorespiratory disease, hypocalcemia, and other biochemical abnormalities. Plasma glucose levels should be determined in an infant exhibiting these symptoms. Plasma or blood glucose levels (plasma levels are 15% higher than whole blood levels) also should be obtained frequently in infants at increased risk for hypoglycemia during the first 48 hours of life, whether or not they have symptoms of hypoglycemia. A number of methods for estimating ranges of blood glucose which can be performed at the bedside are available.

Table 19
Causes of Hypoglycemia

Causes Resulting in Diminished Hepatic Glucose Output	Causes Resulting in Increased Peripheral Uptake of Glucose	Miscellaneous Causes
Diminished glyco-gen stores in liver Immaturity Intra-uterine malnutrition, small-for-date infant Postnatal starva-tion	Pancreatic islet cell tumor Pancreatic islet cell hyperplasia Nesidioblastoma Maternal diabe-tes Erythroblastosis	Idiopathic trans-ient hypogly-cemia Central nervous system dis-eases or anomalies Salicylate poisoning

Causes Resulting in Diminished Hepatic Glucose Output	Causes Resulting in Increased Peripheral Uptake of Glucose	Miscellaneous Causes
Hypothermia; asphyxia Chronic diarrhea Hepatocellular disease Glycogen synthetase deficiency Monosaccharide intolerance Defective glucose release or defective new glucose formation in liver Liver glycogen disease (especially Type I or glucose-6-phosphatase deficiency) Galactosemia Hereditary fructose intolerance Fructose-1, 6-diphosphate deficiency Pyruvate carboxylase or phosphoenolpyruvate carboxykinase deficiencies Growth hormone deficiency Adrenocortical insufficency	Beckwith's syndrome or the "infant giant" Hereditary tyrosinemia Other hyperinsulinemic or possible hyperinsulinemic states Maternal tolbutamide ingestion Abrupt cessation of intravenous glucose infusion Maple syrup urine disease Methylmalonic acidemia Leucine sensitivity	Idiopathic hypoglycemia of childhood Ketotic hypoglycemia Cardiac malformations (especially the hypoplastic left heart syndrome) Tumors Neonatal sepsis

Management

Recognizing the infant at risk of hypoglycemia is important. Early feeding will prevent hypoglycemia in some infants, and the first feeding should be started for these high-risk infants as soon as it is safe to do so. Infants who are too ill to tolerate feedings should receive parenteral glucose. Treatment with intravenous glucose should be started as soon as hypoglycemia is diagnosed. The following steps are recommended in the management of neonatal hypoglycemia:

1. Recognition of high-risk infants, e.g., intra-uterine growth retardation, infants of mothers with diabetes, smaller of twins, erythroblastosis fetalis.

2. Early feeding, starting when the infant is 3 hours old.

3. Frequent monitoring of plasma or blood glucose levels in high-risk infants.

4. If the plasma glucose level is 25 mg/dl or less in low-birth-weight infants or 35 mg/dl or less in normal weight infants, obtain a second blood sample for glucose estimation and administer intravenous glucose immediately without waiting for a second report.

5. Give a 10% glucose solution (2 to 4 ml/kg) into a peripheral vein at a rate of 1 ml per minute. Make sure the needle is in the vein; use caution if the umbilical vein must be used.

6. Continue with 15% glucose in water by intravenous drip, 60 to 70 ml/kg per day (6 to 7 mg glucose per kilogram per minute) for 48 hours; thereafter, if the infant is asymptomatic and plasma glucose is <35 mg/dl, 10% glucose in 30 to 40 mM saline, 100 to 110 ml per kilogram per day. Monitor blood glucose levels every few hours (methods which can be performed at the bedside usually are adequate when quantitative methods are not readily available).*

7. Treat associated conditions, e.g., hypoxia, acidosis, hypocalcemia.

8. If symptoms persist or recur, or if the plasma glucose level is <35 mg/100 ml after 48 hours, consider giving hydrocortisone (2.5 mg per kilogram, intramuscularly every 12 hours) or prednisone (2 mg per kilogram per day orally).

9. Reduce intravenous glucose in a stepwise manner after 1

---

*Some authorities recommend that glucose be administered at a rate of 8 mg per kilogram per minute, equivalent to 11.5 gm per kilogram per day. If a 10% solution of glucose is used, the volume of fluid amounts to 115 ml per kilogram per day; for a 15% solution, it is 77 ml per kilogram per day.

to 3 days if the infant's condition remains satisfactory. The intravenous infusion usually can be discontinued by the fourth or fifth day. **Never stop concentrated glucose intravenous drips abruptly.**

10. Hypoglycemia persisting after 7 days strongly suggests the possibility of a hormone deficiency or excess or an enzyme defect, and a complete investigation should be undertaken to determine the cause.

Prognosis

The prognosis depends on the cause and duration of the hypoglycemia. In preterm infants with symptomatic hypoglycemia, the reported incidence of neurologic sequelae in later childhood has ranged from 25 to 60%. The incidence of complications after asymptomatic hypoglycemia in preterm infants is much less.

Hypoglycemia in the First 5 Years of Life

Possible causes of hypoglycemia in the first 5 years of life are listed in Table 19. These include disorders of hyperinsulinism, glycogenolysis, gluconeogenesis, and a number of less clearly defined clinical syndromes. Of the latter, idiopathic hypoglycemia and ketotic hypoglycemia are the two types most commonly seen in this age group.

Idiopathic hypoglycemia of childhood is not a single entity but a "family" of diseases; many of them have organic hyperinsulinism caused by pancreatic islet cell abnormalities such as hyperplasia or nesidioblastosis (new formation of islet cells from the ductal epithelium). Islet cell adenoma is rare. Approximately one third of children with idiopathic hypoglycemia are leucine sensitive.

Generalized convulsions are the most common symptom. In many patients these convulsions occur in the morning after an overnight fast or after a meal has been delayed. Convulsions may occur at any time of the day, or even during feedings because of leucine sensitivity. Other symptoms include attacks of pallor, sweating, irritability, ataxia, limpness, stupor, and fatigue.

The physician must be alert to the possibility of hypoglycemia in a child with any of the foregoing symptoms, especially if convulsions or other symptoms occur with fasting and are relieved by eating or drinking. A carefully taken history frequently will save many days of laboratory tests. The possibility of hypoglycemia should always be considered in a child with convulsions which respond poorly, or not at all, to anticonvulsant drugs.

Characteristically, the child with ketotic hypoglycemia is a boy, below average in height and weight, with a history of low birth weight, and sometimes with a history of neonatal hypoglycemia. The age of onset of ketotic hypoglycemia is between 12 months and 5½ years, with a peak incidence between 2 and 3 years of age. The disorder remits spontaneously before the child is 6 or 7 years old. Attacks of hypoglycemia are almost always associated with convulsions and occur during fasting, either when a meal has been missed or during episodes of intercurrent illness which may or may not be accompanied by vomiting. Symptoms remit rapidly with the administration of carbohydrate given by mouth.

A history of intermittent convulsions or other neurologic symptoms occurring with fasting in a child with the foregoing characteristics should alert the physician to the possibility of ketotic hypoglycemia. Diagnosis will depend on the demonstration of a low plasma glucose level (e.g., <46 mg/dl) during the attacks or during fasting. Ketonuria is invariably present during the attacks. A provocative ketogenic diet (e.g., high fat, low carbohydrate) will precipitate hypoglycemia in susceptible children and may be used as a diagnostic test. However, the ketosis exhibited by these children is a normal consequence of calorie deprivation, and fasting will precipitate hypoglycemia as well as a ketogenic diet. During attacks, these patients have depleted liver glycogen stores, demonstrated by a lack of a hyperglycemic response to exogenous glucagon. The blood glucose response to glucagon is normal between attacks.

Hypoglycemia in Childhood and Adolescence

In the older child (5 to 15 years old), the hypoglycemic syndromes are similar to those seen in adults (e.g., reactive hypoglycemia in prediabetes and early diabetes, endocrinopathies, and malignancies). The sudden onset of hypoglycemia in an older child who does not have the aforementioned conditions should alert the physician to the possibility of a functioning islet cell adenoma, and vigorous investigation should be pursued.

Fasting plasma insulin levels may not be abnormally elevated, but hyperinsulinism may frequently be demonstrated after a challenge with glucagon, tolbutamide, or leucine. In about one third of the patients, the pancreatic tumor may be visualized by celiac angiography. When the test results are diagnostic or supportive of hyperinsulinism, laparotomy should be undertaken and the pancreas examined for a tumor. Persistence of hypoglycemia after the removal of a pancreatic tumor strongly suggests that one or more additional tumors have been overlooked.

As indicated in Table 19, there are many causes of hypoglycemia. Standard texts should be consulted for additional details concerning diagnosis and management. Proper diagnosis and treatment are essential because hypoglycemia can result in mental impairment.

Reference

1. Cornblath, M., and Schwartz, R.: Disorders of carbohydrate metabolism in infancy, ed. 2. Philadelphia: W. B. Saunders, 1976.

Bibliography

Beard, A., Cornblath, M., Gentz, J., Kellum, M., Persson, B., Zetterström, R., and Haworth, J.C.: Neonatal hypoglycemia: A discussion. J. Pediat., 79:314, 1971.

Haworth, J.C.: Carbohydrate metabolism in the fetus and the newborn; neonatal hypoglycemia. In Gardner, L.I., ed.: Endocrine and Genetic Diseases of Childhood and Adolescence, ed. 2. Philadelphia: W. B. Saunders, pp. 916-930, 1975.

Pagliara, A.S., Karl, I.E., Haymond, M., and Kipnis, D.M.: Hypoglycemia in infancy and childhood, Part I. J. Pediat., 82:365, 1973.

Pagliara, A.S., Karl, I.E., Haymond, M., and Kipnis, D.M.: Hypoglycemia in infancy and childhood, Part II. J. Pediat., 82:558, 1973.

Chapter 27

HYPERLIPIDEMIA

The association between coronary heart disease and blood cholesterol levels noted in both regional and worldwide statistics has made cholesterol and lipid metabolism extremely interesting to physicians and the lay public. Although the incidence of coronary heart disease is now declining in the United States, it remains the leading cause of death in adults in the United States and most industrialized countries. The familial occurrence of coronary heart disease has been known since the nineteenth century; however, the familial risk factors have been delineated only in recent decades. The Framingham study[1] and subsequent studies have identified the following risk factors for coronary heart disease:

1. reduced level of high density lipoprotein (HDL),
2. elevated serum cholesterol level,
3. hypertension,
4. cigarette smoking,
5. impairment of carbohydrate tolerance,
6. lack of physical activity,
7. elevated serum triglycerides.[2]

Not all investigators agree that elevated plasma triglyceride is an independent risk factor for coronary heart disease. Although there is a direct correlation in univariate analysis, this effect is lost when obesity, diabetes mellitus, cholesterol, and high density lipoprotein influences are removed.[1]

In 1972 the Committee on Nutrition, in an attempt to sort out the voluminous literature on cholesterol and lipid metabolism, summarized the following facts:[3]

1. Certain inborn or acquired diseases accompanied by hypercholesterolemia are associated with premature atherosclerosis.

2. Serum cholesterol levels are higher than usual in persons with coronary heart disease.

3. Persons with high serum cholesterol levels develop coronary heart disease more often than those with normal levels.

4. The mortality rate from coronary heart disease in different countries varies in relation to the average blood cholesterol values (and with dietary fat and animal protein intake).

5. Experimentally induced hypercholesterolemia in animals is associated with atherosclerotic deposits.

6. Atherosclerotic plaques contain lipids similar in composition to those in the blood.

Evidence that atherosclerosis begins in childhood includes the following:

1. in autopsies of black and white males and females between 15 and 19 years old, the coronary arteries showed fatty streaks in 71 to 83% and raised atherosclerotic lesions in 7 to 22%;[4]

2. when United States soldiers killed at a mean age of 22 years were examined, 77% of those from the Korean conflict[5] and 45% of those from the Vietnam war showed evidence of coronary vessel atherosclerosis;[6]

3. children with excessively high cholesterol levels may die from coronary heart disease at an early age.

Lipoproteins

The understanding of lipoprotein metabolism has advanced in recent years. Lipoproteins are necessary to make fats soluble so they can be transported in the plasma. All lipoproteins contain an outer polar layer of phospholipid, unesterfied cholesterol, and protein (called an apoprotein). The inner, nonpolar core contains cholesterol ester and triglyceride in varying proportions. The types of lipoproteins are:

1. Chylomicrons, which are formed from dietary fat and enter the plasma via the thoracic duct. They are either removed from the blood by the activity of lipoproteinlipase (LPL) with the fatty acids stored in adipose tissue as triglyceride or are catabolized by the liver. They do not go to form other lipoproteins.

2. Very low density lipoproteins (VLDL, prebeta) are formed from dietary glucose and free fatty acids in the liver and are then secreted into the plasma. The outer surface of VLDL contains apoproteins B-100 and E. The LPL on capillary endothelium of adipose tissue and cardiac and skeletal muscle partially metabolizes the VLDL to free fatty acids for storage or for energy, with a "remnant" remaining. The apoprotein E allows the remnant to be taken up by the liver. Several types of hyperlipoproteinemia have been identified.[7]

3. If the remnant also contains apoprotein B-100, it can be used for synthesis of low density lipoprotein (LDL) in the liver.

4. Low density lipoprotein (LDL, beta lipoprotein) is formed

in the liver from VLDL remnants containing apoprotein B-100. LDL is an important source of cholesterol for peripheral tissues. As will be stated under hyperlipidemia Type IIA, LDL attaches to receptor sites on cell surfaces as an important step in the regulation of cholesterol metabolism.

5. High density lipoprotein (HDL) is secreted by the liver and small intestine. HDL is important in helping to remove cholesterol from cells (high levels are protective; low levels are a strong risk factor for coronary heart disease).

Types of Hyperlipidemia

The hereditary types of hyperlipidemias as classified by Fredrickson et al.[7] and accepted by the World Health Organization sometimes are difficult to separate from the hyperlipidemias secondary to diabetes and other conditions, but an attempt should be made to do so by family studies and other tests.

Type I

Type I hyperlipoproteinemia is found in children and is usually associated with pancreatitis and abdominal pain. The triglycerides in this disorder are primarily chylomicron triglycerides, which stay at the origin on lipoprotein electrophoresis. Lipoprotein lipase activity is diminished or absent, particularly when analyzed 10 minutes after the intravenous injection of 10 U heparin per kilogram body weight. This enzyme is responsible for hydrolysis and removal of chylomicrons from the blood. Thus the pathophysiologic mechanism is decreased triglyceride catabolism. Type I hyperlipoproteinemia is relatively rare; it may occur secondarily in children with lupus erythematosus, pancreatitis, and immunologic disorders.

Type IIA

Type IIA hyperlipoproteinemia, which consists of elevation of the serum cholesterol and LDL (or beta lipoprotein) is probably the most common of the five lipoprotein disorders to become manifest in childhood. The homozygous form can be seen during the first year of life, and the differential diagnosis can be made on the basis of:

1. serum cholesterol above 500 mg/dl,
2. LDL concentrations about twice that of heterozygotes in the same kindred,
3. both parents with elevated serum cholesterol levels,
4. xanthomas appearing before the age of 10 years,
5. vascular disease before age 20 years,
6. exclusion of clinically similar, secondary hyperlipidemias.

In the heterozygous condition, there usually are no skin xanthomas, and the serum cholesterol level is below 500 mg/dl; yet these individuals have a definite predisposition to coronary heart disease in early adult life. The basic metabolic defect is now known to be a lack of functional LDL receptors on the cell membrane, with three different classes of mutations now described.[8] As a result of the LDL not attaching to the cell membrane, cholesterol is not released to suppress the rate-limiting enzyme in cholesterol synthesis, 3-hydroxy 3-methylglutaryl coenzyme A reductase.

Type IIB

Type IIB hyperlipoproteinemia, which includes familial combined hyperlipidemia, consists of elevations of both the triglyceride and cholesterol levels, with concomitant increased LDL and VLDL (prebeta lipoprotein). This is the third most frequent of the types having onset in childhood, but the situation frequently is confusing because the parents may have other types of hyperlipoproteinemia and because of the variations in the cholesterol and triglyceride levels caused by changes in diet and exercise.

Type III

Type III hyperlipoproteinemia, "floating beta," is rare and must be diagnosed by ultracentrifugation techniques, with the LDL having an abnormal density and consisting of an abnormal protein. The onset is usually after age 20 years. The basic defect is thought to be in the conversion of VLDL to LDL (abnormal remnant catabolism) because of an abnormal apoprotein E. Increased remnants, VLDL, chylomicrons, and apoprotein E are all present. Xanthomas may occur, and early coronary and peripheral vascular disease have been reported.

Type IV

Type IV hyperlipoproteinemia is associated with elevated serum triglycerides and is the second most common of the disorders found in children, although the elevation in serum triglycerides may not occur in some patients until a later age. This condition is now frequently referred to as "familial hypertriglyceridemia," which is a monogenic autosomally inherited disorder. It involves an increase in production and secretion of triglyceride-rich VLDL. Elevated triglyceride levels can occur secondary to other factors, such as infrequent exercise, stress, an inadequate period of fasting prior to obtaining blood samples, diabetes, and obesity. It is important to establish that the patient has the genetic disease and that there is not another cause for the elevation. This is best done by studying parents and other family members as well as the patient.

Type V

Type V hyperlipoproteinemia is rare in childhood and is associated with increased triglyceride levels secondary to increased chylomicrons and increased VLDL. This condition may be primarily familial, or it may be secondary to diabetes, nephrotic syndrome, or hypothyroidism. The onset may be similar to Type I, although it occurs in adulthood rather than childhood.

Screening for Hyperlipidemia

Routine screening for hyperlipidemia in children is expensive and probably not indicated. The child must fast for 10 to 14 hours prior to obtaining the blood sample, and routine tests only for serum cholesterol levels may not be sufficient. It would be convenient to screen all infants in the neonatal period as is done for phenylketonuria, but correlations between neonatal lipid levels and levels at later ages have, unfortunately, been poor.[9] Elevated cord triglyceride levels have correlated primarily with maternal-fetal perinatal problems such as anoxia. The 95th percentile value for cord blood cholesterol and triglyceride is 100 mg/dl. After birth, cholesterol levels are higher in infants who are receiving human or cow's milk than in infants who are receiving many of the commercial infant formulas.

When parents are known carriers of Type IIA hyperlipidemia, ultracentrifugation analysis of the LDL cholesterol levels can be used to determine if the infant is affected.[10] However, this is not a practical, routine screening procedure.

Screening is usually best done by first obtaining serum cholesterol and triglyceride levels after a 10- to 14-hour fast. Normal values are shown in Appendix V. HDL cholesterol also should be measured now because this is a separate risk factor from total cholesterol or LDL cholesterol. Values vary between laboratories, but the usual, normal value is 50 ± 20 mg/dl. Some laboratories now use LDL cholesterol rather than total cholesterol. This is slightly more specific because total cholesterol includes the HDL cholesterol. In reality, either is adequate, particularly as a screening test. LDL cholesterol levels vary between the laboratory and method used, but normal values are usually in the range of 100 ± 40 mg/dl.

When elevations in serum total cholesterol (or LDL cholesterol) or triglyceride are detected, the values should be rechecked—emphasizing the importance of the fasting—after waiting at least 2 weeks.

Whom To Screen

It is not yet practical to screen all children for hyperlipidemia; this procedure should be restricted to certain "high-risk" groups: children with high familial risk, children with diabetes, obese children, those on special high-protein athletic diets, and those with certain other childhood diseases.

Children with High Familial Risk

Children whose parents are known to have hyperlipidemia should be tested; likewise, children whose serum is creamy in the fasting state and those with skin xanthomas need to be investigated. The largest group of high-risk children are those whose parents have had an early heart attack. Two of three adults who had a heart attack prior to age 50 had hyperlipidemia.[11] Type IV hyperlipidemia was the most common and was found in 40% of the coronary heart disease victims, Type IIB was found in 14%, and Type IIA was found in 12%. Twenty-nine percent of the children in these families had elevated lipid levels. The most frequent abnormality in the offspring was the Type IV disorder (found in 16%). Type IIA was found in 10%, and Type IIB was found in 3%. Similar findings were described from Cincinnati,[12] where 31% of the offspring of parents who had a heart attack prior to age 50 years were found to have hyperlipidemia. A routine family history always should include information about early heart attacks.

Children with Diabetes

Serum cholesterol and triglyceride levels frequently are elevated in children with insulin-dependent diabetes mellitus,[13] especially in those in poor glucose control. With the known increased risk for atherosclerosis in adults with diabetes, it seems wise to perform blood lipid tests for children with diabetes annually. If elevated lipid levels are found, glucose control should be optimized, and the diet should be evaluated for fat and cholesterol intake.

Obese Children

Obesity in children is a risk factor because of the association between adult obesity and ischemic heart disease and the knowledge that approximately 80% of obese children become obese adults. Studies in obese adults have shown an increased incidence of elevated serum cholesterol and triglyceride levels; and a report from Australia found high triglyceride levels in 18 of 129 obese children and high cholesterol levels in three of them.[14] Others have failed to find such abnormalities in obese children.

Although further studies of the relationship between childhood obesity and hyperlipidemia are indicated, it seems prudent to routinely screen children who are grossly obese, particularly if it is of long duration. Children undergoing a rapid weight change should reach a steady weight level before serum lipids are checked. The same applies to the sedentary child who is to begin an exercise program because triglyceride levels decrease after exercise.

Diets for Athletes

Teen-age boys receiving high-protein diets for various athletic programs are of some concern. They frequently consume large amounts of eggs and protein supplements, in addition to the usual large quantities of meat and milk. Tests for hyperlipidemia are indicated when a history of this type of eating pattern is obtained.[15]

Other Childhood Diseases

The hyperlipidemia of von Gierke's disease can be reduced by continuous nocturnal feedings. Chronic pancreatitis occurs in childhood, and Type I hyperlipoproteinemia with elevated chylomicrons must be excluded.

Children with obstructive liver disease frequently have xanthoma and high cholesterol levels, which sometimes will respond to phenobarbital therapy. Children with nephrotic syndrome and those receiving corticosteroids may have increased cholesterol levels. Hypercholesterolemia also occurs in hypothyroidism and has been found in patients with immunoglobulin deficiency states.

Treatment

Therapy should be initiated after the diagnosis of hyperlipidemia is confirmed by two separate blood tests done at least 2 weeks apart. Dietary therapy is the first mode of treatment in almost all instances whether or not they are of genetic etiology. It is extremely helpful if the patient (or parent if the child is too young) keeps a 3-day diet record prior to suggesting changes; this record should be as typical as possible of the child's usual intake.

Handbooks for the dietary treatment of the different types of hyperlipoproteinemia are available from the National Institutes of Health. However, in recent years there has been a trend toward using one type of diet in the initial treatment of all types of hyperlipidemia.[16] Regardless of which approach is used, some general guidelines apply:

1. Know what the patient is eating.
2. Reduce energy intake to that recommended for age.
3. Reduce total fat to approximately 30% of the energy intake.
4. Reduce cholesterol intake initially to 300 mg per day.
5. Reduce saturated (animal) fat and increase polyunsaturated (vegetable) fat. A ratio of polyunsaturated to saturated fats (P/S ratio) of at least 1.0 is desirable.
6. Increase complex carbohydrates and fiber. This usually means eating more fruits, vegetables, and whole grain foods.

If hypercholesterolemia is present, the intake of total fat (particularly of animal fats) and cholesterol must be decreased. The cholesterol content of foods is shown in Appendix R. Once the P/S ratio is obtained from the initial diet record, suggestions can be made on ways to decrease the saturated fat intake while increasing the polyunsaturated fat intake. In one study, reduction in cholesterol intake alone resulted in a 5% decrease in serum cholesterol levels, while substitution of polyunsaturated fats for saturated fats lowered the level by 22%.[17] Most nutritionists now believe that the reduction in saturated fat is more important than an increase in polyunsaturated fat.

The maximum cholesterol lowering effect of diet is in the range of 25%. Thus, most patients with cholesterol levels higher than 300 mg/dl also will eventually require treatment with drugs. Dietary therapy usually is attempted for a 6-month period; the serum cholesterol levels and 3-day diet records are repeated approximately every 2 months. The beneficial effects of weight loss and daily exercise on lowering triglyceride levels should not be forgotten.

The drug therapy of hyperlipidemia cannot be reviewed thoroughly here. Medications usually are not used in children less than 4 years old unless the hyperlipidemia is severe. This is because of the chance possibility that incorporation of cholesterol into myelin could be lessened. Most advertisements for lipid-lowering agents carry a disclaimer regarding effects on morbidity or mortality from atherosclerosis or coronary heart disease.

Resin therapy (cholestyramine or colestipol) is usually the first medication to be tried. These drugs increase bile acid excretion (the major product of cholesterol breakdown) and prevent the reabsorption of cholesterol substrate.[18] Cholestyramine may bind other medications (thyroid, digitalis, coumadin). Nausea and unpleasant taste are the two major problems.

Clofibrate (Atromid-S or ethylchlorophenoxyisobutyrate) probably acts by decreasing synthesis of cholesterol or triglycerides, although other mechanisms have been suggested. The drug is relatively easy to take (in contrast to cholestyramine). Side effects include nausea and, less commonly, alopecia, leukopenia, agranulocytosis, muscle pain, and increased SGOT or CPK levels. Other medications such as gemfibrozil, nicotinic acid, and dextrothyroxine have been used with less frequency in pediatric patients, although gemfibrozil may soon become the drug of choice for treating hypertriglyceridemia. It decreases serum triglyceride and cholesterol levels and increases the HDL level. It is available in 300 mg capsules; the usual dose is one or two capsules 30 minutes before breakfast and the evening meal. Close laboratory surveillance is necessary.

References

1. Kannel, W.B., Castelli, W.P., and Gordon, T.: Cholesterol in the prediction of atherosclerotic disease: New perspectives based on the Framingham study. Ann. Intern. Med., 90:85, 1979.
2. Carlson, L.A., and Böttinger, L.E.: Ischaemic heart-disease in relation to fasting values of plasma triglycerides and cholesterol: Stockholm prospective study. Lancet, 1:865, 1972.
3. Committee on Nutrition: Childhood diet and coronary heart disease. PEDIATRICS, 49:305, 1972.
4. Strong, J.P., and McGill, H.C., Jr.: The pediatric aspects of atherosclerosis. J. Atheroscler. Res., 9:251, 1969.
5. Enos, W.F., Jr., Beyer, J.C., and Holmes, R.H.: Pathogenesis of coronary disease in American soldiers killed in Korea. J.A.M.A., 158:912, 1955.
6. McNamara, J.J., Molot, M.A., Stremple, J.F., and Cutting, R.T.: Coronary artery disease in combat casualties in Vietnam. J.A.M.A., 216:1185, 1971.
7. Fredrickson, D.S., Goldstein, J.L., and Brown, M.S.: The familial hyperlipoproteinemias. In Stanbury, J.B., Wyngaarden, J.B., and Fredrickson, D.S., ed.: The Metabolic Basis of Inherited Disease, ed. 4. New York: McGraw-Hill Book Company, pp. 604-655, 1978.
8. Goldstein, J.L., and Brown, M.S.: The LDL receptor defect in fa-

milial hypercholesterolemia: Implications for pathogenesis and therapy. Med. Clin. N. Amer., **66**:335, 1982.

9. Darmady, J.M., Fosbrooke, A.S., and Lloyd, J.K.: Prospective study of serum cholesterol levels during first year of life. Brit. Med. J., **2**:685, 1972.

10. Kwiterovich, P.O., Jr., Levy, R.I., and Fredrickson, D.S.: Neonatal diagnosis of familial type-II hyperlipoproteinaemia. Lancet, **1**:118, 1973.

11. Chase, H.P., O'Quin, R.J., and O'Brien, D.: Screening for hyperlipidemia in childhood. J.A.M.A., **230**:1535, 1974.

12. Glueck, C.J., Fallat, R.W., Tsang, R., and Buncher, C.R.: Hyperlipemia in progeny of parents with myocardial infarction before age 50. Amer. J. Dis. Child., **127**:70, 1974.

13. Chase, H.P., and Glasgow, A.M.: Juvenile diabetes mellitus and serum lipids and lipoprotein levels. Amer. J. Dis. Child., **130**:1113, 1976.

4. Court, J.M., Dunlop, M., and Leonard, R.F.: Plasma lipid values in childhood obesity. Austral. Paediat. J., **10**:10, 1974.

15. Committee on Sports Medicine: Sports Medicine: Health Care for Young Athletes. Evanston, Illinois: American Academy of Pediatrics, pp. 161-175, 1983.

16. Connor, W.E., and Connor, S.L.: The dietary treatment of hyperlipidemia: Rationale, technique, and efficacy. Med. Clin. N. Amer., **66**:485, 1982.

17. Anderson, J.T., Grande, F., and Keys, A.: Independence of the effects of cholesterol and degree of saturation of the fat in the diet on serum cholesterol in man. Amer. J. Clin. Nutr., **29**:1184, 1976.

18. Glueck, C.J., Fallat, R., and Tsang, R.: Pediatric familial type II hyperlipoproteinemia: Therapy with diet and cholestyramine resin. PEDIATRICS, **52**:669, 1973.

Chapter 28

OBESITY

Obesity is the most important nutritional disorder in the United States today. Children as well as adults are afflicted, and prevalence figures range from 10 to 30%. Whether obesity is more or less prevalent than in former times is not known, but it has existed throughout recorded history and occurs in many cultures. Present-day concerns about obesity relate both to the social unacceptability and the health hazard. The fact that childhood obesity may persist into the adult years makes the condition especially challenging to those caring for children.

Methods now available for the estimation of body fat content include calculations based on total water or potassium content and densitometry. Because these techniques are too cumbersome for routine use, many investigators use the weight:height ratio, body mass index (W/H^2), or skinfold thickness (caliper measurement of double layer of skin plus subcutaneous tissue) as criteria.

Although weight and weight for height relationship are useful for large scale surveys (see Appendix A), they have the obvious disadvantage of being influenced by the size of the lean body mass and the fat mass. Skinfold thickness, usually measured at the mid-triceps region or at the tip of the scapula, yields an estimate of amount of subcutaneous fat and helps to avoid the problem of intersubject differences in lean weight (see Appendix E).

Humans are among the fattest of mammals. The neonate is about 14% fat, and by 18 years of age the average boy is about 12% fat and the girl about 25% fat. The changes in triceps skinfold thickness which take place during infancy, childhood, and adolescence are shown in Figure 12.

The definition of obesity is arbitrary. For instance, use of the 90th percentile for triceps skinfold thickness automatically means that 10% of the reference population is judged to be obese. However, from the practical standpoint, obesity can be recognized at a glance.

The essential cause of obesity is energy imbalance. Intake of food energy exceeds expenditure, and the excess is stored as fat because adipose tissue is the only organ capable of storing large amounts of energy.* Knittle[2] found that the increase in the amount of adipose tissue in obese children is associated with an increase in both adipocyte size and total adipocyte number, while adult-onset obesity is associated only with increased cell size.[3] Other studies have shown that both cell size and cell number increase in proportion to total body fat content.[4] In the normal, nongrowing individual, the potential energy contained in food is rather precisely converted to kinetic energy (muscle work, metabolic work, and heat), with the result that body weight does not vary more than 1 or 2% over long intervals of time. In the normal child, the accumulation of potential energy represented by the addition of new tissue is likewise a finely regulated process. Despite protestations to the contrary, there is no evidence that the laws of thermodynamics and conservation of energy have been abrogated. The human body must possess a finely tuned set of mechanisms for precisely matching energy balance. Obesity represents a failure of these mechanisms.

The nature of these mechanisms is only partly understood. At the physiologic level there are: (1) the perception of hunger, an innate, unconditioned, physiologic response to the need for food, mediated in part by gastric contractions and the levels of blood glucose and amino acids; and (2) the perception of satiety, which gives a signal that enough food has been consumed for the moment. Studies in experimental animals suggest that both of these are mediated by regions in the hypothalamus.

Another mechanism, most certainly located in centers higher than the hypothalamus, is that of appetite. In contrast to hunger, appetite is a learned psychologic phenomenon involving pleasurable anticipation and is a mechanism for dealing with emotional rather than nutritional needs. In the obese state, appetite phenomena override those of hunger and satiety, and food is consumed in excess of nutritional need.

The contributing causes to obesity are many and are, to a certain extent, a product of modern society. For the first time in centuries, Western society has an abundance of food; and it is food of high biologic quality, widely distributed, and attractively advertised. Economic data show that the individual needs to labor fewer hours to feed a family than in former days. In their zeal to see that no one is underfed, modern nutritionists recommend nutrient intakes higher than those considered

---

*A distinctive form of adipose tissue known as brown fat is present in small quantities in the thoracic region of newborn infants (and even smaller quantities in children and adults); it is responsive to catecholamines, and its principle function is to contribute to nonshivering thermogenesis.

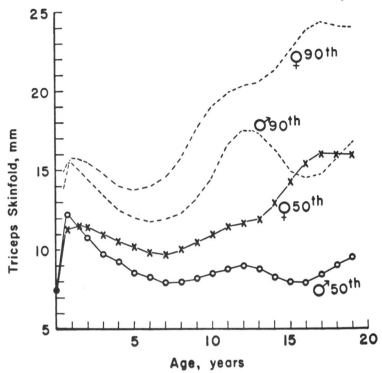

Figure 12. Age changes in subcutaneous fat. Median and 90th percentile values for triceps skinfold thickness (redrawn from Tanner and Whitehouse¹).

the average requirement.† Serious gastrointestional infections, which are known to cause nitrogen wastage, are now relatively infrequent. Breast feeding, which for many infants limits their milk intake, has been less common; and solid foods are offered to infants at an earlier age. School lunch programs are widespread. Although there are individuals who, for one reason or another, are truly in want, the vast majority of individuals in the United States have an abundance of food at their disposal.

Opportunities for significant energy expenditure have declined in recent decades, e.g., suburban living, with its dependence on the automobile; discouragement by heavy traffic of

†When based on data from dietary surveys, the extent of "undernutrition" for any nutrient in any population group is directly proportional to the level of the National Research Council's Recommended Dietary Allowances.

walking and cycling; labor-saving devices of all sorts, both at home and at work; the single story house; high-heeled shoes for women; school buses; and the decline of walking as a pastime. All these factors conspire to make it easier for the modern citizen—adult and child alike—to eat more and exercise less, and hence to achieve a positive energy balance.

A metabolic explanation of obesity has been sought for many years. This search was stimulated in recent years by the discovery of animal models: the obese hyperglycemic mouse, the Zucker rat, the animal with an ACTH-secreting tumor or who is subjected to lesions of the hypothalamus or to injections of gold thioglucose. In humans, hyperadrenocorticism, either induced or the result of disease, leads to excessive accumulation of body fat, as does on occasion hypothyroidism. The Prader-Willi syndrome, associated in some individuals with an abnormality in chromosome 15, includes muscular hypotonia, delayed psychomotor development, hypogonadism, and latent diabetes in addition to obesity. Syndromes of this type account for only a tiny fraction of the total obese population.

Metabolic aberrations have indeed been observed in many obese individuals. These include relative insulin resistance; a blunted plasma growth hormone response to stimuli, such as hypoglycemia and arginine infusion; a modest increase in urinary excretion of adrenocortical steroids; a diabetic-type of oral glucose tolerance curve; and a tendency to high blood levels of insulin and to hypertension. Many of these aberrations can be induced in humans by overeating and will disappear when excess weight is lost. They represent the consequences of obesity, not its cause. It is well to dispel some of the myths which surround the obese state.

1. Food is not diverted to fat in an abnormal fashion; rather, obese individuals have a normal or moderately increased lean weight, and statural growth is slightly accelerated. The relative increment in statural growth is roughly proportional to the degree of obesity. Human obesity thus differs from certain types of experimental obesity; rats subjected to lesions of the hypothalamus have a lower lean weight and are shorter in length than the controls.

2. There is no evidence that the diet of obese individuals involves an abnormal distribution of calories. The mere fact that obese children grow taller and manifest an increase in lean weight is evidence that their diet is adequate in protein and other essential nutrients.

3. Obese individuals lose weight in a predictable fashion when they are subjected to dietary restriction under controlled conditions.

4. There is no incontrovertible evidence that the thermogenic response of obese individuals to food is abnormal.

5. Despite many statements to the contrary, obese individuals eat more than their thin peers when food intake is monitored at home.[4]

A number of factors have been associated with obesity; and, although none have been identified as truly causative, the fact they exist suggests avenues for research. These include (1) social class, to which the prevalence of obesity is inversely related; (2) sex, women and girls are more frequently affected than men and boys; (3) rapid weight gain in infancy, these infants are somewhat more prone to obesity later on;[5] and (4) presence of obesity in the family.

The last factor raises the question of genetic predisposition. Relative fatness in mammals is species dependent, and obese strains have been identified within certain species. Identical twins have a greater degree of concordance for both body weight and skinfold thickness than nonidentical, like-sexed twins. However, feeding habits, and probably exercise habits, may represent the effects of early conditioning by the family, so the relative importance of genetics and environment is hard to quantitate.

A common observation is that some individuals tend to put on weight in certain life situations: cessation of smoking, job or school dissatisfaction, depression, frustrated career goals, emigration, parental or peer disapproval, and so forth. This led to the hypothesis that overeating or normal eating with reduced physical activity, both of which can be construed as abnormal appetite, represent a coping or adaptive mechanism. It may become a compulsion.

As Hilde Bruch so aptly stated, "Whether we like it or not . . . we must learn to recognize that for many people overeating and being fat is a balancing factor in their adjustment to life. Ineffective as it is, it represents the best form of adaptation that such people have been able to make. . . . Without the comfort of eating, life may become so threatening and lacking in any satisfaction there is danger of serious mental illness if reducing is enforced."[6] Later this perceptive student of obesity commented that excessive feeding may have been perceived as cementing the child-mother relationship; and that, for the older child, a large body size may confer a sense of self-importance. These children frequently have been treated as precious possessions from their earliest years bv frustrated, and often obese, parents whose only response to their children's needs was to stuff them with food.

These considerations go far in explaining some of the cardinal features of obesity, namely, the vain hope that help can come without dietary restriction, the tendency to invest "reducing" pills and "fad" diets with magic properties, the high rate of treatment failure, and the proclivity for childhood obesity to continue into adult life. These considerations also help to explain the role of denial in the obese individual's perception of his or her situation by claims such as, "I don't really eat that much," "I must be eating the wrong kind of food," "there must be something wrong with my metabolism," and so on.

Prevention

The tendency for childhood obesity to persist into the adult years is well-known. Recent evidence suggests that overweight infants are more likely to become obese adults than are thin infants.[5] Thus, it is possible to identify at an early age those who are at risk: those born to obese parents, those who gain weight rapidly during infancy, and those whose mothers use food as a means of controlling behavior.

Reasonable, though as yet unproven, preventive measures include: (1) breast feeding;[7] (2) delay in introduction of solid foods and counseling of mothers to give food only in response to hunger, not as a pacifier; a reorientation of family life toward low calorie foods and the ritualization of total mealtime behavior; and (3) the promotion of physical exercise. Incidentally, skimmed milk is an inappropriate food for the young infant because of its high solute to caloric ratio.

Hilde Bruch's advice again deserves careful consideration: Obesity can be prevented, "If a child is fed when hungry, played with when needing attention, and encouraged to be active when restless, he or she is not likely to grow up inhibited and passive, or overstuffed and helpless, unable to control eating because every discomfort is misinterpreted as need to eat."[8]

Treatment

Diet Therapy

Dietary restriction will be necessary for most obese individuals if weight is to be lost. However, even under the best of circumstances, the rate of loss is distressingly slow. Aside from the first few days, obese adults who fast lose only about 0.5 kg per day. Reported experiences with obese adolescents fed 600 to 1,100 kcal diets for several months[9,10] show an average weight loss of 0.16 kg per day. Body fat is a high caloric fuel, with an energy content (per gram) comparable to gasoline.

The caloric requirement depends on the age and sex of the individual. For the relatively inactive adolescent girl, anything over 1,200 kcal is unlikely to result in significant weight loss, whereas a moderately active, adolescent boy may do well and possibly avoid compromise of statural growth on 1,500 kcal. An 800 kcal diet is appropriate for young children. There is no evidence that calorie for calorie the various "fad" diets offer any advantage.

Extremely low-energy diets (300 to 600 kcal per day)— including those which provide generous amounts of protein ("protein-sparing modified fast")—are not without risk. Some lean weight is inevitably lost, and cardiac arrhythmias[11] and sudden death have been recorded in adults.[12]

The lists in Appendix S can be used as a rough guide for dietary advice and as a basis for indoctrinating patients and parents on food values. Special attention should be given to vitamin and mineral needs, especially iron. The advice of a trained dietitian is helpful. It frequently is necessary to involve the entire family in dietary counseling.

Exercise Therapy

Many obese individuals are relatively inactive, and many resist efforts at encouraging exercise. Public schools should provide special programs for obese youngsters. Remember that a brisk walk consumes as much as 250 kcal per hour. See Table 6 on page 61 for energy cost of exercise.

Psychologic Therapy

A prescription of diet and exercise does little good unless the patient can be induced to curb his or her appetite.[13,14]

The child with "situational" obesity developed in response to an immediate stress deserves an understanding of the problem, reassurance and support, emphasis on the potentially satisfying aspects of his or her life, and help in dealing with the problem. The setting of a realistic weight goal may be helpful, and parental counseling is important. Behavior modification, both on an individual and group basis, is currently gaining in popularity. Several recent publications provide details.[15,16] Lay organizations—TOPS, Weight Watchers, Diet Workshop, and so forth—appeal to many adults but, unfortunately, are not geared to children.

Appetite-suppressant drugs and thyroid preparations are of little help.

The "developmental" type of obesity, which so often includes long-established, compulsive eating, is another story. Both Hamburger[17] and Bruch[14] have cautioned against enforced weight loss in these patients because some will then develop more serious emotional disturbances. Attempts to improve physical activity are rarely successful, appetite suppressants have only a temporary effect, and "formula" diets may be resented. This is the "hard core" group whose life adjustment centers around the process of eating and who are caught in the dualistic trap of hyperphagia and inactivity. Psychiatric referral may be necessary. There may be a question about whether a diet should even be attempted. Hamburger stated, "Despite a decreased life expectancy, obesity relating to addiction to food may be a healthier adaptation than addiction to alcohol or other drugs, or to serious depression."[17]

Other Forms of Treatment

Fasting leads to rapid weight loss, as does the intestinal by-pass operation and the gastric stapling procedure. These procedures involve certain hazards, and experience with them in children is limited enough that their use should not be advocated for children, except under extreme circumstances.[18]

Prognosis

Although some weight is lost at first, the long-term success rate for treatment of obesity is poor; and it remains to be seen whether efforts at prevention will be effective.

References

1. Tanner, J.M., and Whitehouse, R.H.: Revised standards for triceps and subscapular skinfolds in British children. Arch. Dis. Child., **50**:142, 1975.
2. Knittle, J.L.: In general discussion. *In* McKigney, J.I., and Munro, H.N., ed.: Nutrient Requirements in Adolescence. Cambridge, Massachusetts: M.I.T. Press, pp. 76-83, 1976.
3. Salans, L.B., Cushman, S.W., and Weismann, R.E.: Studies of human adipose tissue: Adipose cell size and number in non-obese patients. J. Clin. Invest., **52**:929, 1973.
4. Stunkard, A.J., ed.: Obesity. Philadelphia: W.B. Saunders, 1980.
5. Charney, E., Goodman, H.G., McBride, M., Lyon, B., and Pratt, R.: The childhood antecedents of obesity: Do chubby infants become obese adults? New Engl. J. Med., **295**:6, 1976.
6. Bruch, H.: Psychiatric aspects of obesity. Metabolism, **6**:461, 1957.
7. Mann, G.V.: The influence of obesity on health. New Engl. J. Med., **291**:178 and 226, 1974.
8. Bruch, H.: The importance of overweight. *In* Collipp, P.J., ed.: Childhood Obesity. Acton, Massachusetts: Publishing Sciences Group, pp. 75-81, 1975.
9. Archibald, E.H., Harrison, J.E., and Pencharz, P.B.: Effect of a weight-reducing high-protein diet on the body composition of obese adolescents. Amer. J. Dis. Child., **137**:658, 1983.
10. Brown, M.R., Klish, W.J., Hollander, J., Campbell, M.A., and Forbes, G.B.: A high protein, low calorie liquid diet in the treatment of very obese adolescents: Long-term effect on lean body mass. Amer. J. Clin. Nutr., **38**:20, 1983.
11. Lantigua, R.A., Amatruda, J.M., Biddle, T.L., Forbes, G.B., and Lockwood, D.H.: Cardiac arrhythmias associated with a liquid protein diet for the treatment of obesity. New Engl. J. Med., **303**:735, 1980.
12. Isner, J.M., Sours, H.E., Paris, A.L., Ferrans, V.J., and Roberts, W.C.: Sudden, unexpected death in avid dieters using the liquid-protein-modified-fast diet.: Observations in 17 patients and the role of the prolonged QT interval. Circulation, **60**:1401, 1979.
13. Bray, G.A., ed.: Obesity in Perspective. DHEW Publication No. (NIH) 75-708. Washington, D.C.: U.S. Government Printing Office, 1976.
14. Bruch, H.: Eating Disorders: Obesity, Anorexia Nervosa, and the Person Within. New York: Basic Books, 1973.
15. Stuart, R.B., and Davis, B.: Slim Chance in a Fat World: Behavioral Control of Obesity. Champaign, Illinois: Research Press, 1972.
16. Brownell, K.D., and Stunkard, A.J.: Behavioral treatment of obesity in children. Amer. J. Dis. Child., **132**:403, 1978.
17. Hamburger, W.W.: Psychological aspects of obesity, Bull. N.Y. Acad. Med., **33**:771, 1957.

18. Joffe, S.N.: Surgical management of morbid obesity, Gut, **22**:242, 1981.

Bibliography

Garrow, J.S.: Energy Balance and Obesity in Man. New York: North Holland Publishing Company, 1974.
Schemmel, R., ed.: Nutrition, Physiology, and Obesity. Boca Raton, Florida: CRC Press, 1980.

Chapter 29

HYPERSENSITIVITY TO FOOD

Faulty diagnosis of hypersensitivity to food can be a hazard to attainment of optimal nutrition through unwarranted elimination of items from the diet or by failure to identify truly harmful food. Error can be minimized and management of food hypersensitivity made less troublesome by the orderly application of a few rational considerations.

Definition

Hypersensitivity is a term restricted by custom to an immunologic state in which alteration in response to antigenic material has developed after repeated exposure, that is, the individual has become sensitized. The hypersensitivity reactions may depend on elaboration of antibodies or on changed responsiveness of cells. Only reactions to food based on immunologic mechanisms should properly be designated hypersensitivity.

Hypersensitivity and Allergy

The terms hypersensitivity and allergy were once synonymous, but allergy has now been loosely applied to various symptoms claimed to result from foods, additives in foods, or hypothetical derangements of metabolism. Conspicuous among these are ill-defined, largely subjective conditions designated "tension-fatigue" and "hyperactivity." The proponents of this concept have freely used allergy as a descriptive term without providing evidence of an immunologic basis. To separate true hypersensitivity to food from these confusing situations, the term allergy will be avoided. This chapter will cover only genuine hypersensitivity to food on an immunologic basis and to substantiated rather than conjectural manifestations.

Are the Symptoms Caused by Actual Hypersensitivity to Food?

Symptoms associated with ingestion of foods may stem from parasitic or chemical contaminants, deficiencies of digestive enzymes, psychologic aversion, hypersensitivity, and other causes. Before grasping at hypersensitivity as a diagnosis, the physician should consider other possibilities for adverse reactions to food.

Hypersensitivity Reactions to Food

Manifestations commonly ascribed to hypersensitivity to food, but not exclusively due to this cause, are:

1. Systemic—anaphylaxis, failure to thrive.
2. Gastrointestinal—vomiting, abdominal pain, diarrhea, malabsorption, enteropathies.
3. Respiratory—rhinitis, sinusitis, secretory otitis media, cough, wheezing, pulmonary infiltration.
4. Cutaneous—rash, urticaria, atopic dermatitis.

Hypersensitivity reactions to food may be categorized according to the interval between ingestion and appearance of symptoms: immediate (minutes to 2 hours) or delayed (more than 2 hours, usually within 48 hours). According to current hypothesis, these intervals may be associated with corresponding immunologic mechanisms involving IgE (immediate) and, possibly, IgG and IgM and immune complexes containing IgG and IgM (delayed). Any of the manifestations may occur at any period of infancy and childhood.

Diagnosis of Hypersensitivity to Food

A diagnosis of hypersensitivity to food requires: (1) verification that the food in question causes an adverse reaction, (2) exclusion of other causes of adverse reactions, and (3) identification of immunologic sensitization.

Complete delineation of the immunologic basis may be an

elaborate undertaking, which is not essential to practical management but necessary for full comprehension. The practitioner may have to be satisfied with certain signs of an immunologic pathogenesis, as will be discussed later.

Confirmation of Food as the Cause of Symptoms

Various symptoms are commonly ascribed to some food recently eaten. A feeble suspicion readily becomes a strong conviction, especially when no objective test is applied. An unwarranted enthusiasm can lead to overzealous incrimination of foods as the basis of many complaints.

The role of food in the production of symptoms must be confirmed by some arrangement that excludes the bias of the subject and observers. A double-blind food challenge may be necessary if errors in the diagnosis of adverse reactions to food and needless dietary restrictions are to be avoided. In some instances the simpler challenge-withdrawal test will provide the same information.

Food Challenge

With infants and children up to 6 years old, the suspected food may be successfully masqueraded by mixing it with some other food.* For older children, the suspected food or a placebo must be administered in opaque capsules. These are filled by someone other than the subject or observer and designated by a code number. The most common offenders can be obtained in the dry state (e.g., milk, eggs, wheat, peanuts). Wet foods can be freeze-dried and powdered.

Prior to the challenge, the suspected foods are excluded from the diet until symptoms subside. If the foods which may be causing symptoms are unknown, a diet of foods unlikely to cause hypersensitivity may be given (see the Addendum at the end of this chapter). The capsules are swallowed, under close supervision, just before a meal. The restricted diet is provided in regular meals during the period of observation.

---

*Warning: It is unnecessary and unsafe to test a food believed to have caused an anaphylactic reaction.

The test dose in the capsules is chosen according to the impressiveness of the history and ranges from 20 to 2,000 mg as an initial dose. With immediate-type hypersensitivity, symptoms will occur within 2 hours. If no reaction occurs, the amount in the capsules may be increased 2- to 10-fold in subsequent challenges. If 8 gm of a test dose cause no symptoms, usual portions of the food can be added openly to the diet without expectation of an immediate-type reaction. Eight grams of dried food represents between 20 and 160 gm of wet food. If symptoms occur after ingestion of the food capsules, a placebo of glucose-containing capsules usually is not needed. If only subjective complaints or vomiting occur, a challenge with a placebo capsule will be required for clarification. A single, unequivocal reaction in a double-blind challenge may be considered as definitive evidence of an adverse reaction to the food, but it is not necessarily because of an immunologic process.

The oft-repeated dictum that precipitation of symptoms by a food on three occasions can be accepted as evidence of hypersensitivity is misleading. Other mechanisms of adverse reactions, such as deficiency of digestive enzymes, would be expected to produce similar behavior.

With the use of blind food challenges in confirmation of delayed-type reactions, the elimination diet should be continued as long as an adverse reaction is thought to have occurred after ingestion of suspected food. Double-blind food challenge is particularly needed for confirmation of delayed adverse reactions to food because the long interval between ingestion and supposed reaction makes the association prone to error. The elimination diet, although not suitable for long-term use, can be used in the food challenge period without concern.

The testing of suspected foods by double-blind challenges may seem elaborate, yet it can be highly rewarding. In many instances adverse reactions to foods elicited by history will not be confirmed, and incriminated foods can be restored to the diet. Neurotic and subjective complaints are especially susceptible to erroneous association with foods eaten; this can be verified easily through blind challenges.

Differential Diagnosis

When an adverse reaction to a food has been confirmed by blind challenge, the customary procedures to differentiate the various causes of disturbances of the gastrointestinal, respiratory, or cutaneous systems; enzyme deficiencies; cystic fibrosis; infections; and immunologic deficiencies from hypersensitivity disorders must be used. The diagnosis of hypersensitivity must be supported by detection of immunologic sensitization to be conclusive.

Identification of an Immunologic Basis for an Adverse Reaction to Food

At present, a convenient technique for identification of a definitive component of the immunologic basis for a hypersensitivity reaction to food is available only for immediate-type hypersensitivity, which may be the commonest type. The immunologic mechanisms responsible for delayed-type hypersensitivity reactions have not been elucidated sufficiently to permit selection of a definitive means of identification.

Symptoms of immediate-type hypersensitivity are caused by release of mediators (histamine) when food antigen combines with specific IgE antibody attached to basophile and mast cells. In children more than 3 years old, this type of hypersensitivity to food may be identified by a specific wheal and flare reaction in the skin induced by injection of antigenic material from a suspected food. Certain precautions have been found necessary to make skin tests with food extracts trustworthy. Commercially prepared extracts must be subjected to verification. This means finding a source of properly prepared extracts and determining the concentration and technique which will cause no reactions in the skin of persons not hypersensitive but which will produce wheal and flare responses in hypersensitive individuals.

Extracts of 20 foods commonly considered to cause hypersensitivity (produced by Greer Laboratories, Lenoir, North Carolina) were examined, and a 3 mm or greater wheal from use of a 1:20 weight:volume concentration in a skin test (puncture technique) detected the degree of hypersensitivity liable to be associated with a clinical reaction on ingestion of the food.[1]

Use of greater concentrations of food extracts or intradermal injections frequently will evoke wheal and flare reactions which may be indicative of hypersensitivity but of too low a degree to be associated with symptoms after ingestion of the food in double-blind challenge. This procedure reduces the need for food challenges to a relatively small number of the individuals suspected of hypersensitivity reactions. Smaller wheal reactions to intradermal skin tests should be viewed as examples of asymptomatic hypersensitivity to food which is of no clinical consequence and does not require dietary restrictions. By use of verified extracts with appropriate concentration and technique—and bearing in mind the distinction between symptomatic and asymptomatic hypersensitivity—the prevalent confusion about "false-positive" skin tests can be avoided. A properly performed, negative skin test with a verified food extract eliminates hypersensitivity to that food as a cause of immediate-type, clinical adverse reactions to the food. A supposed clinical reaction to a food frequently will not be confirmed by a double-blind food challenge; at other times the reaction may be found to be caused by something other than hypersensitivity.

Diagnostic Approach Summarized

When an impressive history of an adverse reaction to a food is obtained:

1. For children more than 3 years old—Apply puncture skin test with 1:20 food extract. If the net wheal response is less than 3 mm in diameter, significant clinical sensitivity to the food does not exist. If the net wheal response is more than 3 mm, perform a double-blind food challenge to ascertain if the reaction is clinically significant.

2. For children less than 3 years old—Perform a double-blind food challenge; and, if positive, perform skin tests as described here to determine if the reaction is based on immediate-type, immunologic sensitization.

---

†The pediatrician's success and pleasure in improving precision in diagnosis and management of hypersensitivity to foods will be greatly enhanced by learning the correct use of extracts of a small number of foods. Verified extracts of the following will probably serve to identify most infants and children with truly clinically significant, symptomatic, immediate-type hypersensitivity to food: cow's milk, whole egg, wheat, peanut (or other nuts), fish mix, shell fish mix. Chocolate is a traditional, rarely convicted suspect. Control tests with extraction fluid and histamine solutions must be applied regularly. **Do not** test with extracts of foods believed to have caused anaphylactic reactions. A careful history may indicate whether additional foods are worthy of consideration.

Other Methods for Diagnosis of Hypersensitivity to Food

Radioallergosorbent Test

Recently the radioallergosorbent test (RAST) was developed for the estimation of specific IgE in serum. The level of specific IgE reflects the degree of sensitization. As with the skin test, RAST reveals that only the higher degrees of hypersensitivity are correlated with clinical symptoms on exposure to the antigen. RAST has no practical advantage over skin tests performed as described here, except when the skin is unsuitable, as in patients with widespread atopic dermatitis. RAST requires the same verification suggested for skin tests, is much more costly, and requires radioactive materials and elaborate instrumentation.

Serum Antibodies

Antibodies to food proteins in serum may be assayed by various methods (e.g., precipitins, hemagglutinations, isotopic labeling) which detect IgG or IgM antibodies. These antibodies appear whenever foreign protein reaches the cells of an immunocompetent person and are prevalent in the sera of normal infants and individuals hypersensitive to any food. Therefore, the interpretation requires caution, even when titers of specific antibodies are high. The tests are not recommended as useful to pediatricians at present, and they are not generally available except in research laboratories.

Treatment

Rational treatment must be based on a correct diagnosis. A clinically significant hypersensitivity to food may be far less common than generally supposed. Probably a relatively small number of foods are responsible for the majority of confirmable hypersensitivity reactions to foods. The long-term elimination of staple items such as milk, eggs, and wheat should be done only when clearly justified by proper diagnostic procedures. For children, an elimination diet free of milk, eggs, wheat, and the most common offenders (see the Addendum at the end of this chapter) can be used empirically as a trial treatment for up to 1 month without concern for nutrition; but, when this type of diet is used for longer periods, it should be supplemented with the daily requirements of calcium, iron, and vitamins. The actual intake of protein and calories should be calculated periodically to ascertain adequacy. Of course, infants may be reared successfully the first 6 months of life with only a commercial infant formula based on soybean protein. Formulas based on digested milk protein also are available. An elemental diet based on amino acids, which contains no antigenic substances, is available for use in extreme instances. Many foods of low nutritional value can be withheld from the diet one or two at a time without threat to optimal nutrition.

Elimination diets, recipes, and special products can be obtained from the sources listed in the Addendum at the end of this chapter.

Exclusion of a food for 2 to 4 weeks should serve to evaluate any contribution it may make to symptoms. Small amounts of a food may be tolerated, but larger quantities of it may cause symptoms.

Reference

1. Bock, S.A., Buckley, J., Holst, A., and May, C.D.: Proper use of skin tests with food extracts in diagnosis of hypersensitivity to food in children. Clin. Allerg., 7:375, 1977.

Bibliography

Bock, S.A., Lee, W.-L., Remigio, L.K., and May, C.D.: Studies of hypersensitivity reactions to foods in infants and children. J. Allerg. Clin. Immunol., 62:327, 1978.
Bock, S.A.: Food sensitivity: A critical review and practical approach. Amer. J. Dis. Child., 134:973, 1980.

Addendum

Elimination Diet (Free of Commonest Causes of Food Hypersensitivity)

(**Note:** Commercial foods may contain additives such as lemon juice in lamb.)

Foods Allowed at Mealtime

Rice
Puffed rice
Rice flakes
Rice Krispies

Pineapple
Apricots
Cranberries   } also juice
Peaches   of these
Pears

Lamb
Chicken

Asparagus
Beets
Carrots
Lettuce
Sweet potato

Tapioca

White vinegar
Olive oil

Honey
Cane sugar (or beet)
Salt
Oleomargarine without milk (Mazola Margarine)
Crisco, Spry
Bubble-Up (a carbonated, dye-free beverage)

Snacks

Rice cereal (midmorning and midafternoon)

Avoid

Any food not on this list
Pepper and spices
Coffee
Tea
Colored beverages
Chewing gum

Other

Medications, only as specifically ordered

Allergy Diets, Recipes, Products

Diets

Ralston Purina Company, Consumer's Services, Checkerboard Square, St. Louis, Missouri 63164 (free).

Recipes

American Dietetic Association, 430 N. Michigan Avenue, Chicago, Illinois 60611 ($1.00).

Products

Cellu Foods. List from Chicago Dietetic Supply, Inc., 405 E. Shawmut Avenue, La Grange, Illinois 60525.

Chapter 30

NUTRITION AND INFECTION

Few biologic systems are more complex than the interaction of man and microbes. Both depend on a constant supply of similar nutrients for survival. The magnitude and closeness of this interaction can be appreciated from the fact that humans are colonized with microbes on all environmentally exposed surfaces from the time of birth until after death. The determinant for infectious disease in the host is the integrity of numerous defense mechanisms matched against the virulence and numbers of microbial agents. The number of variables in such a system is almost inconceivable. In many respects, more is known about the utilization of nutrients in microbes than in humans. Despite volumes of medical literature dealing with human infection and nutrition, sound scientific data are few. Although advances in the methods for the study of host defenses have been formidable in recent years, there still is a dearth of resources on which to base conclusions about the role of dietary intake on the susceptibility to infectious diseases. Furthermore, the impact of infection on the nutritional status of the host adds to the complexity of clinical research. Possibly the only incontrovertible statement to be made here is that additional research is needed to understand this complex ecosystem. Nevertheless, epidemiologic surveys, *in vitro* laboratory studies, utilization of animal models, and clinical observations permit a reasonable grasp of certain concepts.

Effects of Malnutrition on Host Defenses

Integrity of Skin and Mucous Membranes

The importance of the skin as a barrier to microbial invasion and infection is ascertained easily from the patient with thermal burns or severe exfoliative dermatitis. The delayed wound healing with severe protein or zinc deficiencies, the pellagroid dermatitis and thinning of the intestinal mucosa with kwashiorkor, and the various lesions of the skin associated with vitamin A, riboflavin, niacin, and pyridoxine deficiencies may provide a sufficient breach of the integument to permit a portal of entry for infection.

Secretory Antibody System

Secretory immunoglobulin A (IgA) of nasopharyngeal secretions is reduced with protein-calorie malnutrition, and IgA antibody responses to measles and poliovirus vaccines are diminished. Secretory IgA may increase susceptibility at the mucosal surface to colonization and infection.

Cell-mediated Immunity

The cell-mediated immune response has been reasonably well studied in undernourished children and adults, and results in general show significant impairment, especially in patients with kwashiorkor. Furthermore, the serious infectious diseases encountered with protein-calorie malnutrition are those known to occur with abnormalities in T-lymphocyte function. These include life-threatening infections with measles virus, hepatitis viruses, the herpesviruses, opportunistic fungi, tubercle bacilli, *Pneumocystis carinii*, and Gram-negative bacilli.

The importance of observations made over the last several decades on the diminution in size of the thymus and peripheral lymphoid organs can now be appreciated from the highly sophisticated methods for the study of lymphocyte function. The term "nutritional thymectomy" now seems appropriate for physiologic as well as anatomic abnormalities associated with severe protein-calorie malnutrition.

Cellular immunity is mediated by T (thymus-derived) lymphocytes and can be assessed through *in vitro* studies of lymphocyte function, allograph rejection, and skin tests with intradermally injected antigens (delayed hypersensitivity). In the severely malnourished child, the number of T lymphocytes is reduced.[1] The lymphocytes not identifiable as T or B cells, referred to as "null" cells, tend to be increased in number. The non-T/non-B lymphocytes possess suppressor and cytotoxic function. It seems that, because of the decreased number of T lymphocytes, the increased number of T-suppressor cells, or both, the overall function of T lymphocytes is abnormal. Nutritional replenishment has been followed by a return of T lymphocytes to normal numbers.[1] Some studies in marasmic children have revealed normal lymphocyte transformation.[2]

Delayed hypersensitivity to skin test antigens reflects an overall end response of cell-mediated immunity. Both primary and recall responses are impaired with protein-calorie malnutrition[3] and may be reversed with nutritional replenishment.[4]

Chronic zinc deficiency has been associated with impaired T-cell function.[5]

Because of the frequent association of infection with malnutrition, the impact of either one on the measurements of immune response frequently is difficult to ascertain.

Humoral Immunity

The number and distribution of B (bone-marrow) lymphocytes is normal in the malnourished host. Serum immunoglobulins may be normal or elevated. Some studies have suggested that the antibody levels after immunization with certain antigens may be less in patients with protein-calorie malnutrition than in otherwise normal individuals. However, most studies of this type are fraught with confounding variables.

Complement System

With the exception of C_4, the concentration of complement proteins and total hemolytic complement activities is reduced in malnutrition.[6] These abnormalities can be reversed with dietary replenishment.

Phagocytosis

Certain functions of the phagocyte are impaired in malnourished individuals. The significance of these abnormalities and effects of concurrent infection in those under study are not clearly delineated. Delay in early migration of polymorphonuclear leukocytes has been reported.[7] However, the lack of a normal serum chemotactic stimulus, sensitization of T lymphocytes, and release of mediator lymphokines cannot be discounted as causes of impaired phagocyte migration.

Studies of endocytosis (ingestion) have shown the formation of phagocytic vacuoles, phagolysosome fusion, and degranulation to be normal in protein-calorie malnutrition.

Intracellular killing of phagocytized bacteria and fungi is impaired. Malnutrition impedes oxygen consumption, decarboxylation of glucose through the hexose monophosphate shunt, and hydrogen peroxide production by the phagocyte.[8]

Transferrin and Iron

Free iron is an essential requirement for the growth of microbial organisms. Gram-negative bacteria require from 0.3 to 1.8 μM concentrations of iron, and Gram-positive bacteria and fungi need from 0.4 to 4.0 μM of iron.[9] In humans, iron is avidly bound to proteins such as transferrin and lactoferrin in serum and milk and ferritins in tissues, which curtails its availability to microbial invaders. The serum contains approximately 3.0 mg transferrin per milliliter, which can bind approximately 4.2 μg (0.075 μM) of iron. In normal individuals, serum iron is tightly bound to transferrin, which is 25 to 30% saturated with iron.[10] From these calculations, it is obvious that bacteria and fungi find a nutrient-deprived environment for growth. However, microorganisms may synthesize compounds (siderophores) to solubilize and assimilate iron. An additional factor to consider is the bacteriostatic effect of transferrin. Unsaturated transferrin has been shown to inhibit the replication of a variety of bacteria and fungi. This inhibition may be related to the unavailability of the transferrin-bound iron for microbial use. The addition of iron to serum to achieve 80% saturation of transferrin augments the growth of bacteria and fungi. The administration of iron parenterally to experimental rats and mice reduces the number of organisms required to establish infection, and pretreatment of animals with deferoxamine, an iron chelator, is protective.[11] Several studies in lower animals and humans indicate that parenterally administered iron reduces the resistance to bacterial infections.[9] However, when iron is administered orally, the effect is not well delineated.[9]

From the foregoing statements, iron deficiency may appear to be relatively more protective against infection than a state of iron excess. Unfortunately, clinical data to support or discount this theory are lacking. The important concept to appreciate is that no single component of the complex defense mechanisms against infection can be expected to function independently with sufficient magnitude to protect the host completely. Studies in patients with iron-deficiency anemia have revealed evidence of impaired cell-mediated immunity[12] and impaired digestion of phagocytized bacteria,[13] although other studies have shown these components of the immune system to be normal. In iron-deficiency states, it seems reasonable to expect that the protective effects of unsaturated transferrin may be balanced against impaired cellular responses of the host. From the clinical studies available, infections seem to be more frequent in iron-deficient than in otherwise normal infants.

The role of iron excess in the susceptibility to infection is not clearly delineated. Increased susceptibility to bacterial infections in experimental animals treated with parenteral iron, *in vitro* studies showing inhibition of granulocytic function with iron excess, and the high prevalence of Gram-negative septicemia in a study of infants receiving iron-dextrose injections point to the adverse effects of hyperferremia. However, reasonable arguments and data contradict this concept as a clinically significant factor.[14] Fairly substantial evidence indicates that oral iron supplementation does not enhance the risk of infection. Indeed, transferrin saturation in infants receiving supplemental iron does not exceed 30%. At present there is no reason to modify current recommendations on dietary iron intake for infants and children.

Effects of Infection on Nutrition

The anorexia, vomiting, and diarrhea associated with infections serve to reduce intake and augment losses of various nutrients. Energy consumption increases with fever. An increase of 1°C above the normal temperature requires an average increase in metabolism of about 13%. Gluconeogenesis in the liver is increased. As the synthesis of glucose is increased, so is its oxidation, resulting in an imbalance leading to either hyperglycemia or hypoglycemia in cases of sepsis. During septic episodes, the utilization of albumin is increased and its synthesis is decreased;[15] therefore, nitrogen balance is negative. Serum triglycerides and cholesterol generally are increased with serious infections. Free fatty acid plasma levels may increase when Gram-negative bacillary sepsis is mild but decrease when it is severe.

Hypoferremia occurs early in the course of many infections. Sequestered iron is not used for hematopoiesis, and anemia is a consequence of chronic infection. Serum levels of zinc increase and levels of copper decrease with infection.

The Immunocompromised Host

The impact of nutritional therapy on the incidence and course of infections in the immunocompromised host has not been demonstrated adequately. Impaired cell-mediated responses have been restored by nutritional treatment in surgical patients, and these responses were somewhat predictive of the susceptibility to sepsis.[16] Animal studies show that *Pneumocystis carinii* infection, common in the immunosuppressed patient, can be provoked solely by dietary deprivation of protein; moreover, children with this infection who have leukemia are more likely to have evidence of protein-calorie malnutrition than patients without this infection.[17] Whether or not nutritional support regimens might provide protection against such infections is not known.

The use of "total parenteral nutrition" programs in cancer patients is gaining widespread popularity despite the lack of conclusive data on efficacy other than the improvement of values of various laboratory tests of patients undergoing this management. In a recent, randomized, controlled study of cancer patients, no benefit could be defined about recovery from chemotherapy-induced myelosuppression or the frequency of infectious diseases.[18] At present there is no substantial basis for routinely recommending the highly expensive and laboriously administered total parenteral nutrition regimen for children with cancer.

References

1. Chandra, R.K.: Nutritional modulation of immune response. *In* Wedgwood, R.J., Davis, S.D., Ray, C.G., and Kelley, V.C., ed.: Infections in Children. Philadelphia: Harper and Row, 1982.

2. Schlesinger, L., and Stekel, A.: Impaired cellular immunity in marasmic infants. Amer. J. Clin. Nutr., 27:615, 1974.
3. Harland, P.S., and Brown, R.E.: Tuberculin sensitivity following BCG vaccination in undernourished children. East Afr. Med. J., 42:233, 1965.
4. Edelman, R., Suskind, R., Olsen, R.E., Sirisinha, S.: Mechanisms of defective delayed cutaneous hypersensitivity in children with protein-calorie malnutrition. Lancet, 1:506, 1973.
5. Sugarman, B.: Zinc and infection. Rev. Infect. Dis., 5:137, 1983.
6. Sirsinha, S., Suskind, R., Edelman, R., Charupatana, C., and Olson, R.E.: Complement and C3 proactivator levels in children with protein-calorie malnutrition and effect of dietary treatment. Lancet, 1:1016, 1973.
7. Schopfer, K., and Douglas, S.D.: Neutrophil function in children with kwashiorkor. J. Lab. Clin. Med., 88:450, 1976.
8. Keusch, G.T., Douglas, S.D., Braden, K., Geller, S.A.: Antibacterial functions of macrophages in experimental protein-calorie malnutrition. I. Description of the model, morphologic observations and macrophage surface IgG receptors. J. Infect. Dis., 138:125, 1978.
9. Weinberg, E.D.: Iron and suceptibility to infectious disease. Science, 184:952, 1974.
10. Bullen, J.J., Rogers, H.J., and Griffiths, E.: Role of iron in bacterial infection. Curr. Top. Microbiol. Immunol., 80:1, 1978.
11. Lukens, J.N.: Iron deficiency and infection: Fact or fable. Amer. J. Dis. Child., 129:160, 1975.
12. Joynson, D.H.M., Walker, D.M., Jacobs, A., and Dolby, A.E.: Defect of cell-mediated immunity in patients with iron-deficiency anaemia. Lancet, 2:1058, 1972.
13. Chandra, R.K.: Iron and immunocompetence. Nutr. Rev., 34:129, 1976.
14. Pearson, H.A.: Iron and infection. In 82nd Ross Conference on Pediatric Research. Iron-revisited: Infancy, childhood and adolescence. Columbus, Ohio: Ross Laboratories, pp. 66-70, 1981.
15. Cohen, S., and Hansen, J.D.L.: Metabolism of albumin and γ-globulin in kwashiorkor. Clin. Sci., 23:351, 1962.
16. Pietsch, J.R., Meakins, J.L., and MacLean, L.D.: The delayed hypersensitivity response: Application in clinical surgery. Canad. J. Surg., 20:15, 1977.
17. Hughes, W.T., Price, R.A., Sisko, F., Havron, W.S., Kafatos, A.G., Schonland, M., and Smythe, P.M.: Protein calorie malnutrition: A host determinant for Pneumocystis carinii infection. Amer. J. Dis. Child., 128:44, 1974.
18. Shamberger, R.C., Pizzo, P.A., Goodgame, J.T., Jr., Lowry, S.F., Maher, M.M., Wesley, R.A., and Brennan, M.F.: The effect of total parenteral nutrition on chemotherapy-induced myelosuppression: A randomized study. Amer. J. Med., 74:40, 1983.

Chapter 31

ORAL FLUID THERAPY AND POSTTREATMENT FEEDING FOLLOWING ENTERITIS

The 1982-1983 report by UNICEF on the state of the world's children recommended widespread implementation of oral rehydration as one of the four strategies projected to save the lives of 20,000 children each day. In developing countries, oral rehydration has been shown to be an effective, simple, and inexpensive therapy for dehydration caused by severe enteritis in infants.[1,2] The modern concepts of oral fluid therapy for diarrheal diseases evolved in part from the clinical observation that orally administered, glucose-electrolyte solutions can replace diarrheal fluid losses in cholera. Previous laboratory investigation had demonstrated the presence of a cotransport system of sodium with glucose or other actively transported, small, organic molecules in the small intestine in animals and in man. Clinical studies suggest that this sodium-glucose cotransport system remains intact not only when the pathophysiologic agent is an enterotoxin, such as that elaborated by *Vibrio cholerae* or enterotoxigenic strains of *Escherichia coli*, but also with inflammation such as that associated with rotavirus, *Campylobacter jejuni, E. coli,* and *Yersinia enterocolitica.*[1,2] These observations have provided a physiologic rationale for an appropriately efficient ratio of sodium to glucose in formulating solutions for oral use in treating infants in developing countries who have life-threatening diarrheal dehydration.

Those concerned with the health of children in this country are not usually confronted with the problem of obtaining uncontaminated water or management of large numbers of severely malnourished, young infants with multiple health problems. The usual problem is the management of mild, moderate, and (less frequently) severe diarrheal dehydration in an otherwise normal infant. The outstanding, presenting complaints frequently are decreased food and fluid intake and vomiting. The goal of management is to support the infants (and their parents) for the 2 to 3 days of acute illness and avoid complications which might result from dehydration or from the measures to prevent dehydration. Physicians in this country are sensitive to the possibility that the infants under their supervision might develop hypernatremic dehydration as a consequence of decreased fluid intake or as a result of the administration of inappropriate fluids.[3-8] Physicians also are concerned with the cost of hospital care of infants and the potential complications of hospitalization and parenteral fluid therapy *per se*.

With the foregoing points in mind, the following recommendations for oral fluid therapy seem sound for a "developed" country. The recommendations are for patients of all ages; but, in the older patient (those with weights greater than 10 kg), allowance should be made for lower maintenance water requirements per kilogram of body weight. The composition and the indications for use of two types of oral solutions are shown in Table 20.

The World Health Organization's Oral Rehydration Solution (WHO-ORS) is an exceedingly useful product which has probably saved the lives of many thousands of children. The solution, containing 90 mEq/l of sodium, is appropriate for rapid rehydration of dehydrated infants, regardless of the initial osmolality of the infant's body fluids. However, this solution alone is not suitable for provision of water and solute for maintaining fluid balance in the infant with ongoing losses of fluids from the gastrointestinal tract, nor are other solutions with sodium concentrations of 75 to 90 mEq/l suitable alone for meeting maintenance water requirements.

Oral Rehydration Solutions

The oral rehydrating solutions (i.e., solutions with sodium concentrations ranging from 75 to 90 mEq/l and other components as shown in Table 20 may be used to treat significant dehydration secondary to diarrhea, if the patient is not in shock and is able to drink. These solutions should be used only under supervision of physicians or other trained health personnel, preferably in a health care facility. During the rehydration phase, which should rarely exceed 4 to 6 hours, such an oral rehydrating solution should be used alone in volumes roughly calculated to replace the extracellular fluid loss. Continued use of a solution with sodium concentration in the 75 to 90 mEq/l range is potentially dangerous if given alone beyond the period of treatment for acute dehydration. The carbohydrate concentration should not exceed twice the sodium concentration (both in millimolar units) because the excess carbohydrate may produce osmotic retention of water in the intestine, with subsequent fecal losses.

Vomiting is not a contraindication to oral hydration. In particular, when the fluid is administered by spooning rather than through a nipple or from a cup, successful net retention is usually obtained despite small amounts being vomited.

Maintenance of Hydration or Prevention of Dehydration

Solutions with sodium concentrations ranging from 40 to 60 mEq/l and other components as shown in Table 20 can be used to maintain hydration or prevent dehydration. It is preferable to use a prepared solution containing 40 to 60 mEq/l of sodium for the prevention of dehydration in the infant with ongoing gastrointestinal losses (who may or may not have required initial rehydration). The WHO-ORS preparation or other oral rehydration solutions used to treat acute dehydration may be used for the second phase of rehydration by giving them alternately on a 1:1 basis with a no sodium or low sodium fluid such as water, low carbohydrate juices, or human milk. They should **not** be used as the **sole fluid intake.** If human milk is used with an oral rehydrating solution, breast feeding may be given *ad lib* to satisfy thirst and for hunger. The oral rehydration solution may be alternated with human milk or given after two or more periods of breast feeding. The volume of the 75 to 90 mEq/l rehydrating solution ingested should not exceed 75 ml/kg per 24 hours. The same caveat concerning carbohydrate concentration of the early phase applies in the recovery period as well.

Packaging

To ensure proper composition of the final solution, a premixed oral solution is preferred to a powder which must be diluted by the person caring for the child. Home mixing is fraught with hazards of inaccurate dilution, variation in sodium content because of the use of water softeners, and, in some areas, contamination. However, the powder form has the advantages of longer shelf life, reduced bulk for shipping and storage, convenience, and inherently lower cost. Although the prediluted electrolyte solution is preferable to the powder form, the latter is acceptable if distributed with a container of the appropriate volume and if the physician is confident that the powder will be properly diluted.

Reintroduction to Food

The predominant teaching in this country has advocated a delay in the reintroduction of usual feedings in an infant recovering from acute gastroenteritis.[9,10] In hospitalized patients receiving intravenous hydration, the infant's bowel frequently has been permitted to "remain at rest" for 24 to 48 hours, and suboptimal nutrition has been permitted to continue for several more days because of the persistence or recurrence of loose stools. Recognition of the deleterious effects of starvation, especially in the poorly nourished infant, has led some physicians to urge the early introduction of parenteral nutritional support. Many physicians in this country now question the value of withholding usual feedings for a significant period after acute dehydration has been corrected.

There are many opinions but few data on which to base recommendations for reintroduction of food to infants recovering from acute diarrhea.[11,12] The ingestion of food increases fecal volume during the recovery period; but there is a question whether the infant benefits with a net nutritional gain in spite of increases in the losses. There are actually two separate issues here: (1) the replacement of fluid and electrolytes so dehydration and the associated complications do not recur, and (2) the provision of adequate nutrition.

There is general agreement that usual foods, including milk and formula, should be withheld if there is significant dehydration, severe vomiting, or severe gastric or intestinal distension. Clinical experience suggests that human milk frequently is well tolerated when other foods are not, although the reason for this is not clear.[11,12] There are two areas of concern with the early reintroduction of cow's milk or formula feeding, other than increased vomiting and stool losses. The first area of concern relates to the observations showing that the absorption of macromolecules and whole protein may be great in the infant recovering from acute enteritis. The immunologic and clinical significance of this is not known. The second area of concern centers on the occurrence of carbohydrate intolerance after acute enteritis. The incidence and clinical significance of transient disaccharide intolerance after diarrhea is not known. When clinically evident as a problem for a specific patient, the offending carbohydrate should be avoided. The current data do not suggest that lactose should be routinely eliminated from the diet of infants recovering from diarrhea, although some experienced clinicians make this recommendation.

Table 20
Recommendations for the Use of Oral Solutions for Treating
Pediatric Patients with Gastrointestinal Fluid Losses

Name	Rehydration Solution	Maintenance Solution
Purpose	Treatment of acute dehydration (extracellular volume contraction)	Prevention of dehydration caused by diarrhea or maintenance of hydration after treatment of dehydration.
Sodium	75-90 mEq/l	40-60 mEq/l
Potassium	20 mEq/l	20 mEq/l
Anions	20-30% of anions as base (acetate, lactate, citrate, or bicarbonate) and the remainder as chloride	20-30% of anions as base (acetate, lactate, citrate, or bicarbonate) and the remainder as chloride
Carbohydrate	Glucose: 2.0-2.5% (110-140 mM/l)	Glucose: 2.0-2.5% (110-140 mM/l)
Administration	Volume given to equal estimated fluid deficit: usually 40-50 ml/kg to be given over about 4 hr; reevaluate clinical status and therapy after 3-4 hr	Daily volume should not exceed 150 ml/kg per 24 hr; if additional fluid is needed to satisfy thirst, a low-solute fluid such as water or human milk should be used

Here, as in most areas where quality health care is the goal, individualized management of patients is important. Attention should be focused on the clinical state of hydration and on nutrition after acute dehydration is corrected. Stool watching *per se* should not guide management. A reasonable approach to the reintroduction of food is that, in the absence of a specific contraindication, the reintroduction of feeding should not be delayed more than 24 hours in the infant with acute diarrhea. Human milk may be reintroduced as such, but formula or milk feeding should be reintroduced gradually by starting with dilute mixtures. The older infant or child might be offered rice cereal, bananas, potatoes, or other nonlactose, carbohydrate-rich food shortly after successful rehydration. The infants must be followed closely to detect dehydration because this appears to impair the tolerance to food and may contribute to the development of a chronic illness.[11]

References

1. Santosham, D., Daum, R.S., Dillman, L., *et al.*: Oral rehydration therapy of infantile diarrhea: A controlled study of well-nourished children hospitalized in the United States and Panama. New Engl. J. Med., **306**:1070, 1982.
2. Pizarro, D., Posada, G., and Mata, L.: Treatment of 242 neonates with dehydrating diarrhea with an oral glucose-electrolyte solution. J. Pediat., **102**:153, 1983.
3. Finberg, L., and Harrison, H.E.: Hypernatremia in infants. An evaluation of the clinical and biochemical findings accompanying this state. PEDIATRICS, **16**:1, 1955.
4. Weil, W.B., and Wallace, W.M.: Hypertonic dehydration in infancy. PEDIATRICS, **17**:171, 1956.
5. DeYoung, V.R., and Diamond, E.F.: Possibility of iatrogenic factors responsible for hypernatremia in dehydrated infants. J.A.M.A., **173**:1806, 1960.
6. Colle, E., Ayoub, E., and Raile, R.: Hypertonic dehydration (hypernatremia): The role of feedings high in solutes. PEDIATRICS, **22**:5, 1958.
7. Franz, M.N., and Segar, W.E.: The association of various factors and hypernatremic diarrheal dehydration. Amer. J. Dis. Child., **97**:298, 1959.
8. Paneth, N.: Hypernatremic dehydration of infancy: An epidemiologic review. Amer. J. Dis. Child., **134**:785, 1980.
9. Darrow, D.C., Pratt, E.L., Flett, J., Jr., Gamble, A.H., and Wiese, H.F.: Disturbances of water and electrolytes in infantile diarrhea. PEDIATRICS, **3**:129, 1949.

10. Marriott, W.K., and Jeans, P.C.: Infant Nutrition, ed. 3. St. Louis: C.V. Mosby Co., 1941.
11. Klish, W.J.: The refeeding of acute gastroenteritis. *In* Diagnosis and Management of Acute Diarrhea, Report of the Thirteenth Ross Roundtable on Critical Approaches to Common Pediatric Problems. Columbus, Ohio: Ross Laboratories, pp. 45-54, 1982.
12. Finberg, L., Harper, P.A., Harrison, H.E., and Sack, R.B.: Oral rehydration for diarrhea. J. Pediat., **101**:497, 1982.

Chapter 32

DIET IN THE PREVENTION OF DISEASE IN HEALTHY CHILDREN*

The science of nutrition has nearly accomplished its task of understanding and preventing specific nutritional deficiencies. Recently there has been more understanding of some of the relationships between nutrients, how to use nutritional knowledge to manage metabolic disease, and the problems of excessive intake of specific nutrients. The challenge for the future is the refinement of the knowledge for use in the prevention of the common lethal diseases of later life such as obesity, atherosclerosis, hypertension, and cancer. These are complex illnesses in which there may be a significant nutritional component. Genetic, environmental, and behavioral components also exist. The development of these complex illnesses may be nearly lifelong and may well begin in infancy or childhood. Because of the chronicity of some pathologic processes, it takes many years to test the effects of any suggested intervention. Evaluation of suggested preventive measures in a scientifically rigorous manner, with suitable control groups and single variables, has not been feasible for both economic and ethical reasons. Although epidemiologic methods do not prove causality, they can demonstrate strong interrelationships between factors and suggest possible preventive or remedial measures.

Cancer

". . . what we eat during our lifetime strongly influences the probability of developing certain kinds of cancer . . ." is a statement made recently by the National Research Council.[1] In an extensive report this group has collected, analyzed, and weighed all the human and experimental evidence. Only where epidemiologic evidence, supported by cohort and case

*Adapted from Woodruff, C.W.: Diet in the prevention of disease in otherwise healthy children. *In* Walker, A.W., and Watkins, J.B., ed.: Nutrition in Pediatrics—Basic Science and Clinical Aspects. Boston: Little, Brown and Company, 1985 (used with permission).

control studies, agrees with animal experimental data has the group made any firm recommendations.

Although it is impossible to separate nutrition from other environmental factors, blacks and Japanese living in the United States acquire malignancies in the same pattern as others living in this country rather than in the pattern seen in Africa and Japan.[2] Some relationships meriting recommendations have been found. Although there are no specific pediatric guidelines, the following information relates to the population as a whole and can be applied to children when they consume the same foods as their families.

A high total fat intake is correlated with an increased incidence of cancer of the colon and breast in both epidemiologic and animal studies.[2-5] The recommendation is a reduction in fat intake to about 30% of calories. Because protein intakes tend to parallel fat intakes, the specific effect of protein cannot be defined at present.

Although the hypothesis that high fiber intakes are associated with a low incidence of cancer of the bowel is supported by epidemiologic data,[6] cohort and case control studies give variable results.[7,8] Some workers have estimated total fiber content of the diet; others have worked with high fiber foods and different components which make up the total fiber content of the diet. No conclusive evidence is available from a large number of animal studies. Therefore, the National Research Council[1] made no firm recommendations.

Vitamin A and its precursor carotene must be considered together. There is epidemiologic evidence that diets low in vitamin A and carotene are associated with an increased incidence of cancer of the lung, bladder, and larynx.[9-11] It is not clear whether this increased incidence is caused by a lack of vitamin A and carotene or the presence of some other factor in foods such as liver or green and yellow vegetables containing the vitamin. Other than meeting the Recommended Dietary Allowance for vitamin A (including carotene), the only specific suggestion is to avoid large doses of preformed vitamin A because of its known toxicity.

There is less cancer in some geographic areas where selenium is abundant in the local food supply.[12] Only extremely high doses of selenium have a protective effect in animals. Intakes of selenium greater than the safe and adequate range suggested by the Recommended Dietary Allowance (not more than 200 μg daily for adults) should be avoided.

Some substances in foods cannot be classified as nutrients. They may occur naturally in foods, be added during processing, or be formed during food preservation or preparation. There is epidemiologic evidence that vegetables high in carotene content (dark green or yellow) and cruciferous vegetables such as cabbage and brussels sprouts may contain unidentified substances—both nutrient and nonnutrient—which inhibit carcinogenesis.[13] Consequently, the daily diet should include a cruciferous vegetable. Foods are specified rather than nutrients because the data are based on the intake of specific foods rather than their nutrient content.

Ames[14] has published an extensive review of the numerous compounds in edible plant foods which are carcinogenic or mutagenic for animals. Many of these substances are "nature's pesticides," synthesized by the plants as a defense against bacterial, fungal, and insect predators. Ames estimates that the human dietary intake [of these compounds] is likely to be several grams per day—probably at least 10,000 times higher than the dietary intake of man-made pesticides. Moreover, plants and other foods contain compounds which may protect against cancer because of their antioxidant properties: tocopherol, carotene, ascorbic acid, glutathione, and selenium. This is a challenge for investigators.

Many food additives are now widely used (see Chapter 35). The only substance in the marketplace which has been found to be carcinogenic in animals is saccharin, and its effects on humans have not been analyzed.

Processing and preparation of foods can produce substances which are mutagenic for bacteria and suspect as carcinogens. The charring of fish and meat during cooking at high temperatures (e.g., over charcoal) is one example; the smoking of foods is another. It is not known whether these substances are carcinogenetic for humans. In some parts of the world, large amounts of food preserved by smoking or cured with salt (including salt-pickling), which also produces higher levels of polycyclic aromatic and N-nitroso compounds, are consumed; and a higher incidence of cancer of the esophagus and stomach is found. The consumption of foods preserved by these methods should be minimized.

The recommendations by the National Research Council[1] are limited to adults; there is little information about the influence of diet in early life on cancer prevalence, except as it applies to the various ethnic and cultural groups into which children are born. However, serious students such as Doll are of the opinion that many cancers have an extremely long latent period,[15,16] and dietary manipulations which result in a lessened cancer incidence and increased longevity in rats are most effective when undertaken early in life.[17-19]

A reduction in total food intake has decreased the age-specific incidence of cancer in laboratory animals. However, most studies of this nature have involved a reduction of all nutrients, and it is not known if the lower tumor incidence resulted from a lower intake of a specific nutrient (such as fat) or a lower total energy intake.

The Committee on Diet, Nutrition, and Cancer[1] considered a number of other dietary factors which may have carcinogenic or anticarcinogenic potential; however, the evidence for the role of these factors is not sufficiently documented to justify firm recommendations.

Hypertension

In 1972 the suggestion was made by Dahl[20] that high-sodium intakes in infancy might predispose to the later development of hypertension. Dahl suggested that salt be removed from infant foods. A subcommittee of the Food Protection Committee of the Food and Nutrition Board (NAS-NRC)[21] noted that the average sodium intake of infants was several times the minimum requirement and commented that the evidence relating sodium intake to hypertension in later life was ambiguous. They recommended that the sodium content of infant foods be reduced to a maximum of 0.25%, and this was soon accomplished. In 1974 the Committee on Nutrition[22] pointed out that this reduction in sodium applied only to infants less than 8 months old because cow's milk and table foods contain more sodium than commercial infant formulas and infant foods. In 1977 the infant food industry adopted a policy of "no added salt." By 1979, the increase in breast feeding and the more prolonged use of commercial infant formula and infant foods further reduced the sodium intake of infants 2 to 12 months old. These data were collected in a series of surveys made in 1972, 1977, and 1979[23] and are presented in Figure 13. Although there has been a reduction in the total sodium intake from 36 to 20 mEq per day (mean intakes from 3 to 2 mEq of sodium per kilogram per day), table foods and cow's milk are now the major sources of sodium in the diet of infants less than 12 months old. Older infants and children share the same food sources as adults. With an increased consumption of processed foods, which frequently contain added sodium, even the omission of salt in cooking and from table use will be less and less helpful in achieving a low-sodium intake.

Breast-fed infants thrive on a sodium intake averaging about 1 mEq per kilogram per day, which is close to the minimum requirement calculated from data on growth and dermal losses. Intakes as high as 9 mEq of sodium per kilogram per day appear to be well tolerated. In the only prospective study available on the effects of sodium intake on blood pressure,[24] infants were fed either a low-sodium formula or the same formula with added salt and selected supplemental foods. The intakes approximated the goals of 1 and 9 mEq of sodium per kilogram per day. These diets were begun when the infants were 3 months old and continued for 5 months. During this period, there was no difference in blood pressure, anthropometric measures, extracellular fluid volumes, or serum sodium concentrations. The renin-aldosterone system was activated on the low-sodium diet. From the age of 8 months to 9 to 11 years, when the children were restudied, there were no differences in growth, blood pressure, or preference for salting foods according to the parents. Urine sodium excretions at 9 to 11 years of age were not different. This study demonstrated that 5 months of high-sodium intake in the first year of life had no influence on blood pressure when the children were 9 to 11 years old or on the habitual use of salt at the table.

Because parents buy and feed infant foods as well as prepare food at home, the parents' taste preferences might determine the amount of salt fed to infants. Recent studies on the ability of infants to taste salt[25] showed that infants less than 6 months

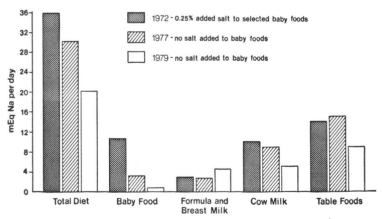

Figure 13. Sodium distribution of the diet of infants age 2 to 12 months old by food group.

old accept salt solutions of 50, 100, and 150 mM/l; by the age of 2 years, they showed a preference for plain water. The available evidence suggests that infants may not have a well developed sense of taste for salt at an age when sucrose is preferred to plain water. The factors responsible for the high-sodium preferences in some individuals are not clearly known. The influence of dietary habits learned during infancy and childhood on the lifelong intake of such substances as salt have never been clearly defined. There are individual differences among members of the same family. At present, education and advertising probably have at least some influence on eating habits in this country.

The etiology and pathogenesis of hypertension have been subject over the years to enthusiastic theories which initially were believed to explain 25% of the incidences but actually explain a much smaller percentage.[26] There currently is no firm evidence for a genetic predisposition to hypertension nor any detailed knowledge concerning the mechanisms by which a high-sodium intake might precipitate clinical disease. However, hypertension affects one of five adults in the United States, and much more than the minimum requirement of sodium is consumed. Many individuals are requested by their physician to reduce their sodium intake for reasons other than hypertension. However, sodium is present in an increasing number of processed foods for which the sodium content is not listed on the label, and this makes limiting sodium intake more difficult. A program of voluntary labelling has been initiated and criteria have been established for "low salt" and "no salt added" foods by the Food and Drug Administration.

There is no conclusive evidence that high-sodium intakes during infancy and childhood are detrimental to the health of even the one fifth of children likely to develop hypertension as adults. But high-sodium intakes are unnecessary, and parents and children should have the opportunity to avoid inapparent sources of sodium in the food supply.

Atherosclerosis

Atherosclerosis, with its clinical manifestations of myocardial infarction, affects one in five men less than 60 years old in the United States. Postmortem studies of young males from the

United States killed in recent wars[47,48] showed that some of them had evidence of significant coronary artery disease. A total of nine principal risk factors have been identified by epidemiologic studies:[27] hyperlipidemia, hypertension, smoking, sedentary living habits, obesity, psychosocial tensions, hyperglycemia, and a family history of premature atherosclerotic or hypertensive disease. Although the long-term, controlled studies necessary to prove that these risk factors are etiologically related to the clinical manifestations of the disease in adults have not been carried out, and probably never will be, there is reason to believe they also apply to children. The earliest manifestation of the disease, fatty streaks in the aorta, appears in the first two decades of life. Although the mechanisms by which these streaks are converted to plaques which produce obstruction of the arteries is not completely known, it is sensible to retard this process from its onset rather than try to reverse it in later life. Because hyperlipidemia, particularly an elevated serum cholesterol, has a high correlation with coronary heart disease, a major emphasis should be placed on dietary management.

Reducing the saturated fat in the diet of adults and increasing the polyunsaturated fat (P/S ratio) has been shown to lower the serum cholesterol, particularly in persons in whom it is elevated. One relatively long-term study also has shown a decrease in the clinical manifestations of atherosclerosis.[28] A recent Finnish study[29] is a good example of the temporary effect of diet on the serum cholesterol because the serum cholesterol values rose again when the subjects were returned to their usual diets. Apparently a lifelong dietary regime is necessary in individuals in whom elevated serum lipids are a risk factor for the development of clinical disease.

Studies in Infants

The relationship between fat intake and serum lipoproteins in infants and school-aged children has received much attention. One major assumption in infant nutrition is that the breast-fed infant of a healthy mother is in better health than the infant fed the best commercial infant formula yet devised. At birth the cholesterol concentration in the serum is low, about 50 to 70 mg/dl. It rises after feeding is begun. The amount of cholesterol fed appears to have an influence on the subsequent serum level because it is higher in breast-fed infants than in infants fed commercial infant formulas containing little cholesterol and larger amounts of linoleic acid. The assumption that this difference is caused entirely by the higher concentration of cholesterol in human milk must be questioned. Apparently the infant's serum lipids are particularly susceptible to dietary influences. As first shown by Insull and co-workers,[30] changes in the lipid composition of human milk readily follow changes in the source of fatty acids available to the mammary gland. When the linoleic acid concentration in the milk is increased, the infant has both an increase in serum linoleate approaching that of the formula-fed infant and a fall in serum cholesterol. In another study, Potter and Nestel[31] showed a similar influence of a high-linoleate intake by the mothers on the serum cholesterol in the infants.

Feeding formulas high in cholesterol and saturated fats compared to feedings low in cholesterol and high in polyunsaturated fat to infants again shows how rapidly they respond to dietary changes.[32] Feeding cow's milk and eggs, which raised the cholesterol intake to a range of 165 to 469 mg per day from practically zero, increased the serum cholesterol concentration by 56 mg/dl.

One theory derived from a large body of animal work, but not substantiated in all species studied, was that a high cholesterol intake in early life would somehow condition the organism so it could metabolize cholesterol more efficiently as an adult. For some time this theory has been applied to the relatively high cholesterol concentration in human milk. If humans react as rats, breast feeding would result in a lower cholesterol concentration than formula feeding. Two studies are available. One study[33] showed that the serum cholesterol concentration when the children were 7 to 12 years old was statistically lower in the formula-fed group. In another cross-sectional study[34] infants were weaned to skimmed milk when they were 4 to 6 months old and their parents advised to avoid giving eggs; the breast-fed group had significantly higher serum cholesterol concentrations when they were 2 to 4 months and 12 months old than those fed commercial infant formula, but there was no difference when these children were 18 to 24 months and 15 to 19 years old. The available human evidence fails to show clear-cut evidence that the intake of cholesterol during the nursing period has an effect on subsequent serum cholesterol concentrations.

Studies in School-aged Children

The results of many studies of the correlation between dietary intake and serum lipids in school-aged children have been reviewed by West and Lloyd[35] and Glueck and Morrison.[36] Two monographs on the pediatric aspects of atherosclerosis have appeared.[37,38] Some trends are evident, such as a probable fall in serum cholesterol concentration during the puberal growth spurt, the observation of a correlation between the serum lipids of children and those of their parents (either genetic or environmental), and a hyperlipoproteinemia of affluence may make the definition of "normal" extremely difficult; but conclusions concerning either the recognition of risk factors or the appropriate dietary responses are far from clear.

Studies on genetically determined diseases involving the apolipoproteins of the high-density lipoproteins (HDL) category[39] have shown that at least seven have been characterized in the low HDL syndromes, which frequently are associated with premature atherosclerosis. Almost nothing is known about either pharmacologic or dietary means for raising HDL proteins, assuming that the HDL component has a protective effect in atherosclerosis. Even this assumption appears to be in doubt.

Problems in Prevention

If atherosclerosis is accepted as a common disease, that it takes many years for the development of clinical manifestations, that a major risk factor is an elevated serum cholesterol, and that dietary manipulations can reduce the serum cholesterol, how should infants and children be fed so atherosclerosis can be prevented? At what age should the diet be altered in fat composition from past practices? Can this be done in such a way that normal growth and development are not endangered and unanticipated nutritional deficiencies avoided? Does the entire population need to be involved, or can susceptible individuals be found by some screening process?

The situation here is analogous to that for cancer: a reduction in total food intake when begun early in life results in less vascular disease in adult animals.[17-19] However, the concept of ideal body weight (Metropolitan Life Insurance Company) which has been developed on actuarial grounds for adults has not been shown to pertain to children.

The Senate's Select Committee on Nutrition and Human Needs,[40] after much study, developed a series of dietary goals:

1. avoid overweight by consuming only as much energy as expended;

2. increase consumption of complex carbohydrates and "naturally occurring" sugars from about 28% of energy intake to about 48%;

3. reduce consumption of refined and processed sugars by about 45% to account for about 10% of total energy intake;

4. reduce overall fat consumption from approximately 40% to about 30% of energy intake;

5. reduce saturated fat consumption to about 10% of total energy intake, and balance this with polyunsaturated and monounsaturated fats, each at about 10% of total energy intake;

6. reduce cholesterol consumption to about 300 mg per day; and

7. reduce salt intake to about 5 gm per day.

The publication of these "goals" has engendered vigorous comments, both pro and con, by responsible nutritionists.[41,42] As pointed out previously, rigorous testing of these recommendations in humans represents an impossible task in view of the multitude of factors involved and the long life span of humans. Dwyer[43] has provided some practical advice for those who wish to emulate these "dietary goals" for children and adolescents.

Before trying to provide answers to the foregoing questions, the questions must be considered in a clinical perspective. Data which may be incomplete and confusing to scientists are the only available basis for decision making by physicians. Waiting until all the facts are known may not be in the best interests of the patients if the recommendations are not shown to be harmful.

With regard to the use of diets low in cholesterol during infancy, there is no evidence that *de novo* synthesis of cholesterol is inadequate to meet the infant's need for synthesis of bile acids, steroid hormones, or myelin. The hypothesis is that early exposure to a high cholesterol intake during the nursing period results in an increased ability to metabolize this substance in later life has received little experimental support. Infants fed skimmed milk in the second 6 months of life do not grow as well as those receiving at least 30% of their calories from fat.[44] The use of 2% milk for infants during this period has not been studied as critically, but other considerations[45] suggest that the use of fresh cow's milk for infants less than 1 year old be avoided. The Committee on Nutrition has recommended,[46] "when breast feeding is unsuccessful, inappropriate, or stopped early, infant formulas provide the best alternative for meeting nutritional needs during the first year of life. Supplementary foods are recommended beginning at 4 to 6 months of age. Dietary fat should not be restricted in this age group."

By the time a child is 1 to 2 years old, any hazard of a diet restricted in saturated fat and cholesterol probably would be the same as those found in adults, but amplified by the relatively greater nutrient needs of children for growth. A variety of conventional foods, including the four basic food groups,† is the major assurance that the nutritional needs of the growing child are met. A gradual transition to complex carbohydrates and a decrease in animal fat would appear to present little hazard. In an industrialized society, the proliferation of processed foods such as substitutes for eggs, cheese, and meat can be anticipated, and some are already available. The use of fabricated foods should not be condemned. Increased effort is needed to evaluate the nutritional adequacy of these foods in animal and clinical studies before widespread use, particularly in children.

A Moderate Approach

The Committee on Nutrition advises moderation in feeding normal children in view of the diet-heart hypothesis.[46] Specific recommendations are:

"After 1 year of age, a varied diet from each of the major food groups is the best assurance of nutritional adequacy.

"Detection of obesity by measuring height and weight and detection of hypertension by measuring blood pressure according to the schedules published by the Academy will permit the early recognition and treatment of obesity and hypertension.

"Maintenance of ideal body weight, a regular exercise program, and, in teenagers, counseling concerning the dangers of smoking should be a routine part of all health supervision visits.

"The family history for every patient should include infor-

---

†I. Meat, fish, poultry, egg; II. dairy products—milk, cheese, milk products; III. fruits and vegetables; IV. cereal grains, potatoes, rice.

mation about family members who have had premature heart attacks or strokes (when the patient is 60 years old or less), hypertension, obesity, and hyperlipidemia.

"Screening of children more than 2 years old who are at risk because of family history should consist of at least two serum cholesterol measurements. The high-density lipoprotein cholesterol should be measured in those who consistently have levels above the 95th percentile for age and sex. If high-density lipoprotein cholesterol is not the cause of the hypercholesterolemia, the patient should be treated with an appropriate diet and/or medication.

"Current dietary trends in the United States toward a decreased consumption of saturated fats, cholesterol, and salt and an increased intake of polyunsaturated fats should be followed with moderation. Diets that avoid extremes are safe for children."

Conclusion

This chapter has focused on the role of diet in the prevention of cancer, hypertension, and atherosclerosis in healthy children. Obesity is discussed in Chapter 28. Hyperactivity may not be a disease, and controlled studies have not demonstrated a consistent relationship with food additives or salicylates (Chapter 35). Other diseases have not been considered in this discussion.

Promotion of health rather than the prevention of disease is perhaps a better term to describe the role played by those giving pediatric care. The promotion of breast feeding is one of the first goals. When the infant is ready to make a transition to foods consumed by the family, the emphasis should be on being fed (and later learning to choose) foods from the four basic groups.† Processed foods play an increasingly important role in the food supply in the United States. There is not yet enough experience with many of these foods to be sure they equal less processed foods in nutritional composition and element bioavailability. Commercial infant formulas have been used successfully for many years, but there have been episodic problems in product composition and quality control. Traditional diets of major population groups throughout the world have maintained survival and reproduction for centuries, and major dietary changes need careful evaluation.

Changes in the foods now available are occurring relatively

rapidly. The prevalence of the diseases discussed also is changing. Although some correlations have been found between diet and certain diseases, causality has not been proven to the satisfaction of the most critical scientists. Screening techniques have been proposed, but neither their economic impact on society nor their psychologic impact on children has been studied.

During the first year or so of life, changes in present feeding recommendations are not indicated. When the child begins to share table food, the amount of fat intake should be limited. A vegetable from the dark green, yellow, or cruciferous family should be included with reasonable frequency. Avoiding an excess of smoked or pickled foods may eventually reduce the prevalence of some types of cancer. Salt is consumed in amounts in excess of need, and there is no evidence that high-sodium intakes are necessary. A moderate approach to the prevention of hyperlipidemia has been given (Chapter 27).

References

1. National Research Council, Committee on Diet, Nutrition and Cancer, Assembly of Life Sciences, National Research Council: Executive summary: Diet, nutrition, and cancer. Nutr. Today, July/August, pp. 20-25, 1982.
2. Armstrong, B., and Doll, R.: Environmental factors and cancer incidence and mortality in different countries, with special reference to dietary practices. Int. J. Cancer, 15:617, 1975.
3. Gray, G.E., Pike, M.C., and Henderson, B.E.: Breast-cancer incidence and mortality rates in different countries in relation to known risk factors and dietary practices. Brit. J. Cancer, 39:1, 1979.
4. Reddy, B.S., Cohen, L.A., McCoy, G.D., Hill, P., Weisburger, J.H., and Wynder, E.L.: Nutrition and its relationship to cancer. Adv. Cancer Res., 32:237, 1980.
5. Silverman, J., Shellabarger, C.J., Holtzman, S., Stone, J.P., and Weisburger, J.H.: Effect of dietary fat on X-ray induced mammary cancer in Sprague-Dawley rats. J. Natl. Cancer Inst., 64:631, 1980.
6. Burkitt, D.P., and Trowell, H.C.: Refined Carbohydrate Foods and Disease: Some Implications of Dietary Fibre. London: Academic Press, 1975.
7. Hill, M., MacLennan, R., and Newcombe, K.: Diet and large-bowel cancer in three socioeconomic groups in Hong Kong. Lancet, 1:436, 1979.
8. Lyon, J.L., and Sorenson, A.W.: Colon cancer in a low-risk population. Amer. J. Clin. Nutr., 31:S227, 1978.
9. Graham, S., Mettlin, C., Marshall, J., Priore, R., Rzepka, T., and

Shedd, D.: Dietary factors in the epidemiology of cancer of the larynx. Amer. J. Epidemiol., 113:675, 1981.

10. Mettlin, C., Graham, S., and Swanson, M.: Vitamin A and lung cancer. J. Natl. Cancer Inst., 62:1435, 1979.

11. Shekelle, R.B., Liu, S., Raynor, W.J., Jr., Lepper, M., Maliza, C., Rossof, A.H., Paul, O., Shryock, A.M., and Stamler, J.: Dietary vitamin A and risk of cancer in the Western Electric Study. Lancet, 2:1185, 1981.

12. Schrauzer, G.N., White, D.A., and Schneider, C.J.: Cancer mortality correlation studies—III: Statistical associations with dietary selenium intakes. Bioinorg. Chem., 7:23, 1977.

13. Graham, S., Dayal, H., Swanson, M., Mittleman, A., and Wilkinson, G.: Diet in the epidemiology of cancer of the colon and rectum. J. Natl. Cancer Inst., 61:709, 1978.

14. Ames, B.N.: Dietary carcinogens and anticarcinogens. Oxygen radicals and degenerative diseases. Science, 221:1256, 1983.

15. Doll, R.: An epidemiological perspective of the biology of cancer. Cancer Res., 38:3573, 1978.

16. Cook, P.J., Doll, R., and Fellingham, S.A.: A mathematical model for the age distribution of cancer in man. Int. J. Cancer, 4:93, 1969.

17. McCay, C.M., Crowell, M.F., and Maynard L.A.: The effect of retarded growth upon the length of life span and upon the ultimate body size. J. Nutr., 10:63, 1935.

18. McCay, C.M., Maynard L.A., Sperling, G., and Barnes, L.L.: Retarded growth, life span, ultimate body size and age changes in the albino rat after feeding diets restricted in calories. J. Nutr., 18:1, 1939.

19. Ross, M.H.: Nutrition and longevity in experimental animals. In Winick, M., ed.: Nutrition and Aging, Vol. 4. New York: Wiley and Sons, 1976.

20. Dahl, L.K.: Salt and hypertension. Amer. J. Clin. Nutr., 25:231, 1972.

21. Filer, L.J., Jr.: Salt in infant foods. Nutr. Rev., 29:27, 1971.

22. Committee on Nutrition: Salt intake and eating patterns of infants and children in relation to blood pressure. PEDIATRICS, 53:115, 1974.

23. Committee on Nutrition: Sodium intake of infants in the United States. PEDIATRICS, 68:444, 1981.

24. Whitten, C.F., and Stewart, R.A.: The effect of dietary sodium in infancy on blood pressure and related factors.: Studies of infants fed salted and unsalted diets for five months at eight months and eight years of age. Acta Paediat. Scand. (Suppl. 279), p. 3, 1980.

25. Beauchamp, G.K.: The development of taste in infancy. In Bond, J.T., Filer, L.J., Jr., Leveille, G.A., Thomson, A.M., and Weil, W.B., Jr., ed.: Infant and Child Feeding. New York: Academic Press, pp. 413-426, 1981.

26. Mendlowitz, M.: Some theories of hypertension: Fact and fancy. Hypertension, 1:435, 1979.

27. Multiple Risk Factor Intervention Trial Group: Statistical design considerations in the NHLI Multiple Risk Factor Intervention Trial. (MRFIT). J. Chronic Dis., 30:261, 1977.
28. Dayton, S., Pearce, M.L., Hashimoto, S., Dixon, W.J., and Tomiyasu, U.: A controlled clinical trial of a diet high in unsaturated fat in preventing complications of atherosclerosis. Circulation (Suppl. II), 40:11, July 1969.
29. Ehnholm, C., Huttunen, J.K., Pietinen, P., Leino, U., Mutanen, M., Kostiainen, E., Pikkarainen, J., Dougherty, R., Iacono, J., and Puska, P.: Effect of diet on serum lipoproteins in a population with a high risk of coronary heart disease. New Engl. J. Med., 307:850, 1982.
30. Insull, W., Jr., Hirsch, J., James, T., and Ahrens, E.H., Jr.: The fatty acids of human milk II. Alterations produced by manipulation of caloric balance and exchange of dietary fats. J. Clin. Invest., 38:443, 1959.
31. Potter, J.M., and Nestel, P.J.: The effects of dietary fatty acids and cholesterol on the milk lipids of lactating women and the plasma cholesterol of breast-fed infants. Amer. J. Clin. Nutr., 29:54, 1976.
32. Nestel, P.J., Poyser, A., and Boulton, T.J.C.: Changes in cholesterol metabolism in infants in response to dietary cholesterol and fat. Amer. J. Clin. Nutr., 32:2177, 1979.
33. Hodgson, P.A., Ellefson, R.D., Elvebach, L.R., Harris, L.E., Nelson, R.A., and Weidman, W.H.: Comparison of serum cholesterol in children fed high, moderate or low cholesterol milk diets during neonatal period. Metabolism, 25:739, 1976.
34. Friedman, G., and Goldberg, S.J.: Concurrent and subsequent serum cholesterols of breast- and formula-fed infants. Amer. J. Clin. Nutr., 28:42, 1975.
35. West, R.J., and Lloyd, J.K.: Hypercholesterolemia in childhood. Adv. Pediat., 26:1, 1979.
36. Glueck, C.J., and Morrison, J.A.: Relationships of pediatric nutrients to lipids, lipoproteins and ultimate risk of atherosclerosis. Pediat. Ann., 10:446, 1981.
37. Lauer, R.M., and Shekelle, R.B.: Childhood Prevention of Atherosclerosis and Hypertension. New York: Raven Press, 1980.
38. Strong, W.B., ed.: Atherosclerosis: Its Pediatric Aspects. New York: Grune and Stratton, 1978.
39. Lees, R.S., and Lees, A.M.: High-density lipoproteins and the risk of atherosclerosis. New Engl. J. Med., 306:1546, 1982.
40. Select Committee on Nutrition and Human Needs, U.S. Senate: Dietary Goals for the United States, ed. 2. Washington, D.C.: U.S. Government Printing Office, December 1977.
41. Harper, A.E.: Dietary goals—A skeptical view. Amer. J. Clin. Nutr., 31:310, 1978.
42. Hegsted, D.M.: Dietary goals—A progressive view. Amer. J. Clin. Nutr., 31:1504, 1978.
43. Dwyer, J.: Diets for children and adolescents that meet the dietary goals. Amer. J. Dis. Child., 134:1073, 1980.

44. Fomon, S.J., Filer, L.J., Ziegler, E.E., Bergmann, K.E., and Bergmann, R.L.: Skim milk in infant feeding. Acta Paediat. Scand., 66:17, 1977.
45. Woodruff, C.W.: The science of infant nutrition and the art of infant feeding. J.A.M.A., 240:657, 1978.
46. Committee on Nutrition: Toward a prudent diet for children. PEDIATRICS, 71:78, 1983.
47. Enos, W.F., Jr., Beyer, J.C., and Holmes, R.H.: Pathogenesis of coronary disease in American soldiers killed in Korea. J.A.M.A., 158:912, 1955.
48. McNamara, J.J., Molot, M.A., Stremple, J.F., and Cutting, R.T.: Coronary artery disease in combat casualties in Vietnam. J.A.M.A., 216:1185, 1971.

Dietary Modification

Chapter 33

NUTRITIONAL ASPECTS OF VEGETARIANISM, HEALTH FOODS, AND FAD DIETS

The purpose of this chapter is to discuss some dietary patterns which may be harmful and/or fail to provide the promised or anticipated benefits. These dietary patterns include those based on religion, lifestyle, morality, or ecologic concerns (e.g., vegetarianism and Zen macrobiotics) and those in which special virtues of a particular food, foods, or nutrients are exaggerated (e.g., organic, natural, and health foods, or diets supplemented with massive doses of one or more vitamins).[1] The Committee on Nutrition urges that claims for benefits from eating special diets should be subjected to critical, scientific evaluation before they are accepted by the medical community.

Vegetarian Diets

Various vegetarian diets are popular, especially among adolescents and young adults. These diets may be classified as lacto-ovovegetarian (plant foods with dairy products and eggs), lactovegetarian (plant foods with dairy products), and pure vegetarian (plant foods only). The term "vegan" refers to individuals who not only eat pure vegetarian diets but also share a philosophy and lifestyle. The Zen macrobiotic diet does not fit this classification and will be described separately.

Many individuals and population groups have practiced vegetarianism on a long-term basis and have demonstrated excellent health. Plant-based diets supplemented with milk or with milk and eggs tend to be nutritionally similar to diets containing meat, except for iron. The Food and Nutrition Board of the National Research Council has emphasized that even pure vegetarians can be well nourished if they select their diets carefully to provide sufficient calories, a good balance of essential amino acids, and adequate sources of calcium, riboflavin, iron, vitamin A, vitamin D, and vitamin B_{12}.[2] Indeed, there are some nutritional benefits of a well balanced vegetarian diet, such as the rarity of obesity[2] and a tendency toward lower serum cholesterol levels.[3] However, the more stringent Zen macrobiotic diet is likely to be hazardous and leaves less room for modification.[4]

Pure Vegetarians and Vegans

Vegetarian diets[5-7] tend to be high in bulk; therefore, they may not meet caloric needs. In such circumstances, protein may be used as an energy source, and thus protein nutrition may be compromised. There are several ways to improve protein nutrition. The quantity of protein in the diet is enhanced by using legumes, in which the concentration of protein is high. The quality of vegetable proteins is improved by combining in each meal foods in a manner to provide the essential amino acids in the optimal ratios. For example, cereal grains (such as wheat and rice), which are poor in the essential amino acid lysine, can be effectively combined with legumes (such as varieties of dry beans, soybeans, and peas), which have adequate lysine but little methionine. When the two foods are eaten at the same meal, they provide a mixture of amino acids that is better than either alone.

The risk of other deficiencies is decreased if a variety of foods is used, and undue reliance on a single cereal staple is avoided. An adequate intake of most vitamins, minerals, and other nutrients can be obtained with legumes (including fortified soybean formulas), whole-grain products, nuts, seeds, and dark green, leafy vegetables. Legumes provide B vitamins and iron in addition to relatively concentrated protein. Whole grains are a source of thiamine, iron, and trace minerals as well as carbohydrate and protein. Nuts and seeds contain B vitamins and iron; they also provide fat, which tends to be low in vegetarian diets. Dark green, leafy vegetables help supply adequate calcium and riboflavin, and citrus fruits supply vitamin C. Vitamin B_{12} deficiency occurs in pure vegetarian diets after a variable period because this vitamin is derived exclusively from animal products; and vitamin D must be obtained by exposure to sunlight. The deficiency can be avoided if vitamin B_{12} supplementation is provided in tablet form or in fortified plant foods such as vitamin B_{12}-fortified soy or nut "milks" that are usually available in health food stores. Vitamin supplements are acceptable to most vegans.

Zen Macrobiotic Diet

The Zen macrobiotic diet is perhaps the most dangerous of the current diets for growing children. The goals of this rigid diet are largely spiritual. Ten stages of dietary restriction progress from -3 to +7, with gradual elimination of animal products, fruits, and vegetables. The lower-level diets can meet nutritional needs, but the highest-level diet is composed only of cereals and restricts the nutritional balance that is inherent in more diverse diets. In addition, caloric intake usually is low. Strict adherence to the more rigid diets can result in scurvy, anemia, hypoproteinemia, hypocalcemia, emaciation, growth failure, or even death. Self-treatment of disease is common in individuals following this dietary regimen, and medical consultation is discouraged. In 1971, the Council on Foods and Nutrition of the American Medical Association pointed out the dangers of the Zen macrobiotic diet.[4] Experience with some parents who use the Zen macrobiotic diet has indicated they may be more accepting of nutritional advice for their children than for themselves. If parents are told of their infant's poor growth and of the long-term consequences of protein-calorie undernutrition, they may adopt a lower, more nutritionally diverse and adequate stage of the diet.

Vitamins

Vitamin A

There are unsubstantiated claims that extremely high doses of vitamin A (25,000 to 50,000 IU per day) improve visual acuity in those who work in either bright or dim light. Large doses of vitamin A also are used for the treatment of acne and to prevent infection. High doses of this vitamin can produce serious toxic effects in children, including anorexia, desquamation of the skin, increased intracranial pressure, and radiographic changes in the long bones. Sufficient vitamin A for infants and children is present in most diets. Caffey[8] has warned that the hazards of vitamin A poisoning from the routine prophylactic use of concentrates of vitamins A and D to healthy infants and children who eat adequate diets are considerably greater than the hazards of vitamin A deficiency in healthy infants and children not fed vitamin concentrates. Ingestion of 20,000 IU per day or more for 1 to 2 months is likely to be toxic. Vitamin A toxicity was found in young children fed large amounts of chicken liver, which contains 300 IU vitamin A per gram.[9] Toxic effects similar to those seen in vitamin A poisoning have been reported with the use of large doses of retinoic acid cogeners (1 to 2 mg isotretinoin per kilogram per day; equivalent to 3,330 to 6,670 IU vitamin A per kilogram) for the treatment of cystic acne as well as other dermatologic disorders.[10,11] These adverse reactions also include birth defects.[12]

Vitamin C

Pauling recommended a daily dose of vitamin C, between 1 and 5 gm, for the prophylaxis of the common cold.[13] This advice has resulted not only in a surge of interest in vitamin C but also in its use in enormous quantities to prevent colds. The Committee on Drugs stated in 1971[14] that there was no scientific evidence vitamin C in the doses recommended by Pauling was either safe or efficacious for the prevention of the common cold. Since then, a number of carefully controlled, double-blind studies suggest that the use of vitamin C has, at best, a small effect on severity and duration of symptoms of the common cold. Discrepancies among these studies have been discussed, and large doses of vitamin C have not been proven to have widespread usefulness as a cold remedy.[15] Large doses of vitamin C can interfere with vitamin B_{12} absorption and metabolism in humans, a problem which may not be overcome by extra vitamin B_{12} supplements; and large doses of vitamin C have been associated with nephrolithiasis.[16] Healthy adults can become conditioned to high doses of ascorbate (0.5 to 1.5 gm per day) over a 2-week period, with the result they develop lower-than-normal serum and leukocyte ascorbic acid values on returning to a normal intake.[17] A similar phenomenon in the fetus may explain the development of scurvy in normally fed offspring of mothers who have ingested 400 mg of ascorbic acid daily throughout pregnancy.[18] Until more information is available, people should be cautious in substantially exceeding the RDA for vitamin C.

Vitamin D

Vitamin D in amounts much greater than the RDA of 400 IU daily has been claimed to build stronger bones, especially when the vitamin is taken in its "natural" form in fish liver oil. There is no evidence to support this claim. The RDA provides an ample margin of safety, even without exposure to sunlight. Overuse of vitamin D in Britain and Europe, with intakes between 3,000 and 4,000 IU daily, is believed to be related to the idiopathic hypercalcemia of infants seen relatively frequently during and after World War II.[19] The disease became extremely rare after the dietary intake of vitamin D was reduced to less than 1,500 IU daily.

Vitamin E

Vitamin E has commanded much public attention, and its benefits are controversial. High dietary intakes of vitamin E have been claimed to prolong life, increase sexual potency, and prevent such diseases as mental retardation, heart disease, and cancer. There is little or no basis for these claims. The wide distribution of vitamin E in vegetable oils and cereal grains makes deficiency in humans unlikely. Vitamin E supplements may be necessary for those with intestinal malabsorption,[20] and for preterm infants whose absorption of the vitamin may be decreased for the first 12 months of life.[21] An excess of vitamin E may be harmful in other situations, although the evidence for this is scant. There is evidence, both in humans and experimental animals, that excess vitamin E intake can interfere with vitamin K metabolism, result in a prolonged prothrombin time, and predispose to bleeding.[22] Excessive vitamin E intake in experimental animals decreases the rate of wound healing,[23] and in man it has resulted in gastrointestinal symptoms and creatinuria.[24]

Pyridoxine

Massive doses of pyridoxine (2 to 6 gm daily, or 1,000 times the requirement) have been shown to cause ataxia and sensory neuropathy in adults.[25,26] Studies of nerve conduction and somatosensory-evoked responses showed dysfunction of the distal portions of peripheral sensory nerves, and biopsies demonstrated widespread axonal degeneration.

Health Foods

The terms "organic," "natural," and "health" foods generally carry the following connotations. Organic foods are plant products grown in soil enriched with humus and compost on which no pesticides, herbicides, or inorganic fertilizers have been used, or they are meat and dairy products from animals raised on "natural" feeds and not treated with drugs such as hormones or antibiotics. Natural foods are those made from ingredients of plant or animal origin which are altered as little as possible and contain no synthetic or artificial ingredients or additives. Health food is a general term which seems to encompass natural and organic foods. The term includes conventional foods which have been subjected to less processing than usual (such as unhydrogenated nut butters and whole-grain flours) and less conventional foods such as brewer's yeast, pumpkin seeds, wheat germ, and herb teas.

Nutritional Aspects

The nutritional value of foods that reach the consumer depends not only on the composition of the raw materials but also on various changes which occur during processing, storage, and distribution.[27] Nutritional losses occur whether food is processed commercially or at home or is stored in an unprocessed state.[28] Variations in the nutrient content of raw foods will affect the content of vitamins and minerals in the final food product as much as, and sometimes more than, the processing itself. For example, carrots may vary 100-fold in their concentration of carotene (provitamin A), and samples of fresh tomato juice have shown 16-fold differences in vitamin C content. Although the data are somewhat sketchy, the raw foods being produced today are not significantly different in terms of vitamin content from those produced two or more decades ago. The food preservation techniques in greatest use today minimize the loss of nutritive value of foods and are safe and well standardized.

There is no test to differentiate organically grown and organically processed food from similar commercial products. Long-term studies have failed to show the nutritional superiority of organically grown crops in comparison to those grown under standard agricultural conditions with chemical fertilizers. If the soil is deficient in nutrients, crop yield rather than the nutritional quality of the plant will be primarily affected.

Other concerns about agricultural practices and food processing procedures may have more validity (e.g., residual hormones and antibiotics in meat, and pesticide residue on dairy, fruit, and vegetable products). In addition, the large variety of food additives in commercial use makes complete screening of such products for safety difficult for industry and federal agencies (see Chapter 35). Each of these issues is complicated, unresolved, and beyond the scope of this handbook. But concern about these issues frequently is the reason for the use of health foods despite their high cost.

Organically grown foods cost more than their nonorganic counterparts. In a 1976 survey by the Department of Agriculture in the Washington, D.C., area, a basket of 33 standard foods bought in a supermarket cost $17.49; the same foods labeled "organic" cost from $23.74 to $28.00 in "health" food stores.[29] The difference in cost (one and one-third to one and two-thirds higher) for foods purchased in "health" food stores is of particular concern for low-income families who may have to skimp in quantity or sacrifice other important items in the budget to afford "health" foods. There is no compelling evidence that the high cost of "health" foods results in concomitant benefit to the consumer. There are no standard tests to identify organically grown foods; therefore, the consumer is forced to rely on the integrity of the farmer and distributor for assurance that the products were grown or prepared as claimed.

Protein-sparing Modified Fast

Proponents of the use of low energy diets (600 kcal or less, mostly from protein) for weight reduction initially claimed that body protein was "spared," but subsequent studies have shown that nitrogen balance is negative and body potassium is lost.[30-32] Although less lean tissue is lost than during fasting, these diets are not without hazard. A number of deaths have been reported in adults[33] and Lantigua and co-workers[34] detected potentially serious arrhythmias in three of their six patients.

Miscellaneous Foods

Depending on the variety, herbal teas may contain nicotine, cathartics, hallucinogens, or atropine-like drugs.[35] Botulism has been reported in infants fed honey from certain regions of the country.[36] The Feingold diet is discussed in Chapter 35; this regime involves a change in family lifestyle as well as diet, and controlled studies have shown that, at best, only a small proportion of "hyperactive" children are helped.[37,38]

Megavitamin Therapy for Childhood Psychoses and Learning Disabilities

The consistent opinion of the Committee on Nutrition has been that normal children receiving a normal diet do not need vitamin supplementation over and above the Recommended Dietary Allowances. However, there are a variety of clinical entities in which the daily intake of vitamins needs to be significantly increased, e.g., the use of fat-soluble vitamins A, D, E, and K in steatorrhoea, and the autosomally recessive, selective malabsorption of vitamin B_{12}.[39] Children treated with isoniazid may require increased pyridoxine; and, those treated with diphenylhydantoin sodium (Dilantin) and phenobarbital need increased folic acid and vitamin D.[40] There also are a number of rare inborn errors of metabolism which affect the apoenzyme at the cofactor-binding site or which involve the metabolism of the vitamin itself to its biologically active derivative.[41] In these so-called dependency syndromes, the metabolic defect may completely or partially be overcome by increasing vitamin or cofactor availability.

Because of the widespread public belief in the benefits of vitamins, the accounts of dramatic amelioration of deficiency states, the easy and relatively inexpensive availability of vitamins, and the occasional, remarkable benefit of large doses of vitamins (both in the dependency syndromes and in certain other clinical situations), it is not surprising that a cult developed in the use of large doses of water-soluble vitamins to treat a wide spectrum of disease states. In particular, "megavitamin" therapy came to be applied to the use of large amounts of nicotinic acid or nicotinamide in the treatment of schizophrenia. In 1968, Pauling[42] coined the term "orthomolecular medicine," meaning the treatment or prevention of diseases by altering body concentrations of certain normally occurring substances. Pauling's term now encompasses the additional use of nicotinamide adenine dinucleotide (NAD), riboflavin, ascorbic acid, pyridoxine, calcium pantothenate, vitamin B_{12}, folic acid, and trace minerals in doses considerably in excess of the Recommended Dietary Allowances for a wide range of problems, including arthritis, neuroses, geriatric problems, hyperlipidemia, and depression.

This "orthomolecular" approach has been used primarily in children in the treatment of nonspecific mental retardation, psychoses, autism, hyperactivity, dyslexia, and other learning disorders reminiscent of an earlier advocacy of large doses of glutamic acid for patients with Down's syndrome. The anecdotal evidence of therapeutic benefit in these and other conditions should be viewed with skepticism until substantial evidence of benefit has been obtained and published in peer reviewed journals.

As an example of the "orthomolecular" approach, Cott[43] reports giving niacin (1 to 2 gm per 24 hours), ascorbic acid (1 to 2 gm per 24 hours), pyridoxine (200 to 400 mg per 24 hours), and calcium pantothenate (400 to 600 mg per 24 hours) combined with a sedative to more than 500 children with psychoses and learning disabilities. Cott claimed the treatment showed promising and even dramatic results; however, no precise data were given on which any objective assessment of the results can be made.

Although no comparable evaluation has been done on children with autism and learning disabilities, the claims of orthomolecular psychiatrists in the treatment of adult schizophrenia were carefully examined by a Task Force on Vitamin Therapy in Psychiatry.[44] The conclusions were emphatic that orthodox, properly controlled, and well standardized trials found nicotinic therapy to be without value. Moreover, there is some evidence that long-term administration of high doses of nicotinic acid in humans may lead to persistent skin erythema, pruritis, tachycardia, liver damage, hyperglycemia, and hyperuricemia.[45]

A recent study of megavitamin use in children with attention deficit disorder found no evidence of benefit; instead, attention was drawn to possible hazards because 42% of the subjects had elevations in serum transaminase values.[46]

In some situations, a specific vitamin deficiency can be demonstrated by the use of biochemical tests; the administration of increased doses of vitamins has been shown to resolve these conditions. Vitamin therapy is justified under these circumstances, and more conditions of this type probably will be identified. But megavitamin therapy as a treatment for learning disabilities and psychoses in children, including autism, is not justified on the basis of documented clinical results.

Conclusion

Most individuals who adhere to unusual dietary practices, except for balanced vegetarianism, are aware their ideas are not in the mainstream of medical and nutritional opinion. Some individuals adopt these diets as an expression of disillusion with medicine or the "establishment." Physicians and other health professionals should be prepared to encounter strong resistance if they attempt to reverse unusual dietary practices. Parents are likely to resist the suggestion of major dietary changes; therefore, it may be best to focus on the features of the diet that are of the most potential harm to their children. However, even with the more extreme dietary practices, serious harm usually can be prevented by striving for dietary variety and balance and working within the value system or philosophy of the group or individual.

References

1. Nutrition misinformation and food faddism. Nutr. Rev. (Suppl.), July, 1974.
2. National Research Council, Food and Nutrition Board, Committee on Nutritional Misinformation: Vegetarian diets. Amer. J. Clin. Nutr., 27:1095, 1974.

3. West, R.O., and Hayes, O.B.: Diet and serum cholesterol levels: A comparison between vegetarians and nonvegetarians in a Seventh-Day Adventist Group. Amer. J. Clin. Nutr., 21:853, 1968.
4. Council on Foods and Nutrition: Zen macrobiotic diets. J.A.M.A., 218:397, 1971.
5. Register, U.D., and Sonnenberg, L.M.: The vegetarian diet: Scientific and practical considerations. J. Amer. Diet. Assn., 62:253, 1973.
6. Robson, J.R.K., Konlande, J.E., Larkin, F.A., O'Connor, P.A., and Liu, H.Y.: Zen macrobiotic dietary problems in infancy. PEDIATRICS, 53:326, 1974.
7. Brown, P.T., and Bergan, J.G.: The dietary status of "new" vegetarians. J. Amer. Diet. Assn., 67:455, 1975.
8. Caffey, J.: Chronic poisoning due to excess of vitamin A: Description of the clinical and roentgen manifestations in seven infants and young children. PEDIATRICS, 5:672, 1950.
9. Mahoney, C.P., Margolis, M.T., Knauss, T.A., and Labbe, R.F.: Chronic vitamin A intoxication in infants fed chicken liver. PEDIATRICS, 65:893, 1980.
10. Ellis, C.N., Madison, K.C., Pennes, D.R., Martel, W., and Voorhees, J.J.: Isotretinoin therapy is associated with early skeletal radiographic changes. J. Amer. Acad. Dermatol., 10:1024, 1984.
11. Adverse effects with isotretinoin. FDA Drug Bulletin, 13:21, 1983.
12. Stern, R.S., Rosa, F., and Baum, C.: Isotretinoin and pregnancy. J. Amer. Acad. Dermatol., 10:851, 1984.
13. Pauling, L.C.: Vitamin C and the Common Cold. San Francisco: W. H. Freeman and Company, 1970.
14. Committee on Drugs: Vitamin C and the common cold. Newsletter (American Academy of Pediatrics), 22:2, November 1, 1971.
15. Part VI. Ascorbic acid and respiratory illness. In King, C.G., and Burns, J.J., ed.: Second conference on vitamin C. Ann. N. Y. Acad. Sci., 258:498-539, 1975.
16. Lamden, M.P.: Dangers of massive vitamin C intake. New Engl. J. Med., 284:336, 1971.
17. Rhead, W.J., and Schrauzer, G.N.: Risks of long-term ascorbic acid overdosage. Nutr. Rev., 29:262, 1971.
18. Cochrane, W.A.: Overnutrition in prenatal and neonatal life: A problem? Canad. Med. Assn. J., 93:893, 1965.
19. Committee on Nutritional Misinformation: Hazards of overuse of vitamin D. Amer. J. Clin. Nutr., 28:512, 1975.
20. Farrell, P.M., Bieri, J.G., Fratantoni, J.F., Wood, R.E., and di Sant' Agnese, P.A.: The occurrence and effects of human vitamin E deficiency: A study in patients with cystic fibrosis. J. Clin. Invest., 60:233, 1977.
21. Melhorn, D.K., and Gross, S.: Vitamin E-dependent anemia in the premature infant: II. Relationships between gestational age and absorption of vitamin E. J. Pediat., 79:581, 1971.
22. Hypervitaminosis E and coagulation. Nutr. Rev., 33:269, 1975.
23. Ehrlich, H.P., Tarver, H., and Hunt, T.K.: Inhibitory effects of

vitamin E on collagen synthesis and wound repair. Ann. Surg., 175:235, 1972.
24. Hillman, R.W.: Tocopherol excess in man: Creatinuria associated with prolonged ingestion. Amer. J. Clin. Nutr., 5:597, 1957.
25. Schaumburg, H., Kaplan, J., Windebank, A., Vick, N., Rasmus, S., Pleasure, D., and Brown, M.J.: Sensory neuropathy from pyridoxine abuse. A new megavitamin syndrome. New Engl. J. Med., 309:445, 1983.
26. Rudman, D., and Williams, P.J.: Megadose vitamins: Use and misuse. New Engl. J. Med., 309:488, 1983.
27. Expert Panel on Food Safety and Nutrition and the Committee on Public Information, Institute of Food Technologists: The effects of food processing on nutritional values. Nutr. Rev., 33:123, 1975.
28. Nesheim, R.O.: Nutrient changes in food processing: A current review. Fed. Proc., 33:2267, 1974.
29. Cromwell, C.: Organic Foods: An Update. Family Economics Review. Agricultural Research Services. Washington, D.C.: U.S. Department of Agriculture, pp. 8-11, Summer, 1976.
30. Yang, M.-U., Barbosa-Saldivar, J.L., Pi-Sunyer, F.X., and Van Itallie, T.B.: Metabolic effects of substituting carbohydrate for protein in a low-calorie diet: A prolonged study in obese patients. Internat. J. Obesity, 5:231, 1981.
31. Fisler, J.S., Drenick, E.J., Blumfield, D.E., and Swendseid, M.E.: Nitrogen economy during very low calorie reducing diets: Quality and quantity of dietary protein. Amer. J. Clin. Nutr., 35:471, 1982.
32. Brown, M.R., Klish, W.J., Hollander, J., Campbell, M.A., and Forbes, G.B.: A high protein, low calorie liquid diet in the treatment of very obese adolescents: Long-term effect on lean body mass. Amer. J. Clin. Nutr., 38:20, 1983.
33. Isner, J.M., Sours, H.E., Paris, A.L., Ferrans, V.J., and Roberts, W.C.: Sudden, unexpected death in avid dieters using the liquid-protein-modified-fast diet: Observations in 17 patients and the role of the prolonged QT interval. Circulation, 60:1401, 1979.
34. Lantigua, R.A., Amatruda, J.M., Biddle, T.L., Forbes, G.B., and Lockwood, D.H.: Cardiac arrhythmias associated with a liquid protein diet for the treatment of obesity. New Engl. J. Med., 303:735, 1980.
35. Toxic reactions to plant products sold in health food stores. Medical Letter, April 6, 1979.
36. Johnson, R.O., Clay, S.A., and Arnon, S.S.: Diagnosis and management of infant botulism. Amer. J. Dis. Child., 133:586, 1979.
37. Forbes, G.B.: Nutrition and hyperactivity. J.A.M.A., 248:355, 1982.
38. Forbes, G.B.: Food fads: Safe feeding of children. Pediatrics in Review, 1:207, 1980.
39. Bell, M., Harries, J.T., Wolff, O.H., Dawson, A.M., and Waters, A.H.: Familial selective malabsorption of vitamin B_{12}. Arch. Dis. Child., 48:896, 1973.
40. Christiansen, C., Rødbro, P., and Nielsen, C.T.: Iatrogenic os-

teomalacia in epileptic children: A controlled therapeutic trial. Acta Pediat. Scand., **64**:219, 1975.

41. Scriver, C.R.: Vitamin-responsive inborn errors of metabolism. Metabolism, **22**:1319, 1973.
42. Pauling, L.: Orthomolecular psychiatry. Science, **160**:265, 1968.
43. Cott, A.: Megavitamins: The orthomolecular approach to behavioral disorders and learning disabilities. Acad. Ther., **7**:245, 1972.
44. American Psychiatry Association, Excerpts from the Report of the Task Force on Vitamin Therapy in Psychiatry: Megavitamin and orthomolecular therapy in psychiatry. Nutr. Rev. (Suppl.), **32**:44, July, 1974.
45. Winter, S.L., and Boyer, J.L.: Hepatic toxicity from large doses of vitamin B₃ (nicotinamide). New Engl. J. Med., **289**:1180, 1973.
46. Haslam, R.H.A., Dalby, J.T., and Rademaker, A.W.: The effects of megavitamin therapy on children with attention deficit disorder (ADD). Pediat. Res. (Abst.), **17**:363A, 1983.

Chapter 34

FAST FOODS

The extent to which so-called fast foods are a factor in the nutritional status of an individual depends on several variables: the nutritive quality of the menu items, the customer's selection of menu items to constitute a meal, the frequency with which those meals are eaten, and the amounts consumed. The popularity of fast food establishments is evident from the fact that 1 of every 10 food dollars currently is spent on fast foods; the total yearly fast foods sales exceeds $20 billion.[1] The extensive patronage of these outlets is aided by the fast service provided and the cost, which is lower than that of most traditional restaurants.

The variety of establishments and frequency of changes within the industry make it difficult to place definitive values on the nutritive quality of all fast foods; however, a number of studies have provided information from which some general conclusions about the nutritive value of fast foods can be drawn.

In 1975 *Consumer Reports* published a study based on assay results of the nutrient content of a typical meal at outlets featuring Colonel Sanders' chicken, Pizza Hut pizza, Arthur Treacher's breaded fish, and sample meals from the three leading hamburger chains.[2] The study included a beverage with all meals and a serving of potatoes with all but the pizza meal.

One characteristic common to all the meals analyzed was a low density of some nutrients relative to energy; however, the protein to energy ratio was adequate (Tables 21 and 22). All meals contained a number of nutrients in quantities equal to or greater than one third of the Recommended Dietary Allowances used by *Consumer Reports* as a standard for adequacy, but half or more of the daily caloric allowance had to be consumed to acquire them. Extra calories were a problem with meals which included soft drinks (the most frequently purchased beverage by diners less than 17 years old[3]) and "shakes" common to fast food restaurants. These "shakes" include some calcium from milk derivatives, but enough sugar is added to make them an inefficient source of calcium relative to caloric content.

The general tendency for low nutrient density in the standard portion size could be magnified when fast foods are used for children. A single meal of hamburger, French fries, and Coca Cola could provide up to 36% of the caloric needs of a 6-year-old child according to the Recommended Dietary Allowances. The need for calcium by children entering an age range when high intakes of calcium are required might not be met within recommended calorie parameters when eating at a fast food outlet.

Sodium and iodine also were found in disproportionately high amounts in most meals analyzed. The 10 in. pizza contained 1½ teaspoons of salt, or the entire daily allowance for many restricted diets. The hamburger, chicken, and roast beef meals tested had nearly 1 teaspoon of salt, but Arthur Treacher's meal had negligible sodium.

The studies also uncovered a number of general deficiencies that were common among the fast food meals. The amount of vitamin A was highly variable. Inadequacies were found for biotin, folacin, pantothenic acid, iron, and copper. Beans; dark green, leafy vegetables; yellow vegetables; and a variety of fresh fruits were recommended as sources of nutrients that could be consumed at other meals to offset the inadequacies. These foods also would compensate for the fiber deficiency common with fast food meals. In addition, bran cereals, whole grain breads, nuts, and seeds will provide a variety of nutrients and fiber.

Some members of the fast food industry already have responded to heightened consumer interest in nutrition since the studies were done in the mid-1970's, e.g., salad bars have been

Table 21
Sample Meals

Foods	Calories	Protein (gm)	CHO (gm)	Fat (gm)	Sodium (mg)
Meal I					
Burger, "fries," cola	612	16	91	20	638 (28 mEq)
percent of calories	–	11	60	29	–
Meal II					
Burger, "fries," "shake"	792	27	107	28	887 (39 mEq)
percent of calories	–	14	54	32	–

Table 22
Comparison of Energy and Protein Content with RDA

Age	% RDA Energy		% RDA Protein	
(yr)	Meal I	Meal II	Meal I	Meal II
1-3	47	61	71	118
4-6	36	47	55	90
7-10	26	33	48	80
11-14 (M)	23	29	36	60
11-14 (F)	28	36	36	59
15-18 (M)	22	28	29	48
15-18 (F)	29	38	36	59

added to improve the nutritional balance of their menu. In addition, there is increasing activity among those trying to combine a fast food and family restaurant format with more nutritionally sound menus and preparation procedures.

Results of the studies cited here also support the assertion that the nutritive value of a meal depends heavily on the food items selected. Milk, pure fruit juice, or water can be substituted for soft drinks or "shakes," for example. Impromptu portion control might be used to reduce the effects of low-nutrient density, high-calorie foods on children. A "shake" or French fries could be shared with a parent or sibling, for example; and part or all of a bun can be removed so the amount of calories is reduced.

After nutritive quality and item selection, frequency is the third major variable in determining the effect fast food dining has on an individual's nutritional status. The National Restaurant Association indicates that 79% of the families in the United States are in the eating-away-from-home market, with the average family studied eating out more than four times a week.[3] Other statistics indicate that individuals 17 years old or younger visit fast food restaurants more often than any other restaurant type—about two meals a week.[4] Based on these figures, the frequency of fast food dining would not be difficult to offset with complementary foods at home, school, or other types of eating establishments. No doubt the frequency of fast food meals is much higher for some individuals, and excesses or deficiencies not offset elsewhere will be cumulative in proportion to their frequency. However, a consumer who is aware of the tradeoffs and can compensate for the peculiarities of fast food dining should be able to enjoy the convenience of fast food dining without ill effects, unless there is a specific restriction against an unavoidable by-product such as the common high sodium consumption. Fast foods are not necessarily off limits to children on restricted diets, but some planning, forethought, and education are required. Assistance can be obtained from a registered dietitian.

Summary

1. With the exception of the fast food industry's "shake" substitute milk shake, research has found no appreciable difference in the nutrient quality of raw materials used in fast food items and their prepared-at-home equivalents.

2. Existing studies of fast food menus demonstrate the potential for some excesses and deficiencies. Although these might be exaggerated in those 17 years old or younger, for the most part they are relatively easy to correct, except for individuals on a salt-restricted diet.

3. Much of the nutritional quality of a fast food meal depends on the selection of menu items.

4. Unless excesses or deficiencies are compensated for at other meals, their effect will be cumulative in proportion to the frequency that fast food meals are eaten.

References

1. Ross Laboratories, Dietetic Currents, Vol. 8, March-April, 1981.
2. How nutritious are fast food meals? Consumer Reports, May, 1975, pp. 278-281.
3. National Restaurant Association News, p. 36, January, 1983.
4. National Restaurant Association News, p. 30, November, 1982.

Chapter 35

FOOD ADDITIVES

As defined by regulation, a food additive is a substance, or blend of substances, deliberately added to foods through production, processing, storage, or packaging. An additive need not be synthetic to fall within this definition. Many additives, such as spices, are natural products; and certain substances, such as pesticides, may have been added inadvertently.

Thousands of agents may be added deliberately to food. Some are exotic molecular handiworks of the chemist's craft. Others may be as commonplace as sugar and table salt. In the United States, all additives are governed by labeling regulations prescribed by the Food and Drug Administration. The broad categories of food additives are listed in Table 23. For the physician, the foremost questions about food additives hinge on safety and the clinical entities that may reflect adverse effects.

Types of Additives

Flavors

The largest single group of additives are flavorings. There are more than 2,000 flavorings. Of these, about 500 are extracted from natural sources; the rest are synthesized. Sucrose and sodium chloride frequently are added to processed foods to restore flavor lost in processing. Many flavors are mixtures; for example, there are 17 ingredients in artificial pineapple flavor.

Colors

Although coloring agents from natural sources are readily available, synthetic dyes are preferred because of their stability during processing and their strong coloring potency. Only a few synthetic colors are widely used in food. Each batch is certified by Food and Drug Administration chemists for adherence to prescribed standards of purity.

Preservatives

Food spoilage is a serious problem for both economic and health reasons. The more traditional treatments such as smoking, drying, fermenting, heating, and cooling are used primarily to inhibit microbiologic spoilage; few chemical preservatives are used, and their use is decreasing. Antioxidants, such as butylated hydroxytoluene (BHT) and butylated hydroxyanisole (BHA) help prevent rancidity in products containing fats (e.g., oil, lard, potato chips, and crackers). Sulfur dioxide is used to inhibit wild yeasts in wine and maintain the color of such products as dried fruit.

Antibiotics such as penicillin, streptomycin, or tetracycline are not used in human food. Antifungal agents are used in dairy products. Molds are inhibited in bread by the use of calcium propionates, which extend the shelf life of the breads.

Nitrates and nitrites combat microbial toxins in products such as sausage and bacon. However, these additives may undergo transformation to nitrosamines under some condi-

Table 23
Intentional Food Additives

Class	Number in Use
Preservatives	33
Antioxidants	28
Sequestrants	45
Surface active agents	111
Stabilizers, thickeners	39
Bleaching and maturing agents	34
Buffers, acids, alkalies	60
Food colors	34
Nonnutritive and special dietary sweeteners	4
Nutritive supplement	117
Flavorings, synthetic	1,610
Flavorings, natural	502
Miscellaneous: yeast foods, texturizers, firming agents, binders, anticaking agents, enzymes	157
Total number of additives	2,764

tions; and questions about their carcinogenic potential have arisen. The Food and Drug Administration has limited nitrites in bacon because of this concern.

Texture Agents

Emulsifiers, stabilizers, and thickening agents probably comprise the greatest amount of additives. They are used in baked goods, ice cream, puddings, toppings, soft drinks, and the new, textured vegetable proteins. Emulsifiers and stabilizers are exemplified by glycerol esters, carboxymethylcellulose, and propylene glycol. Thickeners include modified starches, celluloses, and natural products such as carob bean gum.

Miscellaneous Agents

The list of other agents which might be added to foods is too extensive to be given here, but it includes such substances as those added to control acidity or alkalinity, to bleach and mature flour, to sequester trace metals, to retain moisture, to glaze surfaces, to prevent wilting, and so forth.

Safety Evaluation

The original Food and Drug Act became law in 1906 as a consumer protection measure. In 1938, the Food, Drug, and Cosmetic Act provided an even more comprehensive regulatory framework, which was then expanded by the Food Additives Amendment of 1958. The latter legislation called for prior approval by the Food and Drug Administration of new, commercially added food ingredients on the basis of utility and safety.

Toxicity Tests

The earliest steps in toxicity testing are aimed at providing information about mode of action, species sensitivity, and other data useful in planning further studies. Such acute toxicity determinations generally use at least two test species, frequently three. Long-term studies typically use rodents, although dogs sometimes are used. The main purpose of these studies is to evaluate human exposure. The dominant concern is carcinogenesis, although many other observations also are made. Typical, long-term studies last a minimum of 18 months in mice and 2 years in rats. Modern assessments of toxicity also include reproduction, embryotoxicity, and teratogenicity. These procedures are now fairly standard,[1] although they seldom include immature animals.

Extrapolation to Humans

To provide acceptable risks for humans on the basis of animal studies, a safety factor is introduced. The amount of a substance that can be included in the diet of a group of animals without producing detectable toxic effects is taken as the "no-effect" level. Such a level is an arbitrary, statistical criterion because the chances of finding an outcome such as liver damage depend on the size of the subject sample. A safety factor, typically 100, then provides what is called the acceptable daily intake for humans. However, no additive is permitted at any level if it has been shown to induce cancer in test animals. This stipulation—the Delaney Clause—evokes constant debate because of its strict criteria. There is a continuing development of methods for toxicity testing to strive for better extrapolation to real-life situations.

GRAS

The 1958 food additives amendment exempted prior permits and substances in common use from the new regulatory requirements. These substances became known as GRAS (for "Generally Regarded As Safe") substances. By 1969, enough skepticism had been voiced about the GRAS strategy to provoke a revaluation. This revaluation is now published and represents a landmark document in toxicology.[2] The report expresses skepticism about permitting the use of substances as food additives solely on the basis that proof of harm to humans is absent. To determine that an agent really is innocuous goes beyond the limits of current toxicologic competence.

Laboratory Limitations

Even if current toxicologic protocols are carried out in a meticulous manner, they fail to reflect certain features of the natural environment. The protocols test only one agent at a time, but humans consume hundreds of different agents simultaneously. Also, they rely on healthy animals fed a nutritious diet to evaluate substances consumed by humans who may be malnourished, old, or sick. The basal diet is not irrelevant. Ershoff[3] discovered that rats fed a low-fiber diet died after consuming food colors at levels (500 times the allowable amounts for man) that did not impair the health of rats fed the typical laboratory diet, which is high in fiber and minerals.

Epidemiology

Despite the most prolonged and thorough laboratory study, toxic substances are bound to slip through the screen. Also, allowable intake levels no doubt will occasionally be set at values that induce adverse effects in humans. If epidemiologic data are to act as a sentinel for such possible—even though unlikely—outcomes, patterns of consumption must be monitored; but this information is difficult to obtain. Processors need not file their formulations with the Food and Drug Administration, and it is impossible to monitor actual intakes or all industry practices. Therefore, there is no way to determine the actual consumption of particular additives by various segments of the population.

Adverse Effects

Medical Consequences

Carcinogenesis dominates the toxicologic evaluation of additives and is the sole reason for the Food and Drug Administration's categorical bans on any specific additive. However, adverse effects may take many forms, most of which attract minimal regulatory attention but may pose troublesome problems for the clinician.

Some effects may be life-threatening. Within a 1-month period, nine young infants in a pediatric ward in Israel developed a significant methemoglobinemia.[4] All the affected infants, who had been recovering from acute gastroenteritis, had been fed a soybean formula. The problem was traced to a manufacturer who had switched to a new fat preservative imported from the United States. This additive contained the antioxidants BHT, BHA, and propyl gallate.

Between 1964 and 1967, heavy beer drinkers in certain parts of the United States and Canada fell victim to fulminating heart failure.[5] Cases began to appear about 6 months after cobalt chloride was introduced as an additive to stabilize the foam in beer. A contributing factor was the low protein and high alcohol intake of many of these patients.

In one study conducted with 122 patients suffering from a variety of what were diagnosed as allergic disorders, oral administration of 50 mg of the food dye tartrazine (FD & C Yellow No. 5) evoked reactions such as weakness, heat sensations, palpitations, blurred vision, rhinorrhoea, feelings of suffocation, pruritus, and urticaria.[6] Although a substantial dose, this quantity of tartrazine would be consumed by a person drinking only a few bottles of soft drinks during the day.

Reactions to various emulsifying and texturizing agents also may mimic allergies. Plant gums, such as gum acacia and tragacanth, frequently are used as stabilizers and thickening agents in both foods and drugs. One of the more serious manifestations of toxicity presenting as "allergy" took place in 1960 in the Netherlands.[7] A margarine producer had introduced a new emulsifying agent into a brand occupying about 14% of the market. Shortly afterward, an epidemic of generalized exanthem occurred. The condition came on suddenly, became generalized in 2 to 24 hours, and was accompanied by severe itching. Some patients experienced high fevers, conjunctivitis, sore throat, and swollen lips. The first clue to the source of this epidemic, which involved about 50,000 of the approximately 600,000 persons estimated to have eaten the margarine, was provided by an observant young boy and a dermatologist who took the boy's observation seriously. The boy thought he may have remained free of the condition because, unlike most of his family, he ate butter rather than margarine.

Monosodium glutamate (MSG), the "flavor enhancer," probably deserves a chapter by itself because of the many ramifications generated by the debate about its safety for young children and its capacity to damage the brain of young rodents.

This latter association provoked its removal from prepared infant foods. In adults, MSG is associated with the Chinese restaurant syndrome because of the enthusiasm of Chinese chefs for MSG. The Chinese restaurant syndrome includes symptoms such as burning sensations, chest pressure, and facial pressure. It leads some victims to believe they are experiencing a heart attack. Although at first it was thought that only a small subpopulation was sensitive to MSG, further studies showed sensitivity to it to be widely distributed and dose related. In some individuals, the syndrome might be provoked by 2 to 3 gm of MSG, an amount frequently added to soups. Insensitive individuals might require as much as 20 gm to experience the syndrome. In children, MSG has led to a deceptive diagnosis of epilepsy because of "shudder" attacks in susceptible children.[8] Because of the broad distribution of sensitivity to MSG, it is particularly difficult for the clinician pursuing a diagnosis; the details of exposure and the consistency of responses must be documented carefully if a reliable pattern is to be discerned.

One study[9] showed that the food color tartrazine (FD & C Yellow No. 5) and certain benzoic acid derivatives used as preservatives both can precipitate "allergic" symptoms. Another study[10] found that salicylate intolerance was common in patients suffering from chronic urticaria and that tartrazine also can evoke the complaint in these patients. Overt manifestations of intolerance, such as urticaria, may represent only a fraction of the total spectrum of adverse reactions. The possibility of behavioral aberrations is now the subject of vigorous debate.

The Feingold Hypothesis

The possibility of a link between diet and the loose collection of behavioral disturbances variously called "hyperkinesis," "hyperactivity," "minimal brain dysfunction," and "attention deficit disorder" was first postulated by Feingold, a pediatric allergist in the Kaiser-Permanente system. First in a professional[11] then in a popular book,[12] Feingold asserted that a significant percent of the children with these behavioral disturbances could be treated effectively by removing from their diet synthetic colors and flavors and natural foods containing "salicylates." Most of these natural foods fall within the fruit group (oranges, apples, grapes, plums, and so forth), and a few fall within the vegetable group (cucumbers, tomatoes). They are designated "salicylate containing" because of their link with aspirin sensitivity. However, the fact that salicylates are present in trace quantities in many foods renders this aspect of the hypothesis untenable.

Feingold's assertions were based on clinical experience and parental testimony of the improvement in their children's symptoms when the additives and specified fruits and vegetables were excluded from the diet. However, his book[12] fails to provide the scientific rigor needed for upholding such assertions.[13]

The Feingold hypothesis can be evaluated now on the basis of several double-blind, controlled, clinical trials.[14] Although Feingold's proponents and his critics offer widely differing estimates of the diet's value, some observers now acknowledge that a few children may be helped by the diet and a few respond adversely to synthetic food dyes. Such a conclusion emerged from a conference held at the National Institutes of Health in January 1982. It also is the position adopted by Feingold's critics. For example, Lipton et al.,[15,16] after concluding that the controlled studies do not support the breadth of Feingold's claims, also note that some hyperactive children may benefit from the additive-free diet.

The possibility exists that young children are more vulnerable. Of interest is the recent development of a new toxicologic discipline, behavioral toxicology, which is concerned with the later functional consequences of prenatal and neonatal toxic exposure.

Physician's Role

Physicians bear two responsibilities in dealing with the potential adverse impact of food additives. One is to provide expert nutritional guidance. Most additives probably are safe in the amounts and forms in current use, but additives are most prevalent in foods that make minimal contributions to nutrition. This is particularly true of cosmetic additives, such as synthetic colors and flavors, that serve only to enhance marketability. Cosmetic additives should be distinguished from functional additives, which serve, for example, to inhibit microbial contamination. Physicians also should be receptive to parents experimenting with the Feingold diet. If the diet is considered a collaborative research program between physician and parent, the physician's guidance is more likely to be accepted, his or her role less resented, and the child's welfare advanced.

Physicians also should press for improved labeling regulations. For example, certain foods now exempt from labeling regulations should be required to comply with those regulations. Emulsifying agents, for example, must be labeled in pasteurized cheese food but not in pasteurized processed cheese. The dairy industry is exempt from many other labeling regulations, making it difficult for parents to test constituents possibly linked to allergies and behavioral disorders. In prescribing medications, physicians also need to be aware that many preparations contain synthetic colors and flavors. In sensitive children, these additives may arouse reactions whose etiology will baffle both parents and the physician.

References

1. World Health Organization: Toxicological Evaluation of Certain Food Additives with a Review of General Principles and of Specifications. World Health Organization Technical Report Series, No. 539. Geneva: World Health Organization, 1974.
2. FASEB Select Committee on GRAS Substances: Evaluation of health aspects of GRAS food ingredients: Lessons learned and questions unanswered. Fed. Proc., 36:2525, 1977.
3. Ershoff, B.H.: Effects of diet on growth and survival of rats fed toxic levels of tartrazine (FD & C Yellow #5) and Sunset Yellow FCF (FD & C Yellow #6). J. Nutr., 107:822, 1977.
4. Nitzan, M., Volovitz, B., and Topper, E.: Infantile methemoglobinemia caused by food additives. Clin. Toxicol., 15:273, 1979.
5. Berglund, F.: Food additives. Arch. Toxicol., Suppl. 1, p. 33, 1978.
6. Neuman, I., Elian, R., Nahum, H., Shaked, P., and Creter, D.: The danger of "yellow dyes" (tartrazine) to allergic subjects. Clin. Allerg., 8:65, 1978.
7. Mali, J.W.H., and Malten, K.E.: The epidemic of polymorph toxic erythema in the Netherlands in 1960: The so-called margarine disease. Acta Derm.-Venereol., 46:123, 1966.
8. Reif-Lehrer, L.: Possible significance of adverse reactions to glutamate in humans. Fed. Proc., 35:2205, 1976.
9. Juhlin, L., Michaelsson, G., and Zetterström, O.: Urticaria and asthma induced by food-and-drug additives in patients with aspirin hypersensitivity. J. Allerg. Clin. Immunol., 50:92, 1972.
10. Noid, H.E., Schulze, T.W., and Winkelmann, R.K.: Diet plan for patients with salicylate-induced urticaria. Arch. Dermatol., 109:866, 1974.

11. Feingold, B.F.: Introduction to Clinical Allergy. Springfield, Illinois: Charles C Thomas, 1973.
12. Feingold, B.F.: Why Your Child Is Hyperactive. New York: Random House, 1975.
13. Forbes, G.B.: Nutrition and hyperactivity. J.A.M.A., **248**:355, 1982.
14. Weiss, B.: Food additives and environmental chemicals as sources of childhood behavior disorders. J. Amer. Acad. Child Psychiat., **21**:144, 1982.
15. Lipton, M.A., Nemeroff, C.B., and Mailman, R.B.: Hyperkinesis and food additives. *In* Wurtman, R.J., and Wurtman, J.J., ed.: Nutrition and the Brain, Vol. 4. Toxic Effects of Food Constituents on the Brain. New York: Raven Press, pp. 1-27, 1979.
16. Lipton, M.A., and Mayo, J.P.: Diet and hyperkinesis—an update. J. Amer. Diet. Assn., **83**:132, 1983.

Appendix

Appendix A

Growth Charts

These charts to record the growth of the individual child were constructed by the National Center for Health Statistics in collaboration with the Centers for Disease Control. The charts are based on data from national probability samples representative of children in the general population. Their use will direct attention to unusual body size which may be due to disease or poor nutrition.

Measuring: Take all measurements with the child in minimal indoor clothing and without shoes. Measure stature with the infant 0 to 36 months old supine and the child 2 to 18 years old standing. Use a beam balance to measure weight.

Recording: First take all measurements and record them. Then graph each measurement on the appropriate chart. Find the child's age on the horizontal scale; then follow a vertical line from that point to the horizontal level of the child's measurement (stature or weight). Where the two lines intersect, make a cross mark with a pencil. In graphing weight for stature, place the cross mark directly above the child's stature at the horizontal level of weight. When the child is measured again, join the new set of cross marks to the previous set by straight lines.

Do not use the weight for stature chart for children who have begun to develop secondary sex characteristics.

Interpreting: Many factors influence growth. Therefore, growth data cannot be used alone to diagnose disease, but they do allow you to identify some unusual children.

Each chart contains a series of curved lines numbered to show selected percentiles. These refer to the rank of a measure in a group of 100. Thus, when a cross mark is on the 95th percentile line of weight for age, it means that only 5 children among 100 of the corresponding age and sex have weights greater than that recorded.

Inspect the set of cross marks you have just made. If any are particularly high or low (for example, above the 95th percentile or below the 5th percentile), you may want to refer the child to a physician. Compare the most recent set of cross marks with earlier sets for the same child. If he or she has changed rapidly in percentile levels, you may want to refer him

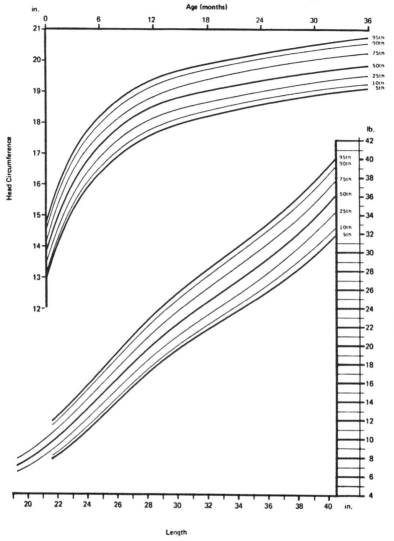

Boys from birth to 36 months; head circumference for age.

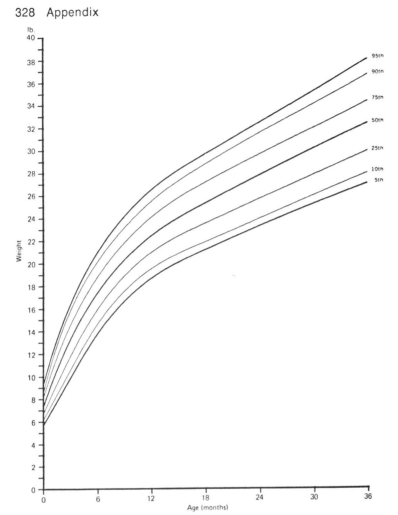

Boys from birth to 36 months; weight for age.

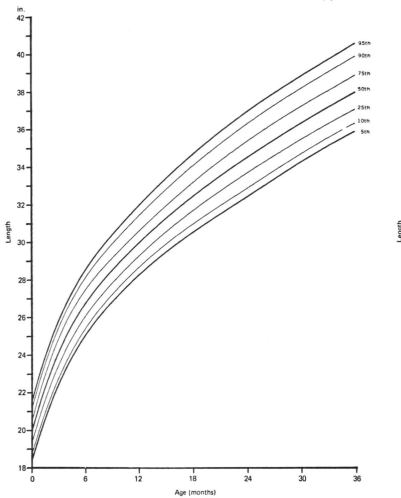

Boys from birth to 36 months; length for age.

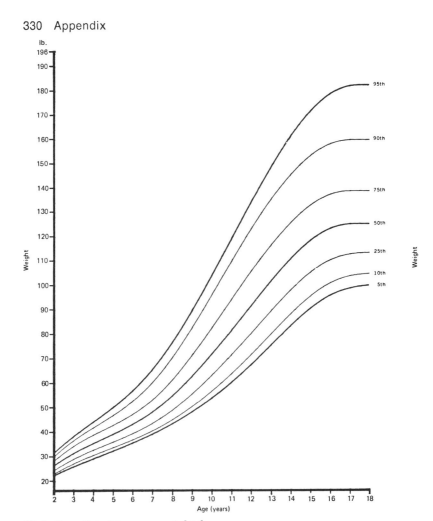

Girls from 2 to 18 years; weight for age.

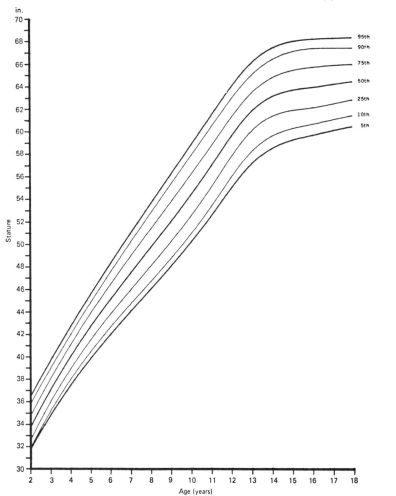

Girls from 2 to 18 years; stature for age.

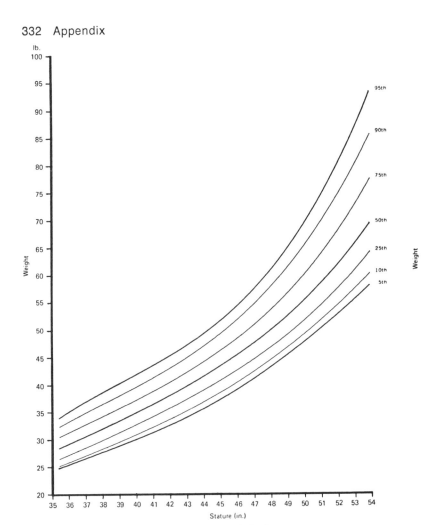

Prepubertal girls from 2 to 10 years; weight for stature.

or her to a physician. Rapid changes are less likely to be significant when they occur within the range from the 25th to the
75th percentile.

In normal teen-agers, the age at onset of puberty varies.
Rises occur in percentile levels if puberty is early, and these
levels fall if puberty is late.

Appendix B

Midparent Stature

Fels Parent-specific Standards for Height:
Children's Stature by Age and Midparent Stature (Boys)*,†

Age (yr)	Parental Midpoint (cm)								
	163	165	167	169	171	173	175	177	178
Birth	47.1	49.7	50.3	50.0	48.3	50.7	50.0	51.5	51.4
0-6 mo	65.1	66.2	66.8	67.4	65.8	70.2	69.0	70.2	70.3
1	73.1	75.6	75.7	75.1	73.4	76.6	77.1	79.6	77.8
2	85.4	87.2	87.0	87.4	87.8	88.0	88.9	92.0	91.3
3	93.2	94.9	96.1	96.0	97.2	98.1	98.3	100.7	99.9
4	99.5	102.2	103.5	103.1	104.6	106.0	106.3	108.0	107.0
5	105.6	108.5	110.6	110.0	111.5	113.2	112.7	114.6	113.8
6	110.9	114.1	116.4	115.4	117.4	119.4	118.7	120.4	119.8
7	116.2	119.7	122.3	121.3	123.2	125.6	124.6	126.4	125.6
8	121.6	125.0	127.8	126.8	128.8	131.6	130.4	132.8	131.6
9	126.9	130.4	133.3	131.9	134.1	138.0	136.0	138.8	137.5
10	132.5	135.8	138.8	137.4	139.8	143.8	141.5	145.3	143.2
11	138.5	141.8	144.1	143.0	145.4	149.9	146.8	151.9	148.9
12	144.7	148.0	149.7	148.4	151.4	155.7	152.4	158.8	154.5
13	151.0	154.2	155.7	154.9	158.0	161.7	159.6	166.3	160.5
14	158.8	161.7	162.3	161.6	165.7	167.6	167.8	173.4	166.9
15	165.8	168.1	169.1	167.9	172.9	173.0	174.7	176.4	175.2
16	169.4	173.3	174.3	172.8	177.3	177.5	176.6	177.4	181.2
17	170.9	174.7	176.8	175.4	179.2	179.4	177.8	177.5	184.3
18	171.5	175.0	177.9	176.2	180.5	180.2	178.6	177.6	186.3

Note: No attempt was made to eliminate sampling fluctuations.

*Midparent stature is calculated by adding the heights of the parents and dividing by 2. Inches can be converted to centimeters by multiplying by 2.54.

†From Garn, S.M., and Rohmann, C.G.: Interaction of nutrition and genetics in the timing of growth and development. Pediat. Clin. N. Amer., **13**:353, 1966.

Fels Parent-specific Standards for Height:
Children's Stature by Age and Midparent Stature (Girls)*,†

Age (yr)	Parental Midpoint (cm)									
	161	163	165	167	169	171	173	175	177	178
Birth	47.3	48.9	49.0	49.2	49.2	48.8	49.7	49.1	49.0	47.5
0-6 mo	64.4	64.7	65.6	65.7	64.6	66.5	66.6	67.4	67.3	65.8
1	72.3	73.0	73.8	74.0	74.0	75.2	75.5	74.6	77.3	73.2
2	84.6	84.0	86.5	87.4	85.5	88.8	88.7	88.2	89.5	87.6
3	93.2	90.4	94.5	95.8	93.8	97.1	96.5	96.5	98.5	96.2
4	100.1	96.8	102.4	103.5	103.9	104.9	104.0	103.8	105.8	104.3
5	106.8	103.5	108.9	109.0	109.1	111.6	110.9	111.0	112.6	111.7
6	113.2	110.2	115.0	116.2	115.0	118.2	117.8	117.3	119.1	118.8
7	118.8	116.5	120.6	122.4	120.2	124.4	124.4	124.0	125.0	125.5
8	124.6	122.4	126.3	128.8	125.8	130.7	130.8	130.2	130.8	132.0
9	130.1	128.6	132.2	134.7	131.4	137.1	136.7	136.6	137.0	138.2
10	136.0	135.1	139.0	140.3	136.9	143.8	142.9	143.1	143.8	143.6
11	141.9	141.6	145.9	146.0	143.4	150.3	149.0	149.6	151.3	149.4
12	148.0	147.8	152.8	151.8	150.3	156.4	155.2	155.8	159.0	154.9
13	152.9	154.2	158.8	157.0	157.0	161.0	161.1	161.7	162.3	160.5
14	155.4	158.8	161.7	160.9	160.4	163.7	165.0	165.9	163.9	164.1
15	155.9	159.8	162.6	163.7	162.2	164.0	167.1	168.4	165.0	166.5
16	156.0	160.5	162.8	165.5	163.4	164.1	167.8	169.7	165.5	168.7
17	156.2	160.8	163.0	166.5	164.0	164.3	167.9	170.9	165.7	170.0
18	156.2	161.0	165.0	167.2	164.3	164.4	167.9	171.8	165.7	170.8

Note: No attempt was made to eliminate sampling fluctuations.

*Midpoint stature is calculated by adding the heights of the parents and dividing by 2. Inches can be converted to centimeters by multiplying by 2.54.

†From Garn, S.M., and Rohmann, C.G.: Interaction of nutrition and genetics in the timing of growth and development. Pediat. Clin. N. Amer., 13:353, 1966.

Appendix C

Perinatal Growth*

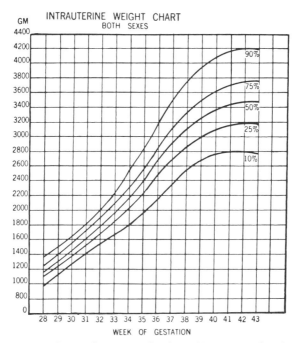

INTRAUTERINE WEIGHT CHART
BOTH SEXES

Fetal body weight percentiles from 28 to 43 weeks of gestation.

*Charts from Naeye, R.L., and Dixon J.B.: Distortions in fetal growth standards. Pediat. Res., **12**:987, 1978.

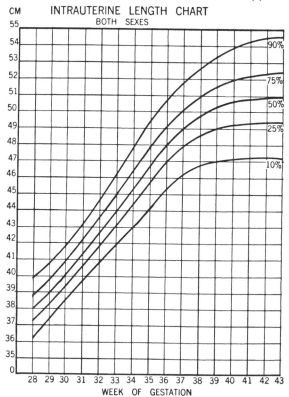

Fetal body length percentiles from 28 to 43 weeks of gestation.

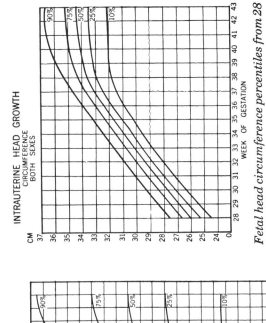

INTRAUTERINE HEAD GROWTH
CIRCUMFERENCE
BOTH SEXES

Fetal head circumference percentiles from 28 to 43 weeks of gestation.

INTRAUTERINE PLACENTAL GROWTH
BOTH SEXES

Placental weight percentiles from 28 to 43 weeks of gestation. In most cases, blood was allowed to drain from the organ and clots were removed before weights were taken.

PERINATAL
GROWTH
CHART

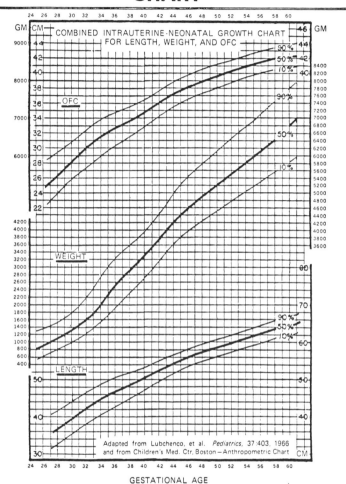

GESTATIONAL AGE

Appendix D

Arm Measurements

Percentiles of Upper Arm Circumference (mm) and Estimated Upper Arm Muscle Circumference (mm) for Whites of the United States Health Examination Survey I of 1971 to 1974*,†

Age (yr)	Arm Circumference (mm)						Arm Muscle Circumference (mm)					
	5th	50th	95th	5th	50th	95th	5th	50th	95th	5th	50th	95th
	Males			Females			Males			Females		
1-1.9	142	159	183	138	156	177	110	127	147	105	124	143
2-2.9	141	162	185	142	160	184	111	130	150	111	126	147
3-3.9	150	167	190	143	167	189	117	137	153	113	132	152
4-4.9	149	171	192	149	169	191	123	141	159	115	136	157
5-5.9	153	175	204	153	175	211	128	147	169	125	142	165
6-6.9	155	179	228	156	176	211	131	151	177	130	145	171
7-7.9	162	187	230	164	183	231	137	160	190	129	151	176
8-8.9	162	190	245	168	195	261	140	162	187	138	160	194
9-9.9	175	200	257	178	211	260	151	170	202	147	167	198
10-10.9	181	210	274	174	210	265	156	180	221	148	170	197
11-11.9	186	223	280	185	224	303	159	183	230	150	181	223
12-12.9	193	232	303	194	237	294	167	195	241	162	191	220
13-13.9	194	247	301	202	243	338	172	211	245	169	198	240
14-14.9	220	253	322	214	252	322	189	223	264	174	201	247
15-15.9	222	264	320	208	254	322	199	237	272	175	202	244
16-16.9	244	278	343	218	258	334	213	249	296	170	202	249
17-17.9	246	285	347	220	264	350	224	258	312	175	205	257
18-18.9	245	297	379	222	258	325	226	264	324	174	202	245
19-24.9	262	308	372	221	265	345	238	273	321	179	207	249
25-34.9	271	319	375	233	277	368	243	279	326	183	212	264
35-44.9	278	326	374	241	290	378	247	286	327	186	218	272
45-54.9	267	322	376	242	299	384	239	281	326	187	220	274
55-64.9	258	317	369	243	303	385	236	278	320	187	225	280
65-74.9	248	307	355	240	299	373	223	268	306	185	225	279

*Adapted from Frisancho, A.R.: New norms of upper limb fat and muscle areas for assessment of nutritional status, Amer. J. Clin. Nutr., **34**:2540, 1981.
†The Lange caliper was used in these studies.

Percentiles for Estimates of Upper Arm Muscle Area (mm²) for
Whites of the United States Health Examination Survey I of
1971 to 1974*,†

| Age (yr) | Arm Muscle Area Percentiles (mm²) | | | | | |
| | 5th | 50th | 95th | 5th | 50th | 95th |
	Males			Females		
1-1.9	956	1,278	1,720	885	1,221	1,621
2-2.9	973	1,345	1,787	973	1,269	1,727
3-3.9	1,095	1,484	1,853	1,014	1,396	1,846
4-4.9	1,207	1,579	2,008	1,058	1,475	1,958
5-5.9	1,298	1,720	2,285	1,238	1,598	2,159
6-6.9	1,360	1,815	2,493	1,354	1,683	2,323
7-7.9	1,497	2,027	2,886	1,330	1,815	2,469
8-8.9	1,550	2,089	2,788	1,513	2,034	2,996
9-9.9	1,811	2,288	3,257	1,723	2,227	3,112
10-10.9	1,930	2,575	3,882	1,740	2,296	3,093
11-11.9	2,016	2,670	4,226	1,784	2,612	3,953
12-12.9	2,216	3,022	4,640	2,092	2,904	3,847
13-13.9	2,363	3,553	4,794	2,269	3,130	4,568
14-14.9	2,830	3,963	5,530	2,418	3,220	4,850
15-15.9	3,138	4,481	5,900	2,426	3,248	4,756
16-16.9	3,625	4,951	6,980	2,308	3,248	4,946
17-17.9	3,998	5,286	7,726	2,442	3,336	5,251
18-18.9	4,070	5,552	8,355	2,398	3,243	4,767
19-24.9	4,508	5,913	8,200	2,538	3,406	4,940
25-34.9	4,694	6,214	8,436	2,661	3,573	5,541
35-44.9	4,844	6,490	8,488	2,750	3,783	5,877
45-54.9	4,546	6,297	8,458	2,784	3,858	5,964
55-64.9	4,422	6,144	8,149	2,784	4,045	6,247
65-74.9	3,973	5,716	7,453	2,737	4,019	6,241

*Adapted from Frisancho, A.R.: New norms of upper limb fat and muscle areas for assessment of nutritional status, Amer. J. Clin. Nutr., **34**:2540, 1981.
†The Lange caliper was used in these studies.

Percentiles for Estimates of Upper Arm Fat Area (mm²) for
Whites of the United States Health Examination Survey I of
1971 to 1974*,†

Age (yr)	Arm Fat Area Percentiles (mm²)					
	5th	50th	95th	5th	50th	95th
	Males			Females		
1-1.9	452	741	1,176	401	706	1,140
2-2.9	434	737	1,148	469	747	1,173
3-3.9	464	736	1,151	473	822	1,158
4-4.9	428	722	1,085	490	766	1,236
5-5.9	446	713	1,299	470	812	1,536
6-6.9	371	678	1,519	464	827	1,436
7-7.9	423	758	1,511	491	920	1,644
8-8.9	410	725	1,558	527	1,042	2,482
9-9.9	485	859	2,081	642	1,219	2,524
10-10.9	523	982	2,609	616	1,141	3,005
11-11.9	536	1,148	2,547	707	1,301	3,690
12-12.9	554	1,172	3,580	782	1,511	3,369
13-13.9	475	1,096	3,322	726	1,625	4,150
14-14.9	453	1,082	3,508	981	1,818	3,765
15-15.9	521	931	3,100	839	1,886	4,195
16-16.9	542	1,078	3,041	1,126	2,006	4,236
17-17.9	598	1,096	2,888	1,042	2,104	5,159
18-18.9	560	1,264	3,928	1,003	2,104	3,733
19-24.9	594	1,406	3,652	1,046	2,166	4,896
25-34.9	675	1,752	3,786	1,173	2,548	5,560
35-44.9	703	1,792	3,624	1,336	2,898	5,847
45-54.9	749	1,741	3,928	1,459	3,244	6,140
55-64.9	658	1,645	3,466	1,345	3,369	6,152
65-74.9	573	1,621	3,327	1,363	3,063	5,530

*Adapted from Frisancho, A.R.: New norms of upper limb fat and muscle areas for assessment of nutritional status, Amer. J. Clin. Nutr., **34**:2540, 1981.
†The Lange caliper was used in these studies.

Percentiles for Triceps Skinfold for Whites of the United States
Health and Nutrition Examination Survey I of 1971 to 1974*.†

Triceps Skinfold Percentiles (mm²)

Age (yr)	Males								Females							
	n	5	10	25	50	75	90	95	n	5	10	25	50	75	90	95
1-1.9	228	6	7	8	10	12	14	16	204	6	7	8	10	12	14	16
2-2.9	223	6	7	8	10	12	14	15	208	6	8	9	10	12	15	16
3-3.9	220	6	7	8	10	11	14	15	208	7	8	9	11	12	14	15
4-4.9	230	6	6	8	9	11	12	14	208	7	8	8	10	12	14	16
5-5.9	214	6	6	8	9	11	14	15	219	6	7	8	10	12	15	18
6-6.9	117	5	6	7	8	10	13	16	118	6	6	8	10	12	14	16
7-7.9	122	5	6	7	9	12	15	17	126	6	7	9	11	13	16	18
8-8.9	117	5	6	7	8	10	13	16	118	6	8	9	12	15	18	24
9-9.9	121	6	6	7	10	13	17	18	125	8	8	10	13	16	20	22
10-10.9	146	6	6	8	10	14	18	21	152	7	8	10	12	17	23	27
11-11.9	122	6	6	8	11	16	20	24	117	7	8	10	13	18	24	28
12-12.9	153	6	6	8	11	14	22	28	129	8	9	11	14	18	23	27
13-13.9	134	5	5	7	10	14	22	26	151	8	8	12	15	21	26	30
14-14.9	131	4	5	7	9	14	21	24	141	9	10	13	16	21	26	28
15-15.9	128	4	5	6	8	11	18	24	117	8	10	12	17	21	25	32
16-16.9	131	4	5	6	8	12	16	22	142	10	12	15	18	22	26	31
17-17.9	133	5	5	6	8	12	16	19	114	10	12	13	19	24	30	37
18-18.9	91	4	5	6	9	13	20	24	109	10	12	15	18	22	26	30
19-24.9	531	4	5	7	10	15	20	22	1,060	10	11	14	18	24	30	34
25-34.9	971	5	6	8	12	16	20	24	1,987	10	12	16	21	27	34	37
35-44.9	806	5	6	8	12	16	20	23	1,614	12	14	18	23	29	35	38
45-54.9	898	6	6	8	12	15	20	25	1,047	12	16	20	25	30	36	40
55-64.9	734	5	6	8	11	14	19	22	809	12	16	20	25	31	36	38
65-74.9	1,503	4	6	8	11	15	19	22	1,670	12	14	18	24	29	34	36

*Adapted from Frisancho, A.R.: New norms of upper limb fat and muscle areas for assessment of nutritional status, Amer. J. Clin. Nutr., 34:2540, 1981.
†The Lange caliper was used in these studies.

Arm muscle circumference (cm) is derived from the arm circumference (ca) and the triceps fat fold (s) using the equation cm = ca − πs. Cross-sectional areas of fat and muscle are more logical measures of energy and protein nutrition than fat fold and arm circumference. The following nomograms for children and adults provide a simple method for calculating the arm muscle circumference and arm muscle area. To obtain the muscle circumference, lay a ruler between the values for arm circumference and triceps fat fold and read the arm muscle circumference and the arm muscle area from the middle line. The fat area = arm area − muscle area. (From Gurney, J.M., and Jelliffe, D.B.: Arm anthropometry in nutritional assessment: Nomogram for rapid calculation of muscle circumference and cross-sectional muscle and fat areas, Amer. J. Clin. Nutr., 26:912, 1973.)

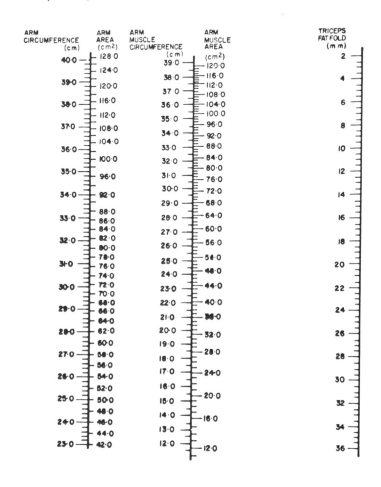

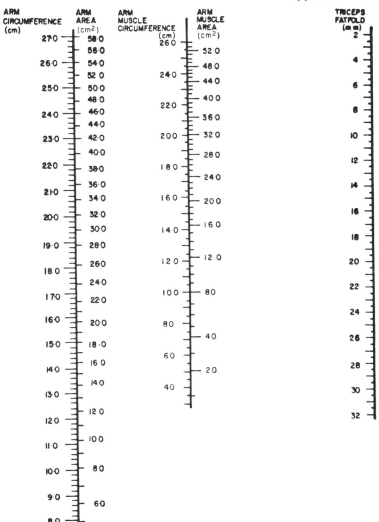

Nomogram for children for calculating arm area, arm muscle circumference, and arm muscle area from measurement of triceps fat fold and arm circumference (arm circumference 8-27 cm).

←

Nomogram for adults for calculating arm area, arm muscle circumference, and arm muscle area from measurement of triceps fat fold and arm circumference (arm circumference 23-40 cm).

Appendix E

Lean Body Mass and Body Fat

(normative means)

Age*	Male			Females		
	LBM (kg)	Fat (kg)	% Fat	LBM (kg)	Fat (kg)	% Fat
Birth	3.06	0.49	14	2.83	0.49	15
6 mo	6.0	2.0	25	5.3	1.9	26
12 mo	7.9	2.3	22	7.0	2.2	24
2 yr	10.1	2.5	20	9.5	2.4	20
4 yr	14.0	2.7	16	13.2	2.8	18
6 yr	17.9	2.8	14	16.3	3.2	16
8 yr	22.0	3.3	13	20.5	4.3	17
10 yr	27.1	4.3	14	26.2	6.4	20
12 yr	34	8	19	32	10	24
14 yr	45	10	18	38	13	25
16 yr	57	9	14	42	13	24
18 yr	61	9	13	43	13	23
20 yr	62	9	13	43	14	25
22 yr	62	10	14	43	14	25

*At nearest birthday.

Appendix F

Body Surface Areas

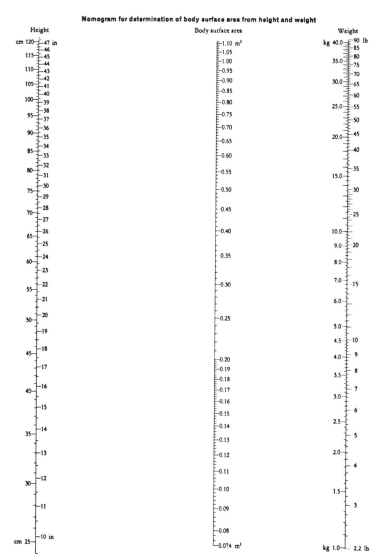

Nomogram for determination of body surface area from height and weight

From the formula of Du Bois and Du Bois, *Arch. intern. Med.*, 17, 863 (1916): $S = W^{0.425} \times H^{0.725} \times 71.84$, or $\log S = \log W \times 0.425 + \log H \times 0.725 + 1.8564$ (S = body surface in cm², W = weight in kg, H = height in cm)

Body surface area of infants and children. (From Documenta Geigy, Basle, Switzerland, pp. 537-538, 1970.)

348 Appendix

Nomogram for determination of body surface area from height and weight

Height	Body surface area	Weight
cm 200 — 79 in	−2.80 m²	kg 150 — 330 lb
— 78	−2.70	145 — 320
195 — 77		140 — 310
— 76	−2.60	135 — 300
190 — 75		130 — 290
— 74	−2.50	— 280
185 — 73	−2.40	125 — 270
— 72		120 — 260
180 — 71	−2.30	115 — 250
— 70	−2.20	110 — 240
175 — 69		105 — 230
— 68	−2.10	100 — 220
170 — 67		
— 66	−2.00	95 — 210
165 — 65	−1.95	90 — 200
— 64	−1.90	
160 — 63	−1.85	85 — 190
— 62	−1.80	
155 — 61	−1.75	80 — 180
— 60	−1.70	
150 — 59	−1.65	75 — 170
— 58	−1.60	— 160
145 — 57	−1.55	70 — 150
— 56	−1.50	
140 — 55	−1.45	65 — 140
— 54	−1.40	
135 — 53	−1.35	60 — 130
— 52	−1.30	
130 — 51	−1.25	55 — 120
— 50	−1.20	
125 — 49	−1.15	50 — 110
— 48	−1.10	— 105
120 — 47		45 — 100
— 46	−1.05	— 95
115 — 45	−1.00	— 90
— 44	−0.95	40 — 85
110 — 43	−0.90	— 80
— 42		35 — 75
105 — 41		— 70
— 40		
cm 100 — 39 in	−0.86 m²	kg 30 — 66 lb

From the formula of Du Bois and Du Bois, *Arch. intern. Med.*, 17, 863 (1916): $S = W^{0.425} \times H^{0.725} \times 71.84$, or
$\log S = \log W \times 0.425 + \log H \times 0.725 + 1.8564$ (S = body surface in cm², W = weight in kg, H = height in cm)

Body surface area of older children and adults. (From Documenta Geigy, Basle, Switzerland, pp. 537-538, 1970.)

Appendix G

Standard Basal Metabolic Rates

Weight (kg)	Male	Female
	kcal/24 hr	
3	140	140
5	270	270
7	400	400
9	500	500
11	600	600
13	650	650
15	710	710
17	780	780
19	830	830
21	880	880
25	1,020	960
29	1,120	1,040
33	1,210	1,120
37	1,300	1,190
41	1,350	1,260
45	1,410	1,320
49	1,470	1,380
53	1,530	1,440
57	1,590	1,500
61	1,640	1,560

Increments or decrements:

1. Add or subtract 12% of above for each degree C (8% for each degree F) above or below rectal temperature of 37.0°C (98.6°F).

2. Add 0 to 30% increments for usual activity: hypo- or hypermetabolic states require greater adjustments.

To determine energy intake for usual activity and growth, multiply basal calories by 1.5 to 2.0.

Appendix H

Dietary Allowances

Food and Nutrition Board, National Academy of Sciences—National Research Council Recommended Dietary Allowances, Revised 1980*,† (Designed for the Maintenance of Good Nutrition of Practically all Healthy People in the United States)

Individual	Age (yr)	Weight (kg)	Weight (lb)	Height (cm)	Height (in.)	Protein (gm)	Fat-soluble Vitamins Vita-min A (μg RE)‡	Vita-min D (μg)§	Vita-min E (mg α-TE)‖	Vita-min C (mg)
Infants	0.0-0.5	6	13	60	24	kg x 2.2	420	10	3	35
	0.5-1.0	9	20	71	28	kg x 2.0	400	10	4	35
Children	1-3	13	29	90	35	23	400	10	5	45
	4-6	20	44	112	44	30	500	10	6	45
	7-10	28	62	132	52	34	700	10	7	45
Males	11-14	45	99	157	62	45	1,000	10	8	50
	15-18	66	145	176	69	56	1,000	10	10	60
	19-22	70	154	177	70	56	1,000	7.5	10	60
	23-50	70	154	178	70	56	1,000	5	10	60
	51+	70	154	178	70	56	1,000	5	10	60
Females	11-14	46	101	157	62	46	800	10	8	50
	15-18	55	120	163	64	46	800	10	8	60
	19-22	55	120	163	64	44	800	7.5	8	60
	23-50	55	120	163	64	44	800	5	8	60
	51+	55	120	163	64	44	800	5	8	60
Pregnant						+30	+200	+5	+2	+20
Lactating						+20	+400	+5	+3	+40

*Adapted from Committee on Dietary Allowances and Food and Nutrition Board: Recommended Dietary Allowances, ed. 9, revised, Washington, D.C.: National Academy of Sciences, 1980.

†The allowances are intended to provide for individual variations among most normal persons as they live in the United States under usual environmental stresses. Diets should be based on a variety of common foods to provide other nutrients for which human requirements have been less well defined.

‡Retinol equivalents. 1 retinol equivalent = 1 μg retinol or 6 μg β-carotene.

§As cholecalciferol. 10 μg cholecalciferol = 400 IU of vitamin D.

‖α-tocopherol equivalents. 1 mg d-α tocopherol = 1 α-TE.

¶1 NE (niacin equivalent) is equal to 1 mg of niacin or 60 mg of dietary tryptophan.

**The folacin allowances refer to dietary sources as determined by Lactobacillus casei assay after treatment with enzymes (conjugases) to make polyglutamyl forms of the vitamin available to the test organism.

††The recommended dietary allowance for vitamin B_{12} in infants is based on average concentration of the vitamin in human milk. The allowances after weaning are based on energy intake (as recommended by the American Academy of Pediatrics) and consideration of other factors, such as intestinal absorption.

‡‡The increased requirement during pregnancy cannot be met by the iron content of habitual diets of people in the United States nor by the existing iron stores of many women; therefore, the use of 30 to 60 mg of supplemental iron is recommended. Iron needs during lactation are not substantially different from those of nonpregnant women, but continued supplementation of the mother for 2 to 3 months after parturition is advisable to replenish stores depleted by pregnancy.

			Water-soluble Vitamins					Minerals			
Thia-min (mg)	Ribo-flavin (mg)	Niacin (mg NE)¶	Vita-min B₆ (mg)	Fola-cin** (µg)	Vita-min B₁₂ (µg)	Cal-cium (mg)	Phos-phorus (mg)	Mag-nesium (mg)	Iron (mg)	Zinc (mg)	Iodine (µg)
0.3	0.4	6	0.3	30	0.5††	360	240	50	10	3	40
0.5	0.6	8	0.6	45	1.5	540	360	70	15	5	50
0.7	0.8	9	0.9	100	2.0	800	800	150	15	10	70
0.9	1.0	11	1.3	200	2.5	800	800	200	10	10	90
1.2	1.4	16	1.6	300	3.0	800	800	250	10	10	120
1.4	1.6	18	1.8	400	3.0	1,200	1,200	350	18	15	150
1.4	1.7	18	2.0	400	3.0	1,200	1,200	400	18	15	150
1.5	1.7	19	2.2	400	3.0	800	800	350	10	15	150
1.4	1.6	18	2.2	400	3.0	800	800	350	10	15	150
1.2	1.4	16	2.2	400	3.0	800	800	350	10	15	150
1.1	1.3	15	1.8	400	3.0	1,200	1,200	300	18	15	150
1.1	1.3	14	2.0	400	3.0	1,200	1,200	300	18	15	150
1.1	1.3	14	2.0	400	3.0	800	800	300	18	15	150
1.0	1.2	13	2.0	400	3.0	800	800	300	18	15	150
1.0	1.2	13	2.0	400	3.0	800	800	300	10	15	150
+0.4	+0.3	+2	+0.6	+400	+1.0	+400	+400	+150	‡‡	+5	+25
+0.5	+0.5	+5	+0.5	+100	+1.0	+400	+400	+150	‡‡	+10	+50

Estimated Safe and Adequate Daily Dietary Intakes of Selected Vitamins and Minerals*·†

Vitamins

Individual	Age (yr)	Vitamin K (µg)	Biotin (µg)	Pantothenic Acid (mg)
Infants	0-0.5	12	35	2
	0.5-1	10-20	50	3
Children and adolescents	1-3	15-30	65	3
	4-6	20-40	85	3-4
	7-10	30-60	120	4-5
	11+	50-100	100-200	4-7
Adults	–	70-140	100-200	4-7

Trace Elements

Individual	Age (yr)	Copper (mg)	Manganese (mg)	Fluoride (mg)	Chromium (mg)	Selenium (mg)	Molybdenum (mg)
Infants	0-0.5	0.5-0.7	0.5-0.7	0.1-0.5	0.01-0.04	0.01-0.04	0.03-0.06
	0.5-1	0.7-1.0	0.7-1.0	0.2-1.0	0.02-0.06	0.02-0.06	0.04-0.08
Children and adolescents	1-3	1.0-1.5	1.0-1.5	0.5-1.5	0.02-0.08	0.02-0.08	0.05-0.1
	4-6	1.5-2.0	1.5-2.0	1.0-2.5	0.03-0.12	0.03-0.12	0.06-0.15
	7-10	2.0-2.5	2.0-3.0	1.5-2.5	0.05-0.2	0.05-0.2	0.10-0.3
	11+	2.0-3.0	2.5-5.0	1.5-2.5	0.05-0.2	0.05-0.2	0.15-0.5
Adults	–	2.0-3.0	2.5-5.0	1.5-4.0	0.05-0.2	0.05-0.2	0.15-0.5

| | | Electrolytes | | |
		Sodium (mg)	Potassium (mg)	Chloride (mg)
Infants	0-0.5	115-350	350-925	275-700
	0.5-1	250-750	425-1,275	400-1,200
Children	1-3	325-975	550-1,650	500-1,500
and	4-6	450-1,350	775-2,325	700-2,100
adolescents	7-10	600-1,800	1,000-3,000	925-2,775
	11+	900-2,700	1,525-4,574	1,400-4,200
Adults	—	1,100-3,300	1,875-5,625	1,700-5,100

*Adapted from Committee on Dietary Allowances and Food and Nutrition Board: Recommended Dietary Allowances, ed. 9, revised, Washington, D.C.: National Academy of Sciences, p. 178, 1980.

†Because there is less information on which to base allowances, these figures are not given in the main table of RDA and are provided here in the form of ranges of recommended intakes.

‡Because the toxic levels for many trace elements may be only several times usual intakes, the upper levels for the trace elements given in this table should not be habitually exceeded.

Recommended Allowances
Summary Examples of Recommended Nutrient Intakes for Canadians*,†,‡

Age	Sex	Weight (kg)	Protein (gm/da)§	Fat-soluble Vitamins			Water-soluble Vitamins			Minerals				
				Vit. A (RE/da)‖	Vit. D (μg/da)¶	Vit. E (mg/da)**	Vit. C (mg/da)	Folacin (μg/da)††	Vit. B₁₂ (μg/da)	Calcium (mg/da)	Magnesium (mg/da)	Iron (mg/da)	Iodine (μg/da)	Zinc (mg/da)
Months														
0-2	Both	4.5	11‡‡	400	10	3	20	50	0.3	350	30	0.4§§	25	2‖‖
3-5	Both	7.0	14‡‡	400	10	3	20	50	0.3	350	40	5	35	3
6-8	Both	8.5	16‡‡	400	10	3	20	50	0.3	400	45	7	40	3
9-11	Both	9.5	18	400	10	3	20	55	0.3	400	50	7	45	3
Years														
1	Both	11	18	400	10	3	20	65	0.3	500	55	6	55	4
2-3	Both	14	20	400	5	4	20	80	0.4	500	65	6	65	4
4-6	Both	18	25	500	5	5	25	90	0.5	600	90	6	85	5
7-9	M	25	31	700	2.5	7	35	125	0.8	700	110	7	110	6
	F	25	29	700	2.5	6	30	125	0.8	700	110	7	95	6
10-12	M	34	38	800	2.5	8	40	170	1.0	900	150	10	125	7
	F	36	39	800	2.5	7	40	170	1.0	1,000	160	10	110	7
13-15	M	50	49	900	2.5	9	50	160	1.5	1,100	220	12	160	9
	F	48	43	800	2.5	7	45	160	1.5	800	190	13	160	8
16-18	M	62	54	1,000	2.5	10	55	190	1.9	900	240	10	160	9
	F	53	47	800	2.5	7	45	160	1.9	700	220	14	160	8
19-24	M	71	57	1,000	2.5	10	60	210	2.0	800	240	8	160	9
	F	58	41	800	2.5	7	45	165	2.0	700	190	14	160	8
25-49	M	74	57	1,000	2.5	9	60	210	2.0	800	240	8	160	9
	F	59	41	800	2.5	6	45	165	2.0	700	190	14¶¶	160	8
50-74	M	73	57	1,000	2.5	7	60	210	2.0	800	240	8	160	9
	F	63	41	800	2.5	6	45	165	2.0	800	190	7	160	8
75+	M	69	57	1,000	2.5	6	60	210	2.0	800	240	8	160	9
	F	64	41	800	2.5	5	45	165	2.0	800	190	7	160	8

Pregnancy (additional)										
1st trimester	15	100	2.5	2	305	1.0	500	15	6	25	0
2nd trimester	20	100	2.5	2	305	1.0	500	20	6	25	1
3rd trimester	25	100	2.5	2	305	1.0	500	25	6	25	2
Lactation (additional)	20	400	2.5	3	120	0.5	500	80	0	50	6

*Adapted from Committee for the Revision of the Dietary Standard for Canada: Recommended Nutrient Intakes for Canadians, Ottawa: Canadian Government Publishing Centre, pp. 179-181, 1983.

†Recommended intakes of energy and of certain nutrients are not listed in this table because of the nature of the variables on which they are based. The figures for energy are estimates of average requirements for expected patterns of activity. For nutrients not shown, the following amounts are recommended: thiamin, 0.4 mg/1,000 kcal (0.48 mg/5,000 kJ); riboflavin, 0.5 mg/1,000 kcal (0.6 mg/5,000 kJ); niacin, 7.2 NE/1,000 kcal (8.6 NE/5,000 kJ); vitamin B_6, 15 µg, as pyridoxine, per gram of protein; phosphorus, same as calcium.

‡Recommended intakes during periods of growth are taken as appropriate for individuals representative of the midpoint in each age group. All recommended intakes are designed to cover individual variations in essentially all of a healthy population subsisting on a variety of common foods available in Canada.

§The primary units are grams per kilogram of body weight. The figures shown here are only examples.

‖One retinol equivalent (RE) corresponds to the biological activity of 1 µg of retinol, 6 µg of β-carotene or 12 µg of other carotenes.

¶Expressed as cholecalciferol or ergocalciferol.

**Expressed as d-α-tocopherol equivalents, relative to which β- and γ-tocopherol and α-tocotrienol have activities of 0.5, 0.1, and 0.3, respectively.

††Expressed as total folate.

‡‡Assumption that the protein is from human milk or is of the same biological value as that of human milk and that between 3 and 9 months adjustment for the quality of the protein is made.

§§It is assumed that human milk is the source of iron up to 2 months of age.

‖‖Based on the assumption that human milk is the source of zinc for the first 2 months.

¶¶After menopause, the recommended intake is 7 mg/day.

Appendix I

Recommended Ranges of Nutrients in Formulas

The following recommendations were prepared by the Committee on Nutrition in March 1983 and submitted to the Food and Drug Administration.

Nutrient (per 100 kcal)	Lowest Adequate	Not to Exceed*
Protein (gm)	1.8† (7.2% of kcal)	4.5 (18% of kcal)
Fat (gm)	3.3 (30% of kcal)	6.0 (54% of kcal)
Including Essential fatty acid (linoleate) (mg)	300.0 (2.7% of kcal)	
Vitamins		
A (μg retinol equivalents)‡	75.0	225.0
D (μg cholecalciferol)§	1.0	2.5
K (μg)	4.0	–
E (mg tocopherol equivalents)‖	0.5	–
C (ascorbic acid) (mg)	8.0	–
B$_1$ (thiamine) (μg)	40.0	–

*Where no upper limit is given, toxicity is not well defined. However, the Committee is concerned that excess concentrations have adverse consequences.

†At least nutritionally equivalent to casein, quality recommended as outlined in: Commentary on breast feeding and infant formulas, including proposed standards for formulas, PEDIATRICS, 57:278, 1976 (see also Chapter 2).

‡Retinol equivalents: 1 RE = 1 μg retinol or 6 μg β-carotene (1 RE = 3.33 IU vitamin activity from retinol).

§Cholecalciferol 1 μg = 40 IU vitamin D.

‖α-tocopherol equivalents.
1 mg of dl-α-tocopherol = 0.74 α-tocopherol equivalent (or 1.1 IU)
1 mg of d-α-tocopherol = 1 α-tocopherol equivalent (or 1.49 IU)
1 mg of d-α-tocopherol acetate = 0.91 α-tocopherol equivalent (or 1.36 IU)
1 mg of d-α-tocopherol succinate = 0.81 α-tocopherol equivalent (or 1.21 IU)
At least 0.5 mg per day α-tocopherol per gram linoleic acid.

Nutrient (per 100 kcal)	Lowest Adequate	Not to Exceed*
B₂ (riboflavin) (µg)	60.0	–
B₆ (pyriodoxine) (µg)	35.0 (with 15 µg/gm protein in formula)	–
B₁₂ (µg)	0.15	–
Niacin (µg)	250.0 (or 0.8 mg niacin equivalents)	–
Folic acid (µg)	4.0	–
Pantothenic acid (µg)	300.0	–
Biotin (µg)	1.5#	–
Choline (mg)	7.0#	–
Inositol (mg)	4.0#	–
Minerals**·††		
Calcium (mg)	60.0‡‡	–
Phosphorus (mg)	30.0‡‡	–
Magnesium (mg)	6.0	–
Iron (mg)	0.15	2.5§§
Iodine (µg)	5.0	75.0
Zinc (mg)	0.5	–
Copper (µg)	60.0	–
Manganese (µg)	5.0	–
Sodium (mg)	20.0 (5.8 mEq/l)	60.0 (17.5 mEq/l)
Potassium (mg)	80.0 (13.7 mEq/l)	200.0 (34.3 mEq/l)
Chloride (mg)	55.0 (10.4 mEq/l)	150.0 (28.3 mEq/l)

#Average present in milk-base formulas; should be included in this amount in other formulas.

**Formula should be manufactured with water low in fluoride to facilitate appropriate fluoride supplementation. (For explanation see: Fluoride supplementation: Revised dosage schedule, PEDIATRICS, 63:150, 1979; see also Chapter 17).

††Selenium is recognized as essential. A minimum amount for infant formulas cannot be established on the basis of currently available information.

‡‡Calcium to phosphorus ratio should be no less than 1.1:1 nor more than 2:1 (mg:mg).

§§Prudence indicates there should be an upper limit for iron. Formula labeled "infant formula with iron" should contain not less than 1 mg iron per 100 kcal.

Appendix J

Guidelines for Essential Nutrients in Nutritionally Complete Liquid Formulas for Oral and Tube Feeding*,† (for use under the age of 4 years)

Mission

At the request of the Bureau of Foods of the Food and Drug Administration, the Committee on Nutrition convened a group of experts in nutrition from both the medical community and industry to determine the rationale, suggested composition, dosage, recommendations for establishing of safety and adequacy, labeling, including information that should be in the package insert, and clinical testing of the proposed formulations to ensure that nutrients are present in sufficient amounts to maintain concentrations within the normal range in blood and urine without causing excessive or deficient tissue concentration of any single nutrient. A task force met on July 22 and 23, 1981, and subsequently approved the following report.

Background

A growing number of nutritionally complete, commercially prepared products for oral and tube feeding is becoming available. These products are generally known as "defined formula diets" or "medical foods," although the latter term has not been precisely defined by the Food and Drug Administration. They are specially formulated products intended for use under medical supervision in the nutritional support or dietary management of patients with various diseases or medical conditions. Most of these products are designed to meet the increased or special nutritional requirements of adults and older children with various diseases or medical conditions, but they also are sometimes used in the nutritional management of infants and children less than 4 years old. The task force limited its discussion to products which were nutritionally complete and to the

---

*Report to the Food and Drug Administration, Department of Health and Human Services, by the Committee on Nutrition, American Academy of Pediatrics, February 1982.
†This study was supported by FDA Contract No. 223-76-2091.

suitability of these products for use in the age groups of 0 to 1 and 1 to 4 years.

Nutritional Considerations

In general, minimum and maximum recommended levels of protein, minerals, and vitamins per 100 kcal as proposed by the Committee for infant formulas are acceptable guidelines for selecting "medical foods" for use in infants and children up to 4 years old. If products which are designed by the manufacturer to be used as a sole source of nutrition do not contain these minimal levels of nutrients, or if they provide nutrients at levels exceeding the maximum recommended amounts per 100 kcal, this information should be included in a label statement and in other product information.

With respect to specific nutrient intakes, it is recognized that the requirements of some infants and children who must use these foods will be greater than the requirements of normal infants and children because of (1) increased metabolic rate incident to stress, (2) increased needs for catch-up growth, or (3) increased needs incident to ongoing nutrient losses (particularly gastrointestinal). With few exceptions, these patients also have increased caloric needs. Consequently, the increased needs for specific nutrients usually will be provided by most "medical foods" which meet the Committee's guidelines for infant formula if the intake of these "medical foods" is sufficient to meet the patients' energy needs.

For infants less than 9 to 12 months old, the addition of water to reduce the caloric density below a maximum of 0.8 kcal/ml is recommended, except when specifically prescribed otherwise by the attending physician. A maximum, acceptable renal solute load of "medical foods" for use in infants and children is not easily defined. Renal solute load is affected primarily by dietary intake of protein, sodium, potassium, and chloride. Products with protein concentrations greater than 18% of the calories exceed the maximum established by the Committee for infant formulas; these products should not be used as the sole dietary item for infants and children less than 4 years old unless specifically indicated by a physician. Adherence to the Committee's guidelines on protein and electrolyte content will minimize the risk of excessive renal solute load in infants and children fed these "medical foods."

In many of the currently available "medical foods," the amounts of vitamin D and calcium per 100 kcal and the calcium:phosphorus may be less than the Committee standard for infant formula. In these instances, the need for a supplement of vitamin D and calcium should be assessed. The iron requirement of infants is high in relation to calories, and dietary iron supplementation may be needed to meet the Committee's recommended intake of 1 mg iron per 100 kcal for infants. Products with a sodium content greater than 60 mg per 100 kcal exceed the Committee's maximum limit for infant formulas; this should be noted on the label and in other product information.

In addition to the nutrients identified in the Committee's standards for infant formulas, "medical foods" used as the sole dietary item also should contain trace elements such as chromium, selenium, and molybdenum. Although the Committee makes no specific recommendations for these trace elements, the estimates of the food and nutrition board, National Academy of Sciences/National Research Council (NAS/NRC), seem appropriate (see Appendix H).

The undetermined anion $(Na + K + Ca + Mg)$ minus $(Cl + 1.8 P)$ should be determined and a recommended range established to avoid the production of metabolic acidosis, especially when the protein component is an amino acid mixture.

Testing and Clinical Monitoring

There is relatively little published information concerning clinical testing of "medical foods" in children less than 4 years old. Consequently, the ability of these products to maintain normal tissue concentrations of essential nutrients when used as the **sole source of calories over prolonged periods of time** has not been well documented, although their approximate composition meets or exceeds the recommended dietary allowances of the NAS/NRC.

Concern over the absence of such data reflects several factors: (1) some patients may have abnormal nutrient losses secondary to certain disease states, and (2) quantitative knowledge concerning nutrient interrelationships is lacking. Future regulations should contain a statement similar to the following: Nutritionally complete medical foods recommended for use in children less than 4 years old should be nutritionally adequate to promote normal growth and development when used in accordance with the directions for use.‡

‡CODEX Alimentarius Commission: Recommended International Standards for Foods for Infants and Children. CAC/RS 72/74-1976. Rome: FAO-WHO, 1976.

Products which contain protein sources such as hydrolysates or mixtures of amino acids or other major ingredients which are not on the GRAS (generally recognized as safe) list should be tested in animals as well as in short-term adult studies prior to use in infants and children. This testing should be done on a product which has been processed in a manner similar to that used in the manufacture of the "medical foods" to evaluate protein quality and bioavailability of other nutrients in the product as it will be used in humans.

The testimony by the Committee to the Food and Drug Administration regarding the clinical testing of infant formulas in June 1980 also seems applicable to the use of "medical foods" in infants and children less than 4 years old.

When defined-formula diets or "medical foods" are used as a sole source of nutrients over a prolonged period of time in infants and young children, careful hematological, biochemical, and developmental testing should be performed to monitor nutrition status because of the possible continuing losses secondary to disease and the demands of growth.

Future Research

Several subjects deserve research in the future. Although interrelationships between nutrients are known to influence requirements, detailed evaluations are not available. Some of these nutrients are not easily measured, and interpretation of available observations is uncertain. Furthermore, the effect of various diseases and medical conditions on nutrient requirements is not well defined. Consequently, as a general rule, nutrients, especially trace elements and the water-soluble vitamins (B complex and C), may be present in amounts consistent with or slightly higher than the RDA. Trace minerals should be in nutritionally appropriate proportions or ratios to each other. All nutrients should be provided in biologically available forms. Studies on quantitative nutrient interrelationships which have predictive values are being carried out, and the results should be considered when these data become available.

Conclusion

The task force felt that, despite multiple needs for further information concerning the suitability of "medical foods" presently on the market for infants and children less than 4 years old, excessively stringent regulations would tend to inhibit the development of products which are needed in the management of disease states in this age group.

Membership of *ad hoc* Committee

Duane Benton, Ph.D., Ross Laboratories
John E. Canham, Ph.D., Cutter Laboratories
Joginder Chopra, M.D., Food and Drug Administration
David Cook, Ph.D., Mead Johnson and Company
William Heird, M.D., Columbia University, New York, New York
Stanley Hellerstein, M.D., Children's Mercy Hospital, Kansas City, Missouri
Parvin Justice, Ph.D., American Academy of Pediatrics
Jean D. Lockhart, M.D., American Academy of Pediatrics
Robert Longley, Ph.D., Doyle Pharmaceuticals
Harold Sandstead, M.D., U.S. Department of Agriculture
Maurice Shils, M.D., Memorial Sloan-Kettering Cancer Center, New York, New York
Lewis Steginek, Ph.D., University of Iowa, Iowa City, Iowa
Philip White, Sc.D., American Medical Association
Calvin Woodruff, M.D., University of Missouri, Columbia, Missouri

Appendix K

Composition of Human Milk: Normative Data

The following table provides composition data on human milk as derived from an extensive review of the current literature. Because of space limitations, only a select bibliography is given. Data from more than 200 publications were considered in constructing the table; however, the values presented should not be taken in a strict statistical sense; rather, they are based on recent data and personal judgment.

Colostrum differs from mature milk in certain respects: energy and fat contents are lower, and protein, sodium, chloride, and iron are higher than in mature milk (as are immunoglobulins and leukocytes).[1] The data in the table are based solely on publications in which it is evident that mature milk from mothers delivering at term was analyzed.

The tables also contain information on the variability of the various constituents. Note that the standard deviations for some are an appreciable fraction of the mean. A recent publication from England documents a wide range of values for many constituents.[2]

Data on composition of milk from mothers who deliver prematurely have recently started to appear, but it is too early to decide on normative values. Some authorities report that nitrogen, sodium, chloride, and magnesium contents are 10 to 30% higher than in milk from mothers who deliver at term;[3-5] others[6] find no difference in nitrogen content. Calcium and phosphorus content are about the same as milk from mothers who deliver at term.

References

1. Committee on Nutrition: Composition of milks. PEDIATRICS, 26:1039, 1960.
2. Hibbard, C.M., Brooke, O.G., Carter, N.D., Haug, M., and Harzer, G.: Variation in the composition of breast milk during the first 5 weeks of lactation: Implications for the feeding of preterm infants. Arch. Dis. Child., 57:658, 1982
3. Atkinson, S.A., Bryan, M.H., and Anderson, G.H.: Human milk: Difference in nitrogen concentration in milk from mothers of term and premature infants. J. Pediat., 93:67, 1978.

4. Gross, S.J., Geller, J., and Tomarelli, R.M.: Composition of breast milk from mothers of preterm infants. PEDIATRICS, 68:490, 1981.
5. Lemons, J.A., Moye, L., Hall, D., and Simmons, M.: Differences in the composition of preterm and term human milk during early lactation. Pediat. Res., 16:113, 1982.
6. Anderson, D.M., Williams, F.H., Merkatz, R.B., Schulman, P.K., Kerr, D.S., and Pittard, W.B., III: Length of gestation and nutritional composition of human milk. Amer. J. Clin. Nutr., 37:810, 1983.

Composition of Mature Human Milk*

Nutrient		$\bar{X} \pm$ S.D.	References
Protein	(gm/100 ml)	1.05 ± 0.20	
Fat	(gm/100 ml	3.90 ± 0.40	
Lactose	(gm/100 ml)	7.20 ± 0.25	
Energy	(kcal/100 ml)	72 ± 5	
Water	(gm/100 ml)	88 ± 1	
Total solids	(gm/100 ml)	12.3 ± 0.6	
Ash	(gm/100 ml)	0.20 ± 0.01	
Proteins (% of total protein)			
Casein		30	1-4
Whey proteins		70	
Total nitrogen (mg/100 ml)		185 ± 20	
Nonprotein nitrogen (mg/100 ml)		41 ± 4	
Nonprotein nitrogen (% of total nitrogen)		22	
pH		7.2 ± 0.1	
Osmolality (mosmol/kg water)		290 ± 5	
Essential Amino acids (mg/100 ml)			
Histidine		23 ± 3	
Isoleucine		58 ± 5	
Leucine		105 ± 5	
Lysine		68 ± 5	
Methionine		20 ± 3	2-6
Phenylalanine		43 ± 4	
Threonine		52 ± 5	
Tryptophan		21 ± 1	
Valine		65 ± 5	

*Adapted from material supplied by B. Lönnerdal, Ph.D.

Nutrient	$\bar{X} \pm$ S.D.	References
Nonessential Amino Acids		
(mg/100 ml)		
Arginine	45 ± 5	
Alanine	37 ± 5	
Aspartic acid	102 ± 5	
Cystein	23 ± 1	
Glutamic acid	210 ± 5	
Glycine	23 ± 3	2-6
Proline	85 ± 5	
Serine	53 ± 5	
Taurine	4 ±2	
Tyrosine	46 ± 5	
Ornithine	0.2 ± 0.1	
Other Nitrogenous		
Compounds (mg/100 ml)		
Ammonia	30 ± 2	
Creatine	3.3	
Creatinine	2.2	
Carnitine	0.7 ± 0.1	
Urea	31	
Uric acid	4.6	
Fatty Acids (% of total)		
6:0 caproic	0.1 ± 0.1	
8:0 caprylic	0.2 ± 0.1	
10:0 capric	1.3 ± 0.2	
12:0 lauric	4.3 ± 0.4	
14:0 myristic	7.8 ± 2.0	
16:0 palmitic	22 ± 2	
16:1 palmitoleic	2.5 ± 0.3	
18:0 stearic	7.2 ± 0.3	2-4, 7-12
18:1 oleic	35 ± 2	
18:2 ω6 linoleic	10 ± 2	
18:3 ω3 linolenic	1.1 ± 0.2	
20:0 arachidic	1.0 ± 0.1	
20:4 ω6 arachidonic	1.0 ± 0.1	
Other Components		
(mg/100ml)		
Cholesterol	15 ± 3	
Lecithin	78 ± 5	
Choline	9 ± 2	

Nutrient		$\bar{X} \pm$ S.D.	References
Vitamins			
Vitamin A	(retinol equivalents/l)	670 ± 200 (2,230 IU/l)	
Vitamin D	(ng/l)	550 ± 100 (22 IU/l)	
Vitamin E	(mg/l)	2.3 ±1.0	
Vitamin K	(μg/l)	2.1 ± 0.1	
Thiamin	(μg/l)	210 ± 35	
Riboflavin	(μg/l)	350 ± 25	
Niacin	(μg/l)	1,500 ± 200	2, 3, 12-20
Pyridoxine	(μg/l)	205 ± 30	
Pantothenate	(μg/l)	1,800 ± 200	
Folacin	(μg/l)	50 ±5	
B_{12}	(μg/l)	0.5 ± 0.2	
Biotin	(μg/l)	4 ± 1	
Vitamin C	(mg/l)	40 ± 10	
Minerals			
Calcium	(mg/l)	280 ± 26 (7 mM/l ± 0.6)	
Phosphorus	(mg/l)	140 ± 22 (4.5 mM/l ± 0.7)	
Magnesium	(mg/l)	35 ± 2 (1.5 mM/l ± 0.1)	
Sodium	(mg/l)	180 ± 40 (7.8 mM/l ± 1.7)	2, 3, 21-24
Potassium	(mg/l)	525 ± 35 (13.4 mM/l ± 0.9)	
Chloride	(mg/l)	420 ± 60 (11.8 mM/l ± 1.7)	
Sulfur	(mg/l)	120 ± 20 (3.7 mM/l ± 0.6)	
Trace Minerals			
Iron	(mg/l)	0.3 ± 0.1	
Zinc	(mg/l)	1.2 ± 0.2	
Copper	(mg/l)	0.25 ± 0.03	
Manganese	(μg/l)	6 ± 2	2, 3, 21, 22, 25-30
Selenium	(μg/l)	20 ± 5	
Chromium	(μg/l)	50 ± 5	
Nickel	(μg/l)	20 ± 2	
Iodine	(μg/l)	110 ± 40	
Fluoride	(μg/l)	16 ± 5	

References

1. Hambraeus, L., Lönnerdal, B., Forsum, E., and Gebre-Medhin, M.: Nitrogen and protein components of human milk. Acta Paediat. Scand., **67**:561, 1978.
2. Nayman, R., Thomson, M.E., Scriver, C.R., and Clow, C.L.: Observations on the composition of milk-substitute products for treatment of inborn errors of amino acid metabolism. Comparisons with human milk. A proposal to rationalize nutrient content of treatment procedures. Amer. J. Clin. Nutr., **32**:1279, 1979.
3. Department of Health and Social Security: Report on Health and Social Subjects: The composition of mature human milk. London: Her Majesty's Stationery Office, 1977.
4. Gaull, G.E., Jensen, R.G., Rassin, D.K., and Malloy, M.H.: Human milk as food. *In* Milunsky, A., Friedman, E.A., and Gluck, L., ed.: Advances in Perinatal Medicine, Vol. 2. New York: Plenum Publishing Corp., 1982.
5. Soupart, P., Moore, S., and Bigwood, E.J.: Amino acid composition of human milk. J. Biol. Chem., **206**:699, 1954.
6. Naismith, D.J., and Cashel, K.N.: Taurine in breast milk: A role in fat utilization. (Abst.) Proc. Nutr. Soc., **38**:105A, 1979.
7. Jensen, R.G., Clark, R.M., and Ferris, A.M.: Composition of the lipids in human milk: A review. Lipids, **15**:345, 1980.
8. Hall, B.: Uniformity of human milk. Amer. J. Clin. Nutr., **32**:304, 1979.
9. Emery, W.B., III, Canolty, N.L., Aitchison, J.M., and Dunkley, W.L.: Influence of sampling on fatty acid composition of human milk. Amer. J. Clin. Nutr., **31**:1127, 1978.
10. Jensen, R.G., Hagerty, M.M., and McMahon, K.E.: Lipids of human milk and infant formulas: A review. Amer. J. Clin. Nutr., **31**:990, 1978.
11. Gibson, R.A., and Kneebone, G.M.: Fatty acid composition of human colostrum and mature breast milk. Amer. J. Clin. Nutr., **34**:252, 1981.
12. Jansson, L., Åkesson, B., and Holmberg, L.: Vitamin E and fatty acid composition of human milk. Amer. J. Clin. Nutr., **34**:8, 1981.
13. Sandberg, D.P., Begley, J.A., and Hall, C.A.: The content, binding, and forms of vitamin B_{12} in milk. Amer. J. Clin. Nutr., **34**:1717, 1981.
14. Tamura, T., Yoshimura, Y., and Arakawa, T.: Human milk folate and folate status in lactating mothers and their infants. Amer. J. Clin. Nutr., **33**:193, 1980.
15. Johnston, L., Vaughan, L., and Fox, H.M.: Pantothenic acid content of human milk. Amer. J. Clin. Nutr., **34**:2205, 1981.
16. Nail, P.A., Thomas, M.R., and Eakin, R.: The effect of thiamin and riboflavin supplementation on the level of those vitamins in human breast milk and urine. Amer. J. Clin. Nutr., **33**:198, 1980.
17. Haroon, Y., Shearer, M.J., Rahim, S., Gunn, W.G., McEnery, G.,

and Barkhan, P.: The content of phylloquinone (vitamin K_1) in human milk, cow's milk and infant formula foods determined by high-performance liquid chromatography. J. Nutr., 112:1105, 1982.

18. Reeve, L.E., Chesney, R.W., and DeLuca, H.F.: Vitamin D of human milk: Identification of biologically active forms. Amer. J. Clin. Nutr., 36:122, 1982.

19. Thomas, M.R., Sneed, S.M., Wei, C., Nail, P.A., Wilson, M., and Sprinkle, E.E., III: The effects of vitamin C, vitamin B_6, vitamin B_{12}, folic acid, riboflavin, and thiamin on the breast milk and maternal status of well-nourished women at 6 months postpartum. Amer. J. Clin. Nutr., 33:2151, 1980.

20. Cooperman, J.M., Dweck, H.S., Newman, L.J., Garbarino, C., and Lopez, R.: The folate in human milk. Amer. J. Clin. Nutr., 36:576, 1982.

21. Vaughan, L.A., Weber, C.W., and Kemberling, S.R.: Longitudinal changes in the mineral content of human milk. Amer. J. Clin. Nutr., 32:2301, 1979.

22. Fransson, G.-B., and Lönnerdal, B.: Zinc, copper, calcium and magnesium in human milk. J. Pediat., 101:504, 1982.

23. Keenan, B.S., Buzek, S.W., Garza, C., Potts, E., and Nichols, B.L.: Diurnal and longitudinal variations in human milk sodium and potassium: Implication for nutrition and physiology. Amer. J. Clin. Nutr., 35:527, 1982.

24. Greer, F.R., Tsang, R.C., Levin, R.S., Searcy, J.E., Wu, R., and Steichen, J.J.: Increasing serum calcium and magnesium concentrations in breast-fed infants: Longitudinal studies of minerals in human milk and in sera of nursing mothers and their infants. J. Pediat., 100:59, 1982.

25. Smith, A.M., Picciano, M.F., and Milner, J.A.: Selenium intakes and status of human milk and formula fed infants. Amer. J. Clin. Nutr., 35:521, 1982.

26. Vuori, E., and Kuitunen, P.: The concentrations of copper and zinc in human milk: A longitudinal study. Acta Paediat. Scand., 68:33, 1979.

27. Siimes, M.A., Vuori, E., and Kuitunen, P.: Breast milk iron—A declining concentration during the course of lactation. Acta Paediat. Scand., 68:29, 1979.

28. Lönnerdal, B., Keen, C.L., and Hurley, L.S.: Iron, copper, zinc, and manganese in milk. Ann. Rev. Nutr., 1:149, 1981.

29. Fransson, G.-B., and Lönnerdal, B.: Iron in human milk. J. Pediat., 96:380, 1980.

30. Vuori, E.: A longitudinal study of manganese in human milk. Acta Paediat. Scand., 68:571, 1979.

Appendix L

Composition of Formulas

Levels of Selected Nutrients in Formulas Used for Feeding Normal, Full-term Infants* Compared with Human and Animal Milks

Nutrient	Per Liter	Mature Human Milk† (21.6 ± 1.5 kcal/oz)	Milk-based Formulas‡ (20 kcal/oz)	Soy Protein-based Formulas (20 kcal/oz)	Whole Cow's Milk (20 kcal/oz)	Skimmed Milk (11 kcal/oz)	Goat's Milk (21 kcal/oz)
Protein	gm	10.5 ± 0.2	15	18-21	34	35	37
Fat	gm	39.0 ± 0.4	36-38	36-39	37	2	43
Carbohydrate	gm	72.0 ± 0.25	69-72.3	66-69	48	50	46
Calcium	mg	280 ± 26	400-510	630-700	1,219	1,270	1,380
Phosphorus	mg	140 ± 22	300-390	420-500	959	1,050	1,140
Sodium	mEq	7.8 ± 1.7	7-10	9-15	22	23	23
Potassium	mEq	13.4 ± 0.9	14-21	19-24	38	44	54
Chloride	mEq	11.8 ± 1.7	11-14	11-15	27	31	44
Iron	mg	0.3 ± 0.1	1.1-1.5 (12-12.7)§	12-12.7	0.4	0.4	0.5
Estimated renal solute load	mosmol	73	92-105	122-138	226	240	269

*Other nutrients meet the recommendations of the Committee on Nutrition for the composition of infant formulas (see Appendix I).
†Average values with standard deviations for comparison. Detailed data in Appendix K.
‡Values listed are subject to change. Refer to product label or packaging for current information. Milk-based formulas contain lactose and soy protein-based formulas do not.
§Iron content of iron-fortified formulas.

Proximate Composition of Formulas for Special Purposes*†

Nutrient		PM 60/40 (Ross)	Nutramigen (Mead Johnson)	Pregestimil (Mead Johnson)	Ross Carbo-hydrate Free (Ross)
Formula (Company)	Per Liter				
Protein source	gm	15.8 whey and casein	22.3 casein hydrolysate	19.0 casein hydrolysate	20 soy protein isolate
Fat source	gm	37.6 coconut and soy oil	26.5 corn oil	27.6 corn oil and MCT	36 soy and coconut oil
Carbohydrate source	gm	68.8 lactose	88.0 sucrose and modified tapioca starch	91.0 corn syrup solids and modified tapioca starch	0 Requires appropriate supplement
Calcium	mg	400	630	630	700
Phosphorus	mg	200	480	420	500
Sodium	mEq	7	14	14	14
Potassium	mEq	15	18	19	20
Chloride	mEq	11	14	17	17
Iron	mg	1.5	12.7	12.7	1.5
Estimated renal solute load	mosmol	96	134	126	131

*Other nutrients meet the recommendations of the Committee on Nutrition for the composition of infant formulas (see Appendix I).
†Values listed are subject to change. Refer to the product label or packaging for current information.

Composition of Special Formulas for Preterm Infants*

Ingredient	Enfamil Premature	SMA "Preemie"	Similac Special Care
Protein (gm/dl)	2.4	2.0	2.2
Fat (gm/dl)	4.1	4.4	4.4
MCT	40%	12%	50%
oleo oil	0	20%	0
corn oil	40%	0	30%
oleic oil	0	25%	0
coconut oil	20%	25%	20%
soy oil	0	18%	0
Carbohydrate (gm/dl)	8.9	8.6	8.6
lactose	40%	50%	50%
glucose polymers	60%	50%	50%
Minerals (mg/dl)†			
calcium	95 [48]	75 [37]	144 [72]
phosphorus	48 –	40 –	72 –
sodium	32 [14]	32 [14]	35 [15]
potassium	90 [23]	75 [19]	100 [26]
chloride	69 [19]	53 [15]	65 [18]
magnesium	8	7	10
zinc	0.8	0.5	1.2
copper	0.073	0.07	0.2
manganese	0.021	0.02	0.02
iron	0.13	0.3	0.3
iodine	0.006	0.008	0.015
Vitamins (per liter)			
A (IU)	2,540	3,200	5,500
D (IU)	507	510	1,200
E (IU)	16	15	30
C (mg)	69	70	300
B_1 (mg)	0.63	0.8	2
B_2 (mg)	0.74	1.3	5
niacin (mg)	10.1	6.3	40
B_6 (mg)	0.53	0.5	2
B_{12} (μg)	2.5	2	4.5
Folic acid (μg)	240	100	300
K_1 (mg)	0.08	0.07	0.1
Osmolality (mosmol/kg water)	300	270	300

*All formulas have a 60:40 whey protein:casein ratio; all contain 81 calories per deciliter.
†Values in brackets are milliequivalents per liter.

Appendix M

Calcium Content of Foods
(mg per serving)

100+	150+	200+	250+
10 Brazil nuts	1 cup ice cream	1 cup beet greens	1 cup almonds
1 med. stalk broccoli	1 cup oysters	1 oz cheddar cheese	1 oz cheese (Swiss or
1 cup instant Farina	1 cup cooked rhubarb	1 cup cottage cheese	Parmesan)
3 oz canned herring	3 oz canned salmon		1 cup cooked collards
1 cup cooked kale	with bones		1 cup cooked
1 tbsp blackstrap	1 cup cooked spinach		dandelion greens
molasses			4 oz self-rising flour
3 tbsp light (regular)			1 cup milk
molasses			3 oz sardines
1 cup cooked navy beans			1 cup cooked turnip greens
1 cup cooked soybeans			
3½ oz soybean curd (tofu)			
3½ oz sunflower seeds			
5 tbsp maple syrup			

Appendix N

Zinc Content of Foods*

1 to 3 mg per serving	3+ mg per serving
Bacon, 3 slices	Beef (ground, flank,
Beans, common, ½	round, rump,
cup	sirloin, veal), 3½ oz
Beef (corned,	Crabs, 3½ oz
tenderloin, stew),	Gizzard, heart
3½ oz	(chicken, turkey),
Bran flakes, 1 oz	3½ oz
Cheese, 1 oz	Lamb (chop, leg), 3½
Chick peas, cow peas,	oz
lentils, ½ cup	Liver, 3½ oz
Chili con carne, ½ cup	Lobster, 3½ oz
Clams, shrimp, 3½ oz	Oysters, 3½ oz
Eggs, 2 medium	Pork (butt, ham,
Nuts (Brazil, pecan,	sausage, loin), 3½
cashews), 1 oz	oz
Wheat flours, whole,	Turkey (dark meat),
80% extraction, 3½	3½ oz
oz	Wheat germ, ⅓ cup
Soups (beef noodle,	
vegetable beef), ½	
cup	
Pizza, 3½ oz	
Lasagna, 7 oz	
Fish (white fillet,	
salmon, tuna), 3½	
oz	
Frankfurters, 2	
Chicken (neck,	
drumstick, wing),	
3½ oz	

*From American Dietetic Association: Handbook of Clinical Dietetics, New Haven, Connecticut: Yale University Press, 1981.

Appendix O

Foods High in Iron*

Good Sources (1-1.5 mg per serving)	Excellent Sources (>1.5 mg per serving)
Egg, 1 medium	Liver, 2 oz
Prunes, 4 medium	Pork, beef, veal, 3 oz
Strawberries, 1 cup	Navy beans, lima
Apple juice, 1 cup	beans, soybeans,
V-8 juice, 1 cup	lentils, split peas, ½
Broccoli, 1 stalk	cup
Collards, 1 cup	Prune juice, ½ cup
Green peas, ½ cup	Tomato juice, 1 cup
Sweet potato, 1	Oatmeal, ¾ cup
medium	Bran flakes with
	raisins, 1 oz
	Cream of Wheat, ¾
	cup
	Spinach, ½ cup
	Molasses, 2 tbsp
	Corn syrup, 2 tbsp
	Wheat germ, 2 tbsp

*From Balogg, J.D., ed.: Diet Manual, ed 5. Loma Linda, California: Seventh Day Adventists, 1978.

Appendix F

Sodium Content of Foods*

Approximate Sodium Content of Certain Food Groups That May Be Calculated into Sodium-restricted Diets

500 mg Na/Serving	250 mg Na/Serving	200 mg Na/Serving	100 mg Na/Serving	50 mg Na/Serving
Scant ¼ tsp salt	1 oz tuna	1 slice regular bakery bread or roll	½ cup of the following unsalted vegetables: beet greens, frozen mixed peas and carrots, Swiss chard	½ cup of the following fresh, frozen, or canned vegetables, canned without salt: 1 artichoke, edible base and leaves
¾ tsp monosodium glutamate	2 oz canned sardines or salmon	2 thin slices bacon, crisp and drained		
½ bouillon cube	½ cup canned or regularly seasoned carrots, spinach, beets, celery, kale, or white turnips	3 oz canned shrimp cooked in salted water		beets
1 cup tomato juice			1 oz fresh kosher meat	carrots
1 average serving ½ cup cooked rice, spaghetti, noodles, hominy, etc., seasoned with salt		½ cup canned or regularly seasoned vegetables not listed elsewhere	1 oz frozen fish fillets	celery
	5 salted crackers (2 in. square)		¾ cup milk (6 oz)	dandelion greens
½ cup drained sauerkraut	½ cup tomato juice	1 day's supply of drinking water if it contains 100 mg Na/qt		kale
1 average frankfurter (1½ oz)	1 day's supply of drinking water if it contains 120 mg Na/qt	½ cup frozen peas or lima beans		mustard greens
				peas, black eyed
1 day's supply of drinking water if it contains 220 mg Na/qt		1 oz natural cheddar cheese		spinach
		1 tbsp catsup		succotash
				turnip greens
				turnip, white
				1 day's supply of drinking water if it contains 40 mg Na/qt

*From American Dietetic Association: Handbook of Clinical Dietetics, New Haven, Connecticut: Yale University Press, 1981.

Appendix Q

Beverages and Alcoholic Drinks—Calories and Selected Electrolytes (per 100 ml)*

Beverage	kcal	Sodium† (mg)	Potassium† (mg)	Phosphorus (mg)
Regular Soft Drinks				
Cola or pepper	40-47	0-7.6	0-5	11-20.7
Decaffeinated cola or pepper	40-47	0-7.6	0-5	11-20.7
Lemon-lime (clear)	37-43	8.3-15.3	0-1	0-0.3
Orange	47-53	3.7-11.7	0-4.7	0-trace
Other citrus	33-50	4.3-13.6	0-6.7	0-0.3
Root beer	40-50	1.0-17.0	0-5.3	0-5.3
Ginger ale	33-40	0-7.6	0-1.0	0-trace
Tonic water	33-37	0-2.7	0-1.0	0
Other	37-53	0-11.7	0-4.0	0-10.7
Diet Soft Drinks				
Diet cola or pepper	0-<1	0-17.3	0-5	7.0-15.7
Decaffeinated diet cola or pepper	0-<1	6.3-20.0	0-5	7.0-15.7
Diet lemon-lime	0-<1	10.0-26.3	0-4.7	0-trace
Diet root beer	0-<1	11.0-28.3	0-4.3	0-5.3
Other diet	0-<1	3.7-25.0	1.0-3.3	0-trace
Club soda, seltzer and sparkling water	0	0-27	0.3-1.7	0-0.3
Apricot nectar	57	trace	150	12.7
Apple juice	48	trace	100	9.7
Cranberry juice	67	trace	9.5	3.2
Grape juice, canned	67	3.16	117	12.7
Grapefruit juice, unsweetened	42	trace	117	12.9
Orange juice, unsweetened or fresh	49	1.1	202	17.1
Pear nectar	51	trace	38.5	6.4
Peach nectar	48	trace	77	9.6
Pineapple juice, unsweetened	54	trace	150	9.6
Tomato juice	20	200.7	227	16.5
Fruit-flavored beverages	45	–	–	–
Beer	43	6.7	26.7	30.0
Gin, rum, vodka, whiskey— 86 proof	250	trace	3.6	–
Dessert wine, 18.5% alcohol/vol.	137	3.3	76.7	–
Table wine, 12.2% alcohol/vol.	86	3.5	93	10.3

*Based on data from What's in Soft Drinks, Soft Drink Ingredient Series, Washington, D.C.: National Soft Drink Association, May 1984. Other data obtained from Agriculture Handbook No. 456, Agriculture Research Service, Washington, D.C.: USDA, 1975.
†Sodium, 23 mg/100 ml = 10 mEq/l; potassium, 39 mg/100 ml = 10 mEq/l.

Appendix R

Saturated and Polyunsaturated Fat and Cholesterol Content of Common Foods*,†

Foods	Quantity	Saturated Fat (gm)	Polyunsaturated Fat (gm)	Cholesterol (mg)	kcal
Almonds (roasted, salted, shelled)	12	2	2	0	100
Bacon (cured, cooked)	2 slices	4	1	30	90
Beef, good, lean	3 oz	4	0	80	170
Bread	1 slice	0	0	0	70
Butter	1 tablespoon	6	1	35	125
Cheese					
Cheddar	1 oz	5	0	30	100
Cottage, creamed	½ cup	2	0	20	55
Cream or spread	1 oz	5	0	30	100
Chicken (with skin)	3 oz	2	1	75	140
Coconut (dried, sweetened)	2 tablespoons	5	0	0	100
Corn oil	1 tablespoon	2	7	0	125
Cottonseed oil	1 tablespoon	3	6	0	125
Egg, whole	1	2	0	275	81
Egg white	1	0	0	5	16
Egg yolk	1	2	0	270	65

*A low-cholesterol, low-fat diet should limit cholesterol intake to 300 mg per day, have less than 35% of calories as fat, and have polyunsaturated fats at least equal to saturated fats.
†Monounsaturated fat, hence total fat, is not included except under kcal.

Foods	Quantity	Saturated Fat (gm)	Polyunsaturated Fat (gm)	Cholesterol (mg)	kcal
Fish (fillet or flounder, sole)	3½ oz	0	0	60	90
Hamburger	3 oz	10	0	80	250
Ice cream (10% fat)	½ cup	5	0	30	100
Lamb (lean leg)	3 oz	4	0	80	170
Lard and other animal fats	1 tablespoon	6	1	12	125
Liver (beef)	3 oz	5	1	400	170
Margarine					
regular (hydrogenated)	1 tablespoon	3	2	6	100
liquid oil	1 tablespoon	4	2	4	100
Milk					
whole	1 cup	5	0.2	30	160
2%	1 cup	2	0.2	20	115
skimmed	1 cup	0	0	5	90
Olive oil	1 tablespoon	1	1	0	125
Oysters (Eastern)	3½ oz	1	1	60	110
Peanut oil	1 tablespoon	2	3	0	125
Pork (lean)	3 oz	5	0	80	180
Safflower oil	1 tablespoon	1	9	0	125
Salmon, King (canned)	3½ oz	4	4	40	200
Shrimp (canned in wet pack)	3½ oz	0	0	150	90
Soybean oil	1 tablespoon	2	7	0	125
Sweetbreads (calf)	3 oz	5	1	400	170
Tuna fish, canned in vegetable oil	3½ oz	0	0	60	90
Turkey (light meat)	3 oz	2	1	75	140
Yogurt, made from whole milk	1 cup	5	0	30	160

Appendix S

Guide for Constructing Diets of Varying Energy Contents
Daily Food Plan

Food	Number of Exchanges Per Day* (45% of energy from carbohydrate, 20% from protein, and 35% from fat)										
	1,000 kcal	1,200 kcal	1,500 kcal	1,800 kcal	2,000 kcal	2,200 kcal	2,400 kcal	3,000 kcal	3,500† kcal	4,000† kcal
Milk, skimmed	2	2	2	3	3	3	3	4	4	5
Fruit	2	3	4	4	5	5	5	6	8	8
Vegetable	1	2	2	2	2	2	3	4	4	6
Bread	4	5	6	8	9	10	11	14	19	22
Meat, lean	5	5	6	7	8	9	10	11	8	8
Fat	4	6	8	9	10	12	13	17	23	26

*Based on American Dietetic Association exchange lists (The American Dietetic Association: Handbook of Clinical Dietetics, New Haven, Connecticut: Yale University Press, p. F20, 1981).
†50% CHO, 15% protein, 35% fat.

Appendix T

Exchange Lists for Diabetic Diets*

Exchange	Carbohydrate (gm)	Protein (gm)	Fat (gm)	Available Glucose (gm)	kcal (approx.)
Milk, skimmed	12	8	—	17	80
1% fat	12	8	2.5	17	100
2% fat	12	8	5	17	135
Vegetable	5	2	—	6	25
Fruit	10	—	—	10	40
Bread	15	2	—	16	70
Meat, lean (1 oz)	—	7	3	4	55
med. (1 oz)	—	7	5.5	4.5	80
high fat (1 oz)	—	7	8	5	100
Fat	0	—	5	0.5	45

*Based on American Dietetic Association exchange lists.

Food Exchange Lists

List 1—Milk Exchange

12 gm of carbohydrate, 8 gm of protein, a trace of fat, and 80 kcal. Asterisked foods are non-fat.

Non-fat, fortified milk
*Skimmed or non-fat milk	1 cup
*Powdered (non-fat dry, before adding liquid)	⅓ cup

Low-fat, fortified milk
1% fat, fortified milk (omit ½ fat exchange)	1 cup
2% fat, fortified milk (omit 1 fat exchange)	1 cup
Yogurt made from 2% fortified milk (plain, unflavored; omit 1 fat exchange)	1 cup
2% sweet acidophilus milk (omit 1 fat exchange)	1 cup
*Canned, evaporated skimmed milk	½ cup
*Buttermilk made with skimmed milk	1 cup
*Yogurt made from skimmed milk (plain, unflavored)	1 cup

Whole milk
(omit 2 fat exchanges)
Whole milk	1 cup
Canned, evaporated whole milk	½ cup
Buttermilk made from whole milk	1 cup
Yogurt made from whole milk	1 cup

List 2—Vegetable Exchanges

5 gm of carbohydrate, 2 gm of protein, and 25 kcal
One exchange is ½ cup.

Asparagus	Greens:	String beans
Bean sprouts	beet	Summer squash
Beets	chard	Tomatoes
Broccoli	collards	Tomato juice
Brussels sprouts	dandelion	Turnips
Cabbage	kale	Vegetable juice
Carrots	mustard	cocktail
Cauliflower	spinach	Water chestnuts
Celery	turnip	Zucchini

The following *raw vegetables* may be used as desired:

Bamboo shoots	Endive	Lettuce	Radishes
Chicory	Escarole	Parsley	Romaine
Chinese cabbage			Watercress

Greens extra column: Cucumbers, Eggplant, Green pepper, Mushrooms, Okra, Onions, Rhubarb, Rutabaga, Sauerkraut

Starchy vegetables are found in the Bread Exchange List

List 3—Fruit Exchanges

10 gm of carbohydrate and 40 kcal

This list shows the kinds and amounts of fruits to use for one fruit exchange—fresh fruits or fruits canned, dried, or frozen, with no sugar added. Foods high in vitamin C are asterisked.

Apple 2" diameter	1 small
Apple juice	1/3 cup
Applesauce	1/2 cup
Apricots, fresh	2 medium
*Apricots, dried	4 halves
Banana	1/2 small
Berries	
blackberries	1/2 cup
blueberries	1/2 cup
raspberries	1/2 cup
Strawberries	3/4 cup
Cherries	10 large
Cider	1/3 cup
Cranberry juice	1/3 cup
Dates	2
Figs, fresh	1
Figs, dried	1
Fruit cocktail	1/2 cup
*Grapefruit	1/2
*Grapefruit juice	1/2 cup
Grapes	12
Grape juice	1/4 cup

Kumquats	3 medium
Mango	1/2 small
*Melon	
cantaloupe	1/4 small
honeydew	1/8 medium
watermelon	1 cup
Nectarine	1 small
Nectars (fruit)	1/4 cup
*Orange	1 small
*Orange juice	1/2 cup
Papaya	3/4 cup
Peach 2 halves or	1 medium
Pear 2 halves or	1 small
Persimmon, native	1 medium
Pineapple, 2 slices or	1/2 cup
Pineapple juice	1/3 cup
Plums	2 medium
Prunes	2 medium
Prune juice	1/4 cup
Raisins	2 tbsp
*Tangerine	1 medium

List 4—Bread Exchanges

(Includes Bread, Cereal, and Starchy Vegetables)

15 gm of carbohydrate, 2 gm protein, and 70 kcal. All are low fat except prepared foods.

Bread	
White (including French and Italian)	1 slice
Whole wheat	1 slice
Rye or pumpernickel	1 slice
Raisin (no icing)	1 slice
Bagel, small	½
English muffin, small	½
Plain roll, bread	1
Frankfurter roll	½
Hamburger bun	½
Dried bread crumbs	3 tbsp
Tortilla, 6"	1
Starchy vegetables	
Corn	⅓ cup
Corn on the cob	1 small
Lima beans	½ cup
Parsnips	⅔ cup
Peas, green (canned or frozen)	½ cup
Potato, white	1 small
Potato, mashed	½ cup
Beans, peas, lentils (dried and cooked)	½ cup
Baked beans, no pork (canned)	¼ cup

Saltines	6
Soda, 2½" square	4
Pumpkin	¾ cup
Winter squash (Acorn or Butternut)	½ cup
Yam or sweet potato	¼ cup
Cereal	
Bran flakes	½ cup
Other ready-to-eat, unsweetened cereal	¾ cup
Puffed cereal (unfrosted)	1 cup
Cereal, cooked	½ cup
Grits, cooked	½ cup
Rice or barley, cooked	½ cup
Pasta, cooked spaghetti, noodles, macaroni	½ cup
Popcorn (popped, no fat added)	3 cups
Cornmeal, dry	2 tbsp
Flour	2½ tbsp
Wheat germ	¼ cup
Prepared foods	
Biscuit 2" dia (omit 1 fat)	1
Bread stuffing (omit 1 fat)	¼ cup
Chinese noodles (omit 1 fat)	½ cup
Corn bread, 2" x 2" x 1" (omit 1 fat)	1

Crackers	
Arrowroot	3
Graham, 2½" square	2
Matzoh, 4" x 6"	½
Oyster	20
Pretzels, 3⅛" long x ⅛" dia	25
Rye wafers, 2" x 3½" (krisps)	3

Corn muffin, 2" dia (omit 1 fat)	1
Muffin, plain, small (omit 1 fat)	1
Potatoes	
French fried 2" to 3½" (omit 1 fat)	8
Potato or corn chips (omit 2 fat)	15
Pancake, 5" x ½" (omit 1 fat)	1
Waffle, 5" x ½" (omit 1 fat)	1

List 5—Meat Exchanges

Lean Meat

7 gm of protein, 3 gm of fat, and 55 kcal. The exchanges that are asterisked are *low in saturated fat and cholesterol.*

No fat or skin. Select half the servings of meat from lean meat.

*Beef: chipped beef, chuck or flank steak, tenderloin plate ribs, skirt steak, round, rump, tripe	1 oz
*Lamb: leg, rib, sirloin, loin, shank, shoulder	1 oz
*Pork: leg, ham, smoked (center slices)	1 oz
*Poultry: (no skin) chicken, turkey, Cornish or guinea hen, pheasant	1 oz
*Fish: any fresh or frozen, canned salmon, tuna, mackerel, crab, and lobster	¼ cup
clams, oysters, scallops, shrimp	5 or 1 oz
sardines, drained	3
*Cheeses containing less than 5% butterfat	1 oz
*Cottage cheese, dry, and 2% butterfat	¼ cup

*Dried beans and peas (omit 1 bread exchange) — ½ cup
*Pig ears (2 lean meat exchanges) — 3 oz
*Hog maws (2 lean meat exchanges) — ¾ cup

Medium-fat Meat

For each exchange of medium-fat meat omit ½ fat exchange.

Beef: ground (15% fat), corned beef (canned), rib eye, round (ground commercial) — 1 oz
Poultry: (with skin) chicken, turkey, Cornish or guinea hen, pheasant — 1 oz
Pork: loin (all cuts tenderloin), shoulder arm (picnic), shoulder blade, Boston butt,
Canadian bacon, boiled ham — 1 oz
Liver, heart, kidney, and sweetbreads (these are high in cholesterol) — 1 oz
Cottage cheese, creamed — ¼ cup
Cheese: Mozzarella, Ricotta, Farmer's cheese, Neufchatel — 1 oz
Parmesan — 3 tbsp
Egg (high in cholesterol) — 1
Egg substitute (low cholesterol) — ¼ cup
*Peanut butter (omit 2 additional fat exchanges) — 2 tbsp

High-fat Meat

For each exchange of high-fat meat, omit 1 fat exchange.

Beef: brisket, corned beef brisket, ground beef (more than 20% fat), hamburger (commercial), chuck (ground commercial), roast (rib), steaks (club and rib) — 1 oz

Lamb: breast	1 oz
Veal: breast	1 oz
Pork: spare ribs, loin (back ribs), pork (ground), country style ham, deviled ham	1 oz
Pig feet	4 oz
Pig tail	3 oz
Brains	½ cup
Cheese: cheddar types	1 oz
Poultry: capon, duck (domestic), goose	1 oz
Frankfurter	
cocktail size	1 small
Cold cuts 4½″ x ⅛″	2 2″
	1 slice

List 6—Fat Exchanges

5 gm of fat and 45 kcal

Fat exchanges with astrisks are *polyunsaturated.*

*Margarine, soft tub or stick†	1 tsp
*Avocado (4″ in dia)‡	⅛
*Non-dairy creamer‡	1 oz
*Oil: corn, cottonseed, soy, safflower, sunflower	
*Oil, olive‡	1 tsp
*Oil, peanut‡	1 tsp
	1 tsp
*Olives‡	5 small

†Made with corn, cottonseed, safflower, soy, or sunflower oil only.
‡Fat content is primarily monounsaturated.

*Almond‡	10 whole
*Pecans‡	2 large, whole
*Peanuts‡	
*Spanish	20 whole
*Virginia	10 whole
*Walnuts	6 small
*Nuts, other‡	6 small
Margarine, regular stick	1 tsp
Butter	1 tsp
Bacon fat	1 tsp
Bacon, crisp	1 strip
Cream, light	2 tbsp
Cream, sour	2 tbsp
Cream, heavy	1 tbsp
Cream substitute, dried	1 tbsp
Cream cheese	1 tbsp
French dressing§	1 tbsp
Italian dressing§	1 tbsp
Lard	1 tbsp
Mayonnaise§	1 tsp
Salad dressing, mayonnaise type§	2 tsp
Salt pork	¾ in. cube
Cracklins	1 round tsp
Chitterlings	1/8 cup

§If made with corn, cottonseed, safflower, soy, or sunflower oil, can be used on modified-fat diet.

Appendix U

Metrication and SI Units

The British Imperial System of Weights used in the United States today derives from a variety of older cultures. A more logical system evolved from the Metre Convention in 1870, to which the United States was a signatory. Although the scientific community has adopted the metric system, the United States still clings to the older system for everyday use. In 1960, the General Conference on Weights and Measures standardized metric units into a system known as SI (le Système International d'Unités); this system has now been adopted by 18 countries, many of whom use these units in scientific publications.

SI is a system of "base units" and "derived units," with each unit defined in specific terms (see the tables in this appendix). It should be noted that, for the sake of convenience, the liter (l = dm³) also is used.

Of interest to nutritionists is the substitution of the joule for the time-honored calorie as the unit of energy. One calorie equals 4.184 joules (J); hence, a 1,000 kilocalorie diet (erroneously termed 1,000 calories by some) equals a 4.184 kJ, or 4.184 MJ, diet.

SI prefixes and values in both conventional and SI units for a number of laboratory determinations are given in the tables in this appendix.

References

1. Committee on Hospital Care: Metrication and SI units. PEDIATRICS, **65**:659, 1980.
2. Young, D.S.: SI units for clinical laboratory data. J.A.M.A., **240**:1618, 1978.
3. Brief History of Measurement Systems with a Chart of the Modernized Metric System, United States. National Bureau of Standards, revised August 1981.

SI Base Units*

Quantity	Name	Symbol
Length	Meter (metre)†	m
Mass	Kilogram	kg
Time	Second	s
Electric current	Ampere	A
Thermodynamic temperature‡	Kelvin	K
Amount of substance	Mole	mol
Luminous intensity	Candela	cd
Supplementary Units		
plane angle	Radian	rad
solid angle	Steradian	sr

*From Committee on Hospital Care.[1]
†Both spellings acceptable.
‡The Celsius temperature scale (formerly called centigrade) is used for most medical and commercial purposes. The Kelvin (the unit for thermodynamic temperature) is the SI unit for temperature. Although their scale origins differ, the degree Celsius equals the Kelvin in magnitude; thus, a rise in body temperature of 1.0 K is equivalent to a rise of 1.0°C. 0°C is defined as 273.15 K, thus 98.6°F = 37°C = 310.15 K.

Some SI Derived Units*

Quantity	Name	Symbol
Area	Square meter	m^2
Volume	Cubic meter	m^3
Velocity	Meter per second	m/s
Wave number	1 per meter	m^{-1}
Density, mass/ volume	Kilogram per cubic meter	kg/m^3
Concentration (amount of substance)	Mole per cubic meter	mol/m^3
Activity (radioactive)	1 per second	s^{-1}
Specific volume	Cubic meter per kilogram	m^3/kg
Luminance	Candela per square meter	cd/m^2
Frequency	Hertz	$Hz = s^{-1}$
Force	Newton	$N = m \cdot kg \cdot s^{-2}$
Pressure	Pascal	$Pa = N/m^2 = m^{-1} \cdot kg \cdot s^{-2}$
Energy, quantity of heat, work	Joule	$J = N \cdot m = m^2 \cdot kg \cdot s^{-2}$
Power	Watt	$W = J/s = m^2 \cdot kg \cdot s^{-3}$
Electric potential, potential difference, electro-motive force	Volt	$V = W/A = m^2 \cdot kg \cdot s^{-3} \cdot A^{-1}$
Electric resistance	Ohm	$\Omega = V/A = m^2 \cdot kg \cdot s^{-3} \cdot A^{-2}$

*From Committee on Hospital Care.[1]

SI Prefixes*

Factor	Prefix		Factor	Prefix	
	Name	Symbol		Name	Symbol
10^{18}	exa-	E	10^{-18}	atto-	a
10^{15}	peta-	P	10^{-15}	femto-	f
10^{12}	tera-	T	10^{-12}	pico-	p
10^{9}	giga-	G	10^{-9}	nano-	n
10^{6}	mega-	M	10^{-6}	micro-	μ
10^{3}	kilo-	k	10^{-3}	milli-	m
10^{2}	hecto-	h	10^{-2}	centi-	c
10^{1}	deca-	da	10^{-1}	deci-	d

*From Committee on Hospital Care.[1]

Laboratory Data in SI Units*

Constituent	Traditional Normal Range	SI Normal Range†
Bilirubin	0.2-1.0 mg/dl	3-17 μmol/l
Calcium	8.9-10.1 mg/dl, 4.5-5.1 mEq/l	2.2-2.5 mmol/l
Cholesterol	150-270 mg/dl	3.9-7.0 mmol/l
Creatinine		
infants	0.2-0.5 mg/dl	18-49 μmol/l
children	0.4-0.7 mg/dl	35-68 μmol/l
adolescents	0.8-1.5 mg/dl	70-133 μmol/l
Glucose	70-105 mg/dl	3.9-5.8 mmol/l
Iron	70-170 μg/dl	12.5-30.4 μmol/l
Lactic acid	3.2-6.8 mg/dl	0.36-0.75 mmol/l
Lead	<30 μg/dl	<1.4 μmol/l
Phosphate (adult values)	3.0-4.5 mg/dl	1.0-1.5 mmol/l
Potassium	3.8-5.0 mEq/dl	38-50 mmol/l
Sodium	135-148 mEq/l	135-148 mmol/l
Thyroxine (total)	4.0-11.0 μg/dl	51-142 nmol/l
Total protein	6.0-8.2 gm/dl	60-82 gm/l
Triglycerides (as triolein)	40-160 mg/dl	0.45-1.80 mmol/l
Uric acid	3.5-7.2 mg/dl	0.21-0.43 mmol/l
Urea	11-28 mg/dl	–
Urea nitrogen	7-18 mg/dl	2.5-6.4 mmol/l (urea)
Vitamin B_{12}	170-760 pg/ml	125-560 pmol/l

*SI indicates International System of Units.
†In SI units.

Conversion Formulas

1 in. = 2.54 cm	1 cm = 0.394 in.
1 ft = 30.5 cm	
1 yd = 91.4 cm	1 m = 39.4 in.
1 lb = 454 gm	1 kg = 2.205 lb
1 qt (liquid) = 0.946 l	
1 oz (liquid) = 29.6 ml	
1 ml = 1.000028 cm³	

1 kilocalorie (kcal) = 4.184 kilojoules (kJ)

Chemical equivalents:

$$mEq = \frac{atomic\ weight\ (mg)}{valence} \qquad mmol = molecular\ weight\ (mg)$$

$$mosmol = particle\ weight\ (mg)$$

Examples:

23 mg Na = 1 mEq, 1 mmol, 1 mosmol
40 mg Ca = 2 mEq, 1 mmol, 1 mosmol
31 mg P = 1 mmol, 1 mosmol
58.5 mg NaCl = 1 mmol, 2 mosmol
39.1 mg K = 1 mEq, 1 mmol
180 mg glucose = 1 mmol, 1 mosmol

(use mmol, never mEq, for compounds)

Appendix V

Laboratory Values

Relation of Serum Protein Levels to Age*†

Age	Total Proteins (gm/100 ml) Mean ± 1 S.D.	Albumin‡ (gm/100 ml) Mean ± 1 S.D.	Alpha-1‡ (gm/100 ml) Mean ± 1 S.D.	Alpha-2‡ (gm/100 ml) Mean ± 1 S.D.	Beta‡ (gm/100 ml) Mean ± 1 S.D.	Gamma‡ (gm/100 ml) Mean ± 1 S.D.
Cord Blood	6.22 ± 1.21	3.23 ± 0.82	0.41 ± 0.10	0.68 ± 0.14	0.74 ± 0.30	1.28 ± 0.23
1-3 mo	5.64 ± 1.04	3.41 ± 0.72	0.24 ± 0.09	0.74 ± 0.24	0.59 ± 0.20	0.66 ± 0.24
4-6 mo	5.43 ± 0.84	3.46 ± 0.36	0.17 ± 0.04	0.67 ± 0.11	0.61 ± 0.14	0.61 ± 0.26
7-12 mo	6.54 ± 0.76	3.62 ± 0.60	0.35 ± 0.15	0.99 ± 0.30	0.79 ± 0.16	0.84 ± 0.36
13-24 mo	6.66 ± 0.93	3.63 ± 0.80	0.31 ± 0.15	0.88 ± 0.42	0.77 ± 0.31	1.09 ± 0.32
25-36 mo	6.98 ± 0.66	4.11 ± 0.78	0.23 ± 0.09	0.89 ± 0.14	0.67 ± 0.14	1.08 ± 0.28
3-5 yr	6.65 ± 0.85	3.95 ± 0.57	0.21 ± 0.08	0.70 ± 0.15	0.67 ± 0.11	1.13 ± 0.31
6-8 yr	6.95 ± 0.55	4.03 ± 0.45	0.22 ± 0.09	0.67 ± 0.10	0.72 ± 0.11	1.31 ± 0.32
9-11 yr	7.43 ± 0.84	4.24 ± 0.79	0.30 ± 0.07	0.75 ± 0.27	0.84 ± 0.16	1.46 ± 0.41
12-16 yr	7.25 ± 0.85	4.26 ± 0.64	0.19 ± 0.07	0.71 ± 0.15	0.68 ± 0.15	1.40 ± 0.31
Adult	7.41 ± 0.96	4.31 ± 0.59	0.23 ± 0.06	0.61 ± 0.14	0.81 ± 0.22	1.45 ± 0.46

*Adapted from Johnson, T.R., Moore, W.M., and Jeffries, J.E., ed.: Children Are Different: Developmental Physiology, ed. 2, Columbus, Ohio: Ross Laboratories, p. 188, 1978.
†Unpublished data by Ellis, E.F., and Robins, J.B.
‡Cellulose acetate electrophoresis.

Estimated Normal Mean Values and Lower Limits of Normal
(Mean Minus 2 S.D.) for Hemoglobin, Hematocrit, and Mean
Corpuscular Volume*

Age (yr)	Hemoglobin (gm/dl)		Hematocrit (%)		Mean Corpuscular Volume (fl)	
	Mean	Lower Limit	Mean	Lower Limit	Mean	Lower Limit
0.5-1.9	12.5	11.0	37	33	77	70
2-4	12.5	11.0	38	34	79	73
5-7	13.0	11.5	39	35	81	75
8-11	13.5	12.0	40	36	83	76
12-14						
female	13.5	12.0	41	36	85	78
male	14.0	12.5	43	37	84	77
15-17						
female	14.0	12.0	41	36	87	79
male	15.0	13.0	46	38	86	78
18-49						
female	14.0	12.0	42	37	90	80
male	16.0	14.0	47	40	90	80

*Adapted from Rudolph, A.M., and Hoffman, J.I.E.: Pediatrics, ed. 17, Nor-
walk, Connecticut: Appleton-Century-Crofts, p. 1036, 1982.

Note: all values are based on data obtained from venous blood by electronic
counter primarily in Caucasian individuals. Selection of the populations in
general was likely to exclude individuals with iron deficiency. The mean ± 2
S.D. can be expected to encompass 95% of the observations in a normal
population.

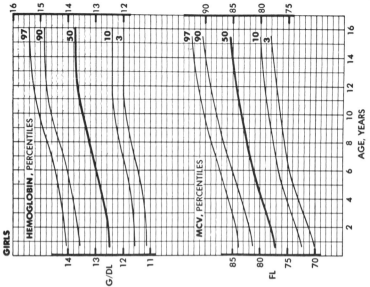

Hemoglobin and MCV percentile curves for girls.

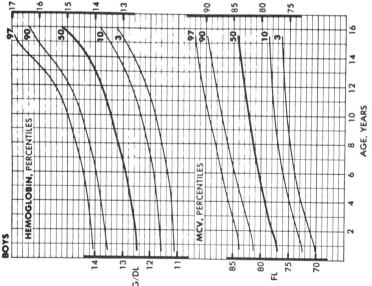

Hemoglobin and MCV percentile curves for boys.

The charts on this page are from: Dallman, P.R., and Siimes, M.A.: Percentile curves for hemoglobin and red cell volume in infancy and childhood, J. Pediat., **94**:26, 1979.

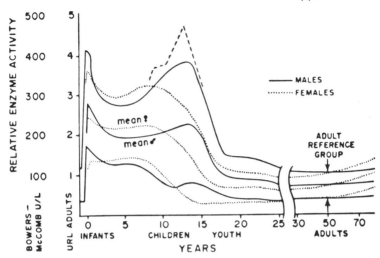

Variation of upper limits, mean, and lower limits of alkaline phosphatase activity with age and sex. (From Meites, S., ed.: Pediatric Clinical Chemistry. A Survey of Reference (Normal) Values, Methods, and Instrumentation, with Commentary, ed. 2. Washington, D.C.: American Association for Clinical Chemistry, p. 69, 1981.)

Normal Fatty Acid Levels in Children*

Fatty Acid	Plasma (mg/dl)	RBC (mg/dl)	Plasma %Total Fatty Acids	RBC's %Total Fatty Acids
Palmitic acid 16:0	46.1 ± 13.1†	36.9 ± 5.7	25.7 ± 2.9	22.7 ± 6.2
Palmitoleic acid 16:1	4.4 ± 1.2	4.8 ± 6.4	2.4 ± 1.1	2.8 ± 3.1
Stearic acid 18:0	20.7 ± 3.5	34.7 ± 10.0	11.6 ± 2.0	21.2 ± 3.4
Oleic acid 18:1	38.8 ± 14.4	26.2 ± 7.9	21.6 ± 4.1	15.9 ± 2.1
Linoleic acid 18:2	53.4 ± 30.8	21.2 ± 6.6	29.4 ± 9.8	12.9 ± 2.9
Eicosatrienoic acid 20:3	3.4 ± 2.5	4.1 ± 2.2	1.8 ± 1.1	2.4 ± 1.2
Arachidonic acid 20:4	12.8 ± 3.9	327.0 ± 11.8	7.2 ± 2.7	19.8 ± 3.5
Linoleic/oleic 18:2/18:1	1.4 ± 0.7	0.8 ± 0.2	–	–

*Data are from Chase, H.P., and Dupont, J.: Abnormal levels of prostaglandins and fatty acids in blood of children with cystic fibrosis, Lancet, **2**:236, 1978.
†± 2 S.D.

Mean and Upper 95th Percentile Values for Fasting Plasma Cholesterol and Triglyceride Levels (mg/dl)*

Age (yr)	Cholesterol		Triglyceride	
	Mean	95th Percentile	Mean	95th Percentile
Males				
0-10	160	200	55	100
10-20	155	200	70	140
20-30	175	230	110	225
30-39	195	260	135	290
40-49	210	270	150	320
50-59	215	275	145	305
60-69	215	275	140	280
>70	205	270	130	260
Females				
0-10	160	200	60	110
10-20	160	200	75	130
20-30	165	220	75	140
30-39	180	235	85	160
40-49	200	260	100	200
50-59	225	295	120	250
60-69	230	300	130	240
>70	230	290	130	235

*Adapted from data derived from cross-sectional plasma lipid distributions among 48,431 Caucasoid participants in Visit 1 of the Lipid Research Clinics Prevalence Study of 11 North American populations (The Lipid Research Clinics Program Data Book: Selected Variables in 11 North American Populations. Vol. 1, Physiologic and Sociodemographic Characteristics, 1979). Ninety-fifth percentile values approximate +2 S.D. above the mean for cholesterol. Because triglyceride levels are not normally distributed, mean values will be higher than median values. Data for females restricted to those not taking estrogen-containing drugs because females taking sex hormones have altered plasma lipid levels.

Index

Index